Guidelines for Transgender Care

Guidelines for Transgender Care has been co-published simultaneously as *International Journal of Transgenderism*, Volume 9, Numbers 3/4 2006.

Guidelines for Transgender Care

Walter O. Bockting, PhD
Joshua M. Goldberg
Editors

Guidelines for Transgender Care has been co-published simultaneously as *International Journal of Transgenderism*, Volume 9, Numbers 3/4 2006.

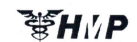

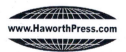

The Haworth Medical Press®
An Imprint of The Haworth Press, Inc.

www.HaworthPress.com

Published by

The Haworth Medical Press®, 10 Alice Street, Binghamton, NY 13904-1580 USA

The Haworth Medical Press® is an imprint of The Haworth Press, Inc., 10 Alice Street, Binghamton, NY 13904-1580 USA.

Guidelines for Transgender Care has been co-published simultaneously as *International Journal of Transgenderism*®, Volume 9, Numbers 3/4 2006.

The development, preparation, and publication of this work has been undertaken with great care. However, the publisher, employees, editors, and agents of The Haworth Press and all imprints of The Haworth Press, Inc., including The Haworth Medical Press® and Pharmaceutical Products Press®, are not responsible for any errors contained herein or for consequences that may ensue from use of materials or information contained in this work. With regard to case studies, identities and circumstances of individuals discussed herein have been changed to protect confidentiality. Any resemblance to actual persons, living or dead, is entirely coincidental.

The Haworth Press is committed to the dissemination of ideas and information according to the highest standards of intellectual freedom and the free exchange of ideas. Statements made and opinions expressed in this publication do not necessarily reflect the views of the Publisher, Directors, management, or staff of The Haworth Press, Inc., or an endorsement by them.

Cover design by Jennifer M. Gaska.

Library of Congress Cataloging-in-Publication Data

Guidelines for transgender care / Walter O. Bockting, Joshua M. Goldberg, editors.
     p. ; cm. – (International journal of transgenderism ; v. 9, no. 3/4 (2006))
   Includes bibliographical references and index.
   ISBN-13: 978-0-7890-3611-7 (soft cover : alk. paper)
   ISBN-10: 0-7890-3611-8 (soft cover : alk. paper)
   1. Transsexuals–Medical care. I. Bockting, Walter O. II. Goldberg, Joshua (Joshua M.) III. Series.
   [DNLM: 1. Transsexualisms. 2. Patient Care. W1 IN791RH v.9 no.3/4 2006 / WM 611 G9464 2006]
RA561.9.T73G85 2006
362.1086´6–dc22
                                               2006038259

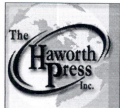

The HAWORTH PRESS Inc

Abstracting, Indexing & Outward Linking

PRINT and ELECTRONIC BOOKS & JOURNALS

This section provides you with a list of major indexing & abstracting services and other tools for bibliographic access. That is to say, each service began covering this periodical during the year noted in the right column. Most Websites which are listed below have indicated that they will either post, disseminate, compile, archive, cite, or alert their own Website users with research-based content from this work. (This list is as current as the copyright date of this publication.)

Abstracting, Website/Indexing Coverage . . . . Year When Coverage Began

- *(CAB ABSTRACTS, CABI)* <http://www.cabi.org> 2006

- **Academic Search Premier (EBSCO)*** <http://search.ebscohost.com> 2006

- **CINAHL (Cumulative Index to Nursing & Allied Health Literature) (EBSCO)***
      <http://www.cinahl.com> 2006

- **CINAHL Plus (EBSCO)*** <http://search.ebscohost.com> 2006

- **International Bibliography of the Social Sciences (IBSS)*** <http://www.ibss.ac.uk> 2006

- **MasterFILE Premier (EBSCO)*** <http://search.ebscohost.com> 2006

- **Psychological Abstracts (PsycINFO)*** <http://www.apa.org> 2006

- **Social Work Abstracts (NASW)*** <http://www.silverplatter.com/catalog/swab.htm> 2005

- *Academic Source Premier (EBSCO)* <http://search.ebscohost.com> 2007

- *Current Abstracts (EBSCO)* <http://search.ebscohost.com> 2007

- *Current Citations Express (EBSCO)* <http://search.ebscohost.com> 2007

- *EBSCOhost Electronic Journals Service (EJS)* <http://search.ebscohost.com> 2005

- *Electronic Collections Online (OCLC)* <http://www.oclc.org/electroniccollections/> 2006

- *Elsevier Eflow-1* 2006

- *Elsevier Scopus* <http://www.info.scopus.com> 2005

- *Family Index Database* <http://www.familyscholar.com> 2005

(continued)

(continued)

Bibliographic Access

- *Cabell's Directory of Publishing Opportunities in Psychology <http://www.cabells.com>*

- *MedBioWorld <http://www.medbioworld.com>*

- *MediaFinder <http://www.mediafinder.com/>*

- *Ulrich's Periodicals Directory: The Global Source for Periodicals Information Since 1932 <http://www. bowkerlink.com>*

Special Bibliographic Notes related to special journal issues (separates) and indexing/abstracting:

- indexing/abstracting services in this list will also cover material in any "separate" that is co-published simultaneously with Haworth's special thematic journal issue or DocuSerial. Indexing/abstracting usually covers material at the article/chapter level.
- monographic co-editions are intended for either non-subscribers or libraries which intend to purchase a second copy for their circulating collections.
- monographic co-editions are reported to all jobbers/wholesalers/approval plans. The source journal is listed as the "series" to assist the prevention of duplicate purchasing in the same manner utilized for books-in-series.
- to facilitate user/access services all indexing/abstracting services are encouraged to utilize the co-indexing entry note indicated at the bottom of the first page of each article/chapter/contribution.
- this is intended to assist a library user of any reference tool (whether print, electronic, online, or CD-ROM) to locate the monographic version if the library has purchased this version but not a subscription to the source journal.
- individual articles/chapters in any Haworth publication are also available through the Haworth Document Delivery Service (HDDS).

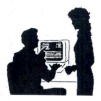

As part of Haworth's continuing committment to better serve our library patrons, we are proud to be working with the following electronic services:

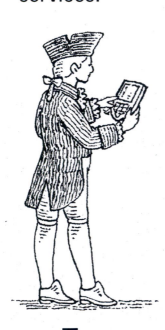

AGGREGATOR SERVICES

EBSCOhost

Ingenta

J-Gate

Minerva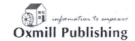

OCLC FirstSearch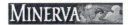

Oxmill

SwetsWise

LINK RESOLVER SERVICES

1Cate (Openly Informatics)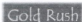

ChemPort (American Chemical Society)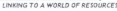

CrossRef

Gold Rush (Coalliance)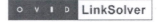

LinkOut (PubMed)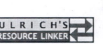

LINKplus (Atypon)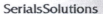

LinkSolver (Ovid)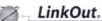

LinkSource with A-to-Z (EBSCO)

Resource Linker (Ulrich)

SerialsSolutions (ProQuest)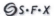

SFX (Ex Libris)

Sirsi Resolver (SirsiDynix)

Tour (TDnet)

Vlink (Extensity, formerly Geac)

WebBridge (Innovative Interfaces)

ABOUT THE EDITORS

Walter O. Bockting, PhD, is a Licensed Psychologist and Associate Professor at the Program in Human Sexuality, Department of Family Medicine and Community Health, University of Minnesota, Minneapolis, USA. He coordinates the University's Transgender Health Services, integrating clinical service, education, and research to promote the health and well-being of the transgender community. Dr. Bockting is a native from the Netherlands and received his PhD from the Vrije Universiteit in Amsterdam. His research interests include transgender identity, intersexuality, sex and the Internet, HIV/STI prevention, and the promotion of sexual health. He has been the recipient of grants from the American Foundation for AIDS Research, the Sisters of Mercy, the Minnesota Department of Health, and the National Institutes of Health. Dr. Bockting is the author of many scientific articles and editor of *Gender Dysphoria: Interdisciplinary Approaches in Clinical Management* (The Haworth Press, Inc., 1992), *Transgender and HIV: Risks, Prevention, and Care* (The Haworth Press, Inc., 2001), *Masturbation as a Means of Achieving Sexual Health* (The Haworth Press, Inc., 2002), and *Transgender Health and HIV Prevention: Needs Assessment Studies from Transgender Communities Across the United States* (The Haworth Press, Inc., 2005). He is a member of the Board of Directors of the Harry Benjamin International Gender Dysphoria Association and a past president of the Society for the Scientific Study of Sexuality.

Joshua M. Goldberg, has been involved in the transgender community since 1996, co-founding three transgender organizations and working on numerous policy, education, research, and legislative initiatives. As a community activist and health researcher, Mr. Goldberg led the community consultation that led to the creation of the Transgender Health Program, and coordinated the program's startup for the Vancouver Coastal Health Authority from 2003-2004. He is currently an Education Consultant for the program, focusing on development of advanced clinical training for health and social service professionals. Mr. Goldberg is the author of numerous publications relating to transgender issues and has been an invited presenter at universities, colleges, and conferences speaking about transgender health and community development. His previous work includes *Making the Transition: Providing Services to Trans Survivors of Violence and Abuse* (Justice Institute of British Columbia, 2006) and *Trans People in the Criminal Justice System: A Guide for Criminal Justice Personnel* (Justice Institute of British Columbia, 2003).

Guidelines for Transgender Care

CONTENTS

Introduction

Transgender people experience multiple barriers to accessing health and social services. This is due in part to a scarcity of transgender services available within public health and social service systems, and a lack of clinical guidance, training, and supportive infrastructure for community-based practitioners (Goldberg, Matte, MacMillan, & Hudspith, 2003). These *Guidelines for Transgender Care* are designed as a tool to guide and train practitioners to meet the needs of transgender people in their community.

The development of these guidelines was part of a new program aiming to improve transgender community access to quality health care and social services throughout British Columbia, Canada. As such, it may serve as a model for promoting transgender health in other communities. The *Transgender Health Program* was created by Vancouver Coastal Health following the closure of the Gender Dysphoria Program at Vancouver Hospital in 2003. Rather than directly providing clinical care, this decentralized, community-based, and peer-driven program developed a network of community-based family physicians, nurses, social workers, counselors, and other clinicians with an interest in transgender care. In addition to serving the transition-related needs of transsexuals, the Transgender Health Program aims to address the broader health issues faced by any person who falls within the following definition of transgender: (a) having a gender identity that is different from the sex assigned at birth, and/or (b) expressing gender in ways that cross or transcend societal expectations for men and women (Kopala, 2003). This broad definition of transgender includes transsexuals, cross-dressers, drag kings/queens, androgynous individuals, Two Spirit individuals, and individuals who are bi- or multi-gendered. The Transgender Health Program is responsible for providing training to the clinicians in the network and assisting with referrals (Knudson, Goldberg, & Hudspith, 2005).

For two decades, community-based clinicians had relied heavily on the Gender Dysphoria Program for the care of transgender individuals. Substantial training and mentorship was needed to be able to take over the care. Building on the World Professional Association for Transgender Health's *Standards of Care for Gender Identity Disorders* (Meyer et al., 2001), basic practice protocols were developed and education was provided to assist community clinicians to meet the transgender community's health needs. In the first year of the program, 33 introductory workshops were provided to clinicians in both rural and urban locations to improve understanding of transgender issues and lay the foundation for sensitive and respectful care. However, more advanced training and clinical guidance was needed to ensure that care was not just trans-positive, but also clinically competent.

With funding from the Canadian Rainbow Health Coalition and Vancouver Coastal Health, the *Trans Care Project* was created to develop advanced practice and training protocols. Local and international clinicians were contracted to partner with transgender community members to create best practice guidelines, frameworks for clinical training, and consumer education materials relating to primary medical care, mental health, care of transgender adolescents, hormone therapy, speech/voice change, sex re-

[Haworth co-indexing entry note]: "Introduction." Bockting, Walter O., and Joshua M. Goldberg. Co-published simultaneously in *International Journal of Transgenderism* (The Haworth Medical Press, an imprint of The Haworth Press, Inc.) Vol. 9, No. 3/4, 2006, pp. 1-2; and: *Guidelines for Transgender Care* (ed: Walter O. Bockting, and Joshua M. Goldberg) The Haworth Medical Press, an imprint of The Haworth Press, Inc., 2006, pp. 1-2. Single or multiple copies of this article are available for a fee from The Haworth Document Delivery Service [1-800-HAWORTH, 9:00 a.m. - 5:00 p.m. (EST). E-mail address: docdelivery@haworthpress.com].

Available online at http://ijt.haworthpress.com
doi:10.1300/J485v09n03_01

assignment surgery, and social and medical advocacy. The clinical guidelines are presented here; the consumer education materials are available at http://www.vch.ca/transhealth/resources/tcp.html.

Improving transgender individuals' access to care requires not only increased clinician awareness of and sensitivity to transgender health concerns, but also assertive and persuasive recruitment of public health professionals to be actively involved in care. From its inception, the Trans Care Project was intended to foster a sense of ownership by local clinicians, and to model clinician-community partnerships as a guiding principle for transgender health care reform. The Transgender Health Program's network of clinicians is limited to one province in Canada. We encourage clinicians and researchers in other regions to work together with local community members to enhance transgender care in the context of their specific health care environment and cultural climate. We hope the *Guidelines in Transgender Care* are useful in stimulating this future work as well as furthering dialogue and research relating to best practices in transgender care.

Walter O. Bockting
Joshua M. Goldberg
Editors

doi:10.1300/J485v09n03_01

REFERENCES

Goldberg, J. M., Matte, N., MacMillan, M., & Hudspith, M. (2003). *Community survey: Transition/crossdressing services in BC–Final report.* Vancouver, BC: Vancouver Coastal Health Authority & Transcend Transgender Support & Education Society.

Knudson, G., Goldberg, J. M., & Hudspith, M. (2005). *From the hospital to the community: A gender program in transition.* Paper presented at the XIX Biennial Symposium of the Harry Benjamin International Gender Dysphoria Association, Bologna, Italy.

Kopala, L. (2003). *Recommendations for a transgender health program.* Vancouver, BC, Canada: Vancouver Coastal Health Authority.

Meyer, W. J., III, Bockting, W. O., Cohen-Kettenis, P. T., Coleman, E., Di Ceglie, D., Devor, H., Gooren, L., Hage, J. J., Kirk, S., Kuiper, B., Laub, D., Lawrence, A., Menard, Y., Monstrey, S., Patton, J., Schaefer, L., Webb, A., & Wheeler, C. C. (2001). *The standards of care for Gender Identity Disorders* (6th ed.). Minneapolis, MN: Harry Benjamin International Gender Dysphoria Association.

Transgender Primary Medical Care

Jamie L. Feldman, MD, PhD
Joshua M. Goldberg

SUMMARY. Transgender medical care involves addressing general medical conditions and those related specifically to transgender issues. This article summarizes existing research in transgender medicine and provides guidance for family physicians and nurses in adapting standard primary care protocols relating to health maintenance, acute illness, and chronic disease management to address trans-specific clinical concerns. Trans-specific issues in physical examination, health history, interpretation of laboratory tests, vaccination, screening, and treatment are explored, and the role of the primary care provider in caring for patients undergoing hormonal or surgical change is discussed. doi:10.1300/J485v09n03_02 *[Article copies available for a fee from The Haworth Document Delivery Service: 1-800-HAWORTH. E-mail address: <docdelivery@haworthpress.com> Website: <http://www.HaworthPress.com> © 2006 by The Haworth Press, Inc. All rights reserved.]*

KEYWORDS. Transgender, primary medical care, primary care, sex reassignment

While there are a number of publications that orient the primary care provider to transgender care (Feldman & Bockting, 2003; Israel & Tarver, 1997; Oriel, 2000; Takata & Meltzer, 2000), there is a paucity of advanced clinical discussion of practice issues in the primary care setting. In this article we summarize empirical evidence relating to transgender medicine, discuss trans-specific primary care concerns, and suggest ways to adapt standard primary care protocols to address trans-specific needs. Trans-specific issues in physical examination, health history, interpretation of laboratory tests, vaccination, screening, and treatment are explored, and the role of the primary care provider in caring for patients undergoing hormonal or surgical change is discussed.

Some of the tasks outlined in this article are specific to physicians' scope of practice, but many are also applicable to advanced practice nursing. As defined by the World Health Organization (1978), *primary health care* includes a

Jamie L. Feldman, MD, PhD, is Assistant Professor in the Department of Family Medicine and Community Health, University of Minnesota Medical School, Minneapolis, MN, USA. Joshua M. Goldberg is Education Consultant of the Transgender Health Program, Vancouver, BC, Canada.

Address correspondence to: Dr. Jamie L. Feldman, Program in Human Sexuality, Department of Family Medicine and Community Health, University of Minnesota Medical School, 1300 South 2nd Street, Suite 180, Minneapolis, MN, USA 55454 (E-mail: feldm010@umn.edu).

This article was adapted from a manuscript created for the Trans Care Project, a joint initiative of Transcend Transgender Support & Education Society and Vancouver Coastal Health's Transgender Health Program, with funding from the Canadian Rainbow Health Coalition. The authors thank Trevor Corneil, Stacy Elliott, Jael Emberley, Eva Hersh, Lori Kohler, Todd Sakakibara, Lukas Walther, and Kathy Wrath for their comments on an earlier draft, and Donna Lindenberg, Olivia Ashbee, A. J. Simpson, and Rodney Hunt for research assistance.

[Haworth co-indexing entry note]: "Transgender Primary Medical Care." Feldman, Jamie L., and Joshua M. Goldberg. Co-published simultaneously in *International Journal of Transgenderism* (The Haworth Medical Press, an imprint of The Haworth Press, Inc.) Vol. 9, No. 3/4, 2006, pp. 3-34; and: *Guidelines for Transgender Care* (ed: Walter O. Bockting, and Joshua M. Goldberg) The Haworth Medical Press, an imprint of The Haworth Press, Inc., 2006, pp. 3-34. Single or multiple copies of this article are available for a fee from The Haworth Document Delivery Service [1-800-HAWORTH, 9:00 a.m. - 5:00 p.m. (EST). E-mail address: docdelivery@haworthpress.com].

doi:10.1300/J485v09n03_02

broad range of social, educational, and political interventions beyond the scope of the family physician or nurse practitioner. We aim not to provide an exhaustive discussion of transgender health, but rather to suggest directions for the range of issues that are, in our experience, commonly of concern to clinicians in the primary medical care setting.

Like every population the transgender community is diverse and health needs vary greatly from patient to patient. As with the non-transgender population, active consideration of biopsychosocial, socioeconomic, and spiritual health is encouraged as part of holistic primary care of transgender patients. It is vital for primary care providers to understand the diversity of the transgender community and to avoid a narrow idea of "transgender health." In this article we have deliberately taken a broad approach to transgender health, but the limits of space prevent a full discussion of all relevant health issues. In-depth guidance relating to endocrinologic, surgical, socioeconomic, and psychosocial care is beyond the scope of this article, but is discussed elsewhere (Bockting, Knudson, & Goldberg, 2006; Bowman & Goldberg, 2006; Dahl, Feldman, Goldberg, Jaberi et al., 2006; de Vries, Cohen-Kettenis, & Delemarre-Van de Waal, 2006; White Holman & Goldberg, 2006a, 2006b).

Our recommendations are consistent with the World Professional Association for Transgender Health (WPATH)'s *Standards of Care* (Meyer et al., 2001). Like the WPATH *Standards*, our suggested protocols are intended to be a flexible framework to guide the treatment of transgender individuals. There is not yet clinical consensus on many of the issues we address, nor is there sufficient empirical evidence to definitively determine best practice. We suggest the recommendations in this document be considered as a step in advancing discussion among experienced practitioners rather than as rigid guidelines. We support the WPATH recommendation that clinical departures from standard practice be recognized as such, explained to the patient, and documented to help the transgender medicine field evolve.

EVIDENCE-BASED DECISION-MAKING IN TRANSGENDER CARE

The recommendations in this document are based on published literature specific to transgender health wherever possible and on clinical experience of primary care clinicians. More research is needed and for this reason some recommendations are based on current practices where the literature is inconclusive or absent.

Currently, few prospective, large scale studies exist regarding transgender health care. The best available evidence comes from a Netherlands historical cohort involving 816 male-to-female (MTF) and 293 female-to-male (FTM) transsexual patients, with use of endocrine agents ranging over 2 months to 41 years (van Kesteren, Asscheman, Megens, & Gooren, 1997). Morbidity and mortality were compared to age-gender specific statistics in the general Dutch population. As the study did not track a specific cohort over a long period of time, particularly into the over age 65 range, the long term health effects of transgender endocrine therapy remain uncertain. Specific results from this study are incorporated into the appropriate sections below. Smaller scale studies on specific issues such as osteoporosis do exist, along with non-trans-specific evidence (i.e., studies involving non-transgender men and women). In many areas, case reports or series are the major source of trans-specific data. Case studies serve to indicate that the condition is possible in the transgender setting; however, further research is needed to determine incidence and clinical significance.

In applying knowledge from the non-transgender setting to transgender patients, the primary care provider should look for rigorous studies that are highly relevant to the clinical context. For example, a large prospective study involving non-transgender women on postmenopausal hormone therapy may be relevant for MTFs over age 50 who are taking similar types of hormones for feminizing purposes. However, care should be taken in applying evidence from studies of natal females to MTFs and studies of natal males to FTMs, as little is known about the ways that physiologic differences between the two populations may affect health outcomes.

Evidence from non-transgender studies can be directly applied to similar transgender patients who have not had surgical or hormonal interventions. For example, studies involving non-transgender women are applicable to individuals in the FTM spectrum who have not taken testosterone or had masculinizing surgery.

RECOGNIZING TRANSGENDER IDENTITY AND EXPERIENCE

Transgender patients are a medically underserved population. Transgender identity and behavior are socially stigmatized, leading many transgender individuals to maintain a traditional gender role while keeping their transgender issues closeted. A Minnesota study of transgender health seminar participants found that 48% had not informed their family physician that they were transgender (Bockting, Robinson, Forberg, & Scheltema, 2005). Experience with transphobia and discrimination in the health care setting, lack of access to transcompetent providers, and (for some) discomfort with the body can lead the transgender patient to avoid medical care altogether (Kammerer, Mason, Connors, & Durkee, 1999). Thus, transgender individuals often lack access to preventive health services and timely treatment of routine health problems.

Patients best explore transgender issues in a setting of respect and trust. This requires referring to the transgender patient by their preferred name and pronoun, reassuring the patient about confidentiality, educating clinic staff and colleagues regarding transgender issues, and respecting the patient's wishes regarding potentially sensitive physical exams and tests such as pelvic examinations or mammograms. Familiarity with commonly used terms and the diversity of gender identities and forms of gender expression within the transgender community–including fluid, non-binary gender identification–is essential.

The transgender patient may present to your office in a variety of ways. Many transgender patients are open about their identity, and may specifically ask about your experience working with the transgender community. The "closeted" transgender patient may avoid elements of the physical exam, such as pelvic or testicular exams.

Even patients who are open about being transgender may act in ways that are incongruous with their self-identification, including wearing clothes, cosmetics, or hairstyle that differ from their sense of self. Transphobia results in many transgender individuals being unable to freely express their identity with loved ones, at school, or in the workplace. Transgender patients who are transitioning to living in the desired gender role, or patients who self-identify as androgynous or bi-gendered, may express some elements of each gender. Patients may also vary their appearance from visit to visit either as part of exploring their identity or due to social pressures (e.g., going to work after their appointment). None of these behaviours necessarily signal ambivalence about being transgender, nor should they be considered a sign of mental illness; in most cases they are simply an accommodation to difficult circumstances.

Asking About Transgender Issues in an Appropriate Manner

While transgender identity is not the only (or necessarily the most) important factor in primary care, knowing a patient is transgender is important in determining effective and appropriate care. Because transgender identity is not always obvious, and many transgender individuals are intensely private or fearful of negative consequences should they disclose this information, sensitive questioning is needed to create an environment conducive to discussion of any concerns relating to transgender issues and transgender-specific assistance that may be required.

While we encourage questions relating to transgender issues, care must be taken not to pressure the patient to discuss transgender concerns or to disclose suspected transgender identity. In some instances, even though you think a patient is transgender, this may be an incorrect assumption. In other cases the patient may not feel that transgender identity is the most relevant or pressing issue.

Transgender experience is not rare in the general population. In a large study of randomly sampled Swedish adults 18-60 years of age, 2.8% of men and 0.4% of women reported having crossdressed for erotic purposes at least once (Langström & Zucker, 2005). Transsexualism is estimated at 1 per 11,900 male-to-female and 1 per 30,400 female-to-male (Bakker, van Kesteren, Gooren, & Bezemer, 1993). Because transgender experience is not uncommon, the primary care provider should be comfortable inquiring about gender concerns on a regular, if not routine, basis.

We recommend an approach that normalizes transgender experience and also establishes questions about transgenderism as routine. For example, the clinician may state, "Because so many people are impacted by gender issues, I have begun to ask everyone about it. Anything you do say about gender issues will be kept confidential. If this topic isn't relevant to you, tell me and I'll move on." Alternatively, the clinician might ask, "Out of respect for my clients' right to self-identify, I ask all clients what gender pronoun they'd prefer I use for them. What pronoun would you like me to use for you?" After establishing that this topic is broached with every patient, the clinician can directly ask, "Do you identify as transgender?"

If you use an intake form, asking a question about gender on the form can be a way to encourage disclosure of transgender identity. Some agencies use "Gender: _____," with the blank to be filled in by the patient. This allows the transgender patient to write in a description of identity such as "transgender," "transsexual," "MTF," "androgynous," or another term. Other agencies use the wording, "Choose as many as apply: M/F/MTF/FTM/other (please specify)."

Recognizing Gender Concerns

Not all transgender individuals struggle with gender issues. Among those who do, there are varying concerns. Some individuals seek help because they are confused about their identity or are struggling with despair, shame, or guilt relating to crossdressing or transgender feelings; others are dysphoric about physical characteristics associated with sex or gender, the perceptions of others relating to gender, or roles associated with gender. Individuals who are questioning their gender or are confused about

gender identity issues may be unsure how to articulate this, or may express their concerns as confusion about sexual orientation. Referral to a mental health professional experienced in gender identity issues is appropriate if distress is negatively impacting mental health or overall functioning (Bockting et al., 2006).

Gender concerns can affect individuals of all ages. MTF transgender patients tend to seek psychological or medical treatment for gender concerns during middle age (Blanchard, 1994), while FTM patients are typically younger. As the transgender population becomes more visible, however, patients ask for assistance at younger ages, including childhood and adolescence. Seniors may also present with previously untreated gender concerns.

TRANSGENDER HEALTH ASSESSMENT

General Medical History

The patient's *general health history* should be reviewed, including all medications and the most recent physical exam (including Pap smear, testicular, and rectal exams, where appropriate). A thorough gynecologic and obstetric history is important in FTM patients, as there may be an increased incidence of polycystic ovarian syndrome in this population (Balen, Schacter, Montgomery, Reid, & Jacobs, 1993; Bosinski et al., 1997; Futterweit, Weiss, & Fagerstrom, 1986).

The patient's *family history* should be reviewed, with particular attention to history of clotting disorders, cardiovascular disease, hypertension, diabetes, and mental illness. Any family history for breast, ovarian, uterine, or prostate cancer should also be noted, as these cancers are known to be influenced by exogenous hormones and may require different or more frequent screening if patients are taking feminizing or masculinizing endocrine agents.

Taking a *sexual health history* is an essential part of good primary care for all patients, not just those who are transgender. Sensitivity is needed in taking a sexual history; discussion should be initiated gradually and pacing should depend on patient comfort. A screening sexual history should cover sexual orientation, risk behaviors related to sexually transmitted infections, and sexual function (Nusbaum & Hamilton, 2002). If the screening history raises concerns, a more detailed sexual history is warranted.

Psychosocial history should be discussed, as a transgender patient's family, economic and larger social environment can be sources of support or stress. Societal stigma associated with transgenderism can make life challenging for the transgender person. Social isolation, rejection by family and community of origin, harassment, and discrimination can significantly impact the transgender individual's health (Goffman, 1963). Transphobia may be internalized, resulting in shame, guilt, and a loathing of oneself or other transgender individuals (Bockting, 2003; Keatley, Nemoto, Operario, & Soma, 2002). While an extended psychosocial evaluation is not within typical scope of practice for the primary care provider, it is useful for the primary care provider to gain a basic understanding of the psychosocial issues facing the patient as a transgender person. Areas to explore include: (a) how the patient feels about being transgender, (b) how the patient feels being transgender has affected areas of life that are important to the patient (e.g., family relationships, social networks, employment), and (c) what supports and resources the patient has to cope with being transgender in a transphobic society.

Psychosocial dynamics may be complicated, especially during gender transition. Referral to peer-based or professional counseling and advocacy resources may be helpful for both the transgender person and loved ones if there are psychosocial concerns.

Social history includes evaluation of poverty and possible homelessness. In North America, as a result of employment discrimination and family abandonment, many transgender people live in poverty in both rural and urban areas, and housing concerns are not uncommon (Goldberg, Matte, MacMillan, & Hudspith, 2003; Lombardi, Wilchins, Priesing, & Malouf, 2001; Mottet & Ohle, 2003). Referral to trans-experienced advocates may be helpful if the patient needs assistance with housing, application for health benefits, or application for social assistance (White Holman & Goldberg, 2006b). For the homeless transgender patient, the American National Health Care for the Homeless Council has published recommendations for modification to clinical practice to address the multiple challenges faced by homeless people in adhering to care plans (Bonin et al., 2004).

History of Feminizing or Masculinizing Interventions

When establishing care with a transgender patient, a thorough history of any hormonal, surgical, or other interventions to bring the body into greater congruence with gender identity is essential. For some transgender patients, hormonal and surgical concerns are less prominent, and this part of the history is accordingly brief. Questions may include:

1. Has the patient ever taken feminizing or masculinizing endocrine agents, and if so, are there any complications or concerns regarding past or current use? Feminizing and masculinizing medications have the potential for numerous drug interactions and the primary care provider needs to be cognizant of these before prescribing anything new. Medically unsupervised use of hormones is common among transgender patients who have limited access to care (Sember, Lawrence, & Xavier, 2000; Sperber, Landers, & Lawrence, 2005). Patients may borrow hormones from friends or buy hormones illicitly. Increasingly, transgender persons are purchasing hormones over the internet, usually with little to no clinician involvement. The primary care provider should also inquire about "herbal hormones"–phytoestrogens or androgen-like compounds sold as dietary supplements. Transgender patients with coexisting chronic medical problems should have closer follow-up once they begin endocrine therapy, as the effects of cross-sex hormones on chronic illnesses such as diabetes and coronary artery disease are not well defined. Potential risks and complications of transgender endocrine therapy are discussed further in the next section of this document and also elsewhere (Dahl et al., 2006).

2. Has the patient undergone any feminizing or masculinizing surgical procedures, and if so, are there any complications or concerns regarding past surgeries? For individuals in the FTM spectrum, surgeries may include chest reconstruction, hysterectomy, salpingo-oophorectomy, vaginectomy, metaidoioplasty or phalloplasty (penile construction), urethroplasty, scrotoplasty, and procedures to masculinize facial and body contours. For individuals in the MTF spectrum, surgery may include breast augmentation, orchiectomy, penectomy, vaginoplasty, facial feminization, tracheal shave, surgery to elevate voice pitch, and procedures to feminize body contours. Complications relating to genital surgery (for both MTFs and FTMs) are not infrequent, particularly in patients who underwent surgery many years ago when techniques were less sophisticated and followup care less consistent. Care of the patient undergoing sex reassignment surgery is discussed elsewhere by Bowman and Goldberg (2006).

3. Does the patient plan to pursue transgender endocrine therapy or surgery in the future? Awareness of future plans is useful in coordinating referrals and planning relating to care for any co-existing medical, social, or psychological concerns.

4. Are there any additional feminizing or masculinizing interventions sought by the patient? Peer-based resources are often useful for assistance relating to appearance (clothing, hairstyle/makeup, footwear, etc.) and change in legal name or sex designation (White Holman & Goldberg, 2006b). Referrals to trans-competent clinicians may be sought for speech change (Davies & Goldberg, 2006), hair removal, or hair transplant. Professional counseling can be useful for the patient who is just starting to explore gender identity or wants support adjusting to changes (Bockting et al., 2006).

Transgender Physical Exam

Physical exams should be structured based on the organs present rather than the perceived gender of the patient. For example, the prostate is not removed in vaginoplasty, and prostate exams should be performed for the MTF patient as discussed below. If the uterus and cervix are present in FTMs, pelvic exams and Pap smears typically need to be done on a regular basis, although these may be deferred for FTMs who have not had penetrative vaginal intercourse (discussed further in a subsequent section).

Transgender patients may be uncomfortable with their bodies and may find some elements of physical examination traumatic. Unless there is an immediate medical need, sensitive elements of the exam–particularly breast, genital and rectal exam–should be delayed until strong clinician-patient rapport has developed. Sensitive exams can be managed in a variety of ways depending on patient preference; some patients prefer the exam to be done as quickly as possible, while others require a slow pace or even light sedation. Discuss with your patients when, where and how you might need to touch. When the purpose of the exam is explained clearly, most patients will understand. The physical exam is an important opportunity to educate patients about their bodies, and the need for ongoing health maintenance.

Clinicians can expect to observe a range of development in patients undergoing transgender endocrine therapy. FTM patients may have beard growth, clitoromegaly, acne, and androgenic alopecia; those who have bound their breasts for numerous years may have rash or yeast infection of the skin under the breasts. MTF patients may have feminine breast shape and size, often with relatively underdeveloped nipples; breasts may appear fibrocystic if there have been silicone injections. Galactorrhea is sometimes present in MTF patients with high prolactin levels, especially among those using breast pumps to stimulate development (Schlatterer, Yassouridis et al., 1998). There may be minimal body hair, with variable facial hair depending on length of time on hormones and manual hair removal treatments such as electrolysis. Testicles may become small and soft; defects or hernias at the external inguinal ring may be present due to the practice of "tucking" the testicles near or into the inguinal canal. Particularly in the absence of endocrine therapy, findings suggestive of intersex conditions should be further evaluated.

Physical findings in post-operative patients will depend on the types of surgeries which have been done, the quality of the surgical work, the impact of post-operative complications, and any revisions that have been performed after the initial surgery (Bowman & Goldberg, 2006). FTM patients after chest surgery will have scar tissue consistent with the type of procedure, and may have large nipples or small grafted nipples depending on the technique used. The FTM neophallus created from the release of an augmented clitoris looks like a very small penis, while a grafted penis constructed by phalloplasty will be adult-sized but more flaccid than in the natal male (erection is obtained through use of a stiffener or pump). MTF patients may have undergone breast augmentation with implants. MTF genital surgery typically involves simultaneous removal of the penis and testicles and creation of a neovagina; some patients may just have the testes removed, prior to or instead of vaginoplasty. There may be varying degrees of labial reconstruction and clitoral hooding, depending on the completion of additional surgery or revisions. The neovagina typically appears less moist than in natal women, and may be stenosed internally if the patient does not dilate daily or is not sexually active.

Laboratory Requisition Forms

Most requisition forms for laboratory tests ask for the sex of the patient, to provide the primary care provider with normal ranges for sex-dependent results and to flag abnormal results. Normal values specifically for transgender individuals who are undergoing or have completed gender transition have not been established for any laboratory test, and there is no consensus about how sex should be recorded on lab requests for the transgender patient. The primary care provider will need to balance consideration of the following issues: (a) the stress placed on the patient going into the lab with a sex on the form that doesn't match their name/ appearance, (b) getting the lab values most appropriate to the patient's physiology, and (c) minimizing lab error in performing the correct test in the correct manner. Interpretation of lab results is dependent on the patient's physiology and the specific test being performed.

As stated in the preceding paragraph, physiologic considerations are not the only factor in determining the sex to be recorded on the requisition form. When physiologic considerations are judged to be of primary importance, the following approach may be taken: (a) for transgender patients who are not taking hormones and have not had surgical gonadal removal, use the natal sex for laboratory reference purposes; (b) for transgender patients who have undergone orchiectomy or oophorectomy and are on a cross-sex hormonal regimen, use the sex opposite to their natal sex (i.e., M for FTMs and F for MTFs); (c) for patients who are currently transitioning or have partially transitioned, one may need to vary the reported sex depending on the lab test–for example, for MTF patients beginning feminizing endocrine therapy male laboratory norms may be more appropriate for creatinine and cholesterol, but female values may be more relevant for testosterone levels.

Regardless of the approach taken, the primary care provider should explain to the patient the challenges involved in laboratory testing and how their sex is coded for lab interpretation purposes. It is helpful to discuss the situation with the laboratory director, so that lab staff can understand the transgender context. Ideally, laboratory forms would include FTM and MTF categorization, as well as a checkbox for "male" or "female" reference ranges.

VACCINATIONS

Recommended vaccinations are the same for transgender and non-transgender patients. It is important to assess whether vaccinations are up to date, as transgender patients may lack regular primary care. While vaccination of all children for Hepatitis B is now recommended, many transgender adults are not immune and could benefit from vaccination, particularly persons with more than one sexual partner in the last six months, patients with a recent sexually transmitted infection, individuals who share needles to inject hormones or other substances, and those residing in or traveling to endemic areas.

In recent years there have public health campaigns targeting gay and bisexual men for vaccination against Hepatitis A and Meningococcal C in response to local outbreaks among men who have sex with men. Mass vaccination campaigns do not depend on assessment of an individual's sexual or social risks; membership in a population considered at risk is sufficient to warrant vaccination, regardless of whether an individual in that population is engaged in the activities that pose risk for transmission. Accordingly, it is recommended that vaccination campaigns for men who have sex with men (MSM) be extended to include transgender individuals (both FTM and MTF) who have sex with men, as transgender individuals who have sex with men (TSM) are at risk for many of the same reasons as MSM (Gay and Lesbian Medical Association, 2001). For joint MSM-TSM vaccination campaigns to be effective, (a) promotional materials must use language that will reach transgender individuals who do not identify as MSM, and (b) primary care providers with TSM patients should discuss vaccination as they would with MSM patients.

GENERAL PRIMARY PREVENTION, SCREENING, AND MANAGEMENT

Risks and recommendations for screening depend on the patient's hormonal and surgical status and on regional primary care protocols. In each section below we give recommendations specific to each population, based on North American primary care protocols. Summaries of recommendations for MTFs and FTMs are available as online supplements at http://www.vch.ca/transhealth/resources/library/tcpdocs/guidelines-primcare.pdf.

Cancer

Breast Cancer

Male-to-female. There is no evidence of increased risk of cancer in MTFs who are not taking feminizing endocrine agents compared to natal male patients, in the absence of other known risk factors (e.g., Klinefelter's syndrome). Routine screening, either in the form of regular breast exams or mammography, is not indicated for these patients.

Currently, there are no long term, prospective studies on the risk of breast cancer among MTF patients who have taken feminizing endo-

crine agents. A retrospective study revealed no breast cancer cases (van Kesteren et al., 1997), but the population may not have been old enough or followed long enough to detect any difference. Published case reports exist regarding breast cancer among MTF transgender patients taking feminizing agents (Ganly & Taylor, 1995; Pritchard, Pankowsky, Crowe, & Abdul-Karim, 1988; Schlatterer, Yassouridis, et al., 1998; Symmers, 1968).

Multiple prospective studies have demonstrated an increased risk of breast cancer among menopausal non-transgender women on hormone replacement therapy (Colditz, 2005; Nelson, Humphrey, Nygren, Teutsch, & Allan, 2002; Rossouw et al., 2002; Schairer et al., 2000). In these studies, risk appears to increase with combined estrogen and progestin use, and with length of therapy over five years. McPherson, Steel, and Dixon (2000) suggest that the risk of breast cancer appears related to age; age at menarche, menopause, and first birth; and family history more so than exogenous hormone use among natal females. Among transgender women, length of time exposed to exogenous estrogens may be more important given the relative lack of endogenous estrogens.

Annual screening with mammography has shown a demonstrated significant benefit for natal women age 50 and over, and a lesser benefit for women ages 40 to 50 years (Humphrey, Helfand, Chan, & Woolf, 2005; Olsen & Gotzsche, 2001; Smith et al., 2003). However, the risk of breast cancer in the MTF population appears substantially lower, with accompanying increased risk of false positive findings resulting in emotional distress, biopsies, and cost to the patient without health insurance. Accordingly, we only recommend screening mammography in MTF patients over age 50 who have used feminizing endocrine agents for over 5 years and have additional risk factors, such as a family history of breast cancer.

Annual clinical breast exam and periodic self-breast exam have not been shown to decrease breast cancer morbidity or mortality in the natal female population. Current Canadian guidelines thus recommend against them as part of routine primary care (Baxter, 2001). However, clinical and self-breast exam may provide an opportunity for education regarding breast health, and this may be valuable for the MTF patient.

Although there are no studies on the long-term effects of saline or silicone breast implants in MTFs, studies in non-transgender women do not suggest an increased risk of breast cancer (Bryant & Brasher, 1995). However, breast implants may impair the accuracy of mammography (Gumucio et al., 1989; Hayes, Vandergrift, & Diner, 1988), and the technician should be informed that the patient has implants so special techniques can be utilized. Despite the lower accuracy of mammography in women with augmentation and thus the potential for delay in diagnosis, there is no evidence that a delay in diagnosis in women with implants has clinical significance in terms of mortality (Brinton et al., 2000; Deapen, Hamilton, Bernstein, & Brody, 2000; Miglioretti et al., 2004).

In summary, MTF patients who have taken feminizing endocrine agents may be at increased risk of breast cancer compared to natal males, but likely have significantly decreased risk compared to natal females. The length of feminizing hormone exposure, family history, BMI greater than 35, and use of progestins may further increase risk. Screening mammography for MTF patients receiving transgender endocrine therapy is advisable in patients over age 50 with additional risk factors, with the technician advised if the patient has breast implants. Annual clinical breast exam and periodic self-breast exam are not recommended for MTFs except as a tool to educate about general breast health.

Female-to-male. Currently, there are no long term, prospective studies on the risk of breast cancer among FTM patients. A retrospective study revealed no breast cancer cases (van Kesteren et al., 1997), but the population may not have been old enough or followed long enough to detect any cases. Case series do exist of breast cancer among FTM patients, post-chest surgery and on testosterone (Burcombe, Makris, Pittam, & Finer, 2003; Eyler & Whittle, 2001). FTM patients who undergo breast reduction or mastectomy retain some degree of breast tissue (Bowman & Goldberg, 2006) and are therefore still at risk of breast cancer.

The incidence of breast cancer among natal males is 1% of the incidence among natal fe-

males. However, the breast cancer risk among men with Klinefelter's syndrome (XXY chromosomes)–who, like FTMs, have lower testosterone levels, higher estrogen levels, higher gonadotropin levels, and increased gynecomastia compared to XY males–is 50 times higher than among non-Klinefelter's men (Hultborn et al., 1997). While Klinefelter's syndrome is not completely analogous to the FTM patient, the apparent relationship between hormone levels and breast growth to breast cancer incidence suggests the possibility of increased risk of breast cancer for FTMs compared to natal males.

There is no strong evidence that testosterone either increases or decreases breast cancer risk. For the FTM patient who has not had chest surgery, regardless of testosterone use breast exams and screening mammography are recommended as for natal females.

Multiple studies in non-transgender women after breast reduction surgery show reduced risk of breast cancer, directly related to the amount of tissue removed (Boice et al., 1997, 2000; Brinton, Persson, Boice, McLaughlin, & Fraumeni, 2001) and age at time of surgery (with the greatest reduction in risk seen when patients had the procedure after age 40). Even after breast reduction, the risk remains higher in natal females than in natal males. Pre-surgical mammography does not appear to significantly improve detection of occult cancers in these patients (Netscher et al., 1999), and we therefore do not recommend mammography before chest surgery unless the FTM patient meets the usual recommendations for mammography in natal females.

Annual clinical breast exam and periodic self-breast exam have not been shown to decrease breast cancer morbidity or mortality in the natal female population. Current Canadian guidelines thus recommend against them as part of routine primary care (Baxter, 2001). However, a yearly examination for chest masses and axillary adenopathy is a low-cost, low risk intervention which provides an opportunity for education regarding breast cancer risks.

In summary, chest exams and screening mammography guidelines for natal females should be applied to FTM patients who have not had chest surgery, regardless of testosterone use. Following chest surgery, yearly chest wall and axillary exams, along with education regarding the small but possible risk of breast cancer, are recommended for FTM patients.

Cervical Cancer

Male-to-female. Cervical Pap smears are generally not indicated for MTF patients because a cervix is generally not present even after vaginoplasty. A case of intraepithelial neoplasia (carcinoma in situ) has been reported in an MTF patient who underwent vaginoplasty with the glans penis used to create a neocervix (Lawrence, 2001). Pap smear of the neocervix should be done routinely in these cases, as (a) the glans appears to be more prone to carcinomatous change than the skin of the penile shaft, and (b) there appears to be greater risk of progression to invasive carcinoma with intraepithelial neoplasia of the glans compared to intraepithelial neoplasia of other penile skin (Lawrence, 2001).

In natal women primary vaginal carcinoma is rare. Accordingly, Pap smear of the vaginal cuff is not indicated in natal women who have no history of cervical abnormality and have had cervical removal as part of hysterectomy (Saslow et al., 2002). There are also concerns that vaginal cytology is a poor screening tool, with a high false positive rate and a low sensitivity to vaginal neoplasia (Lawrence, 2001). In the immunocompromised MTF patient at increased risk for vaginal cancer due to human papilloma virus (HPV) exposure, vaginal Pap smear may be considered.

In summary, following vaginoplasty MTFs should have cervical Pap smears as per recommendations for natal females if the glans penis has been used to create a neocervix, but not if other techniques are used. A regular vaginal Pap smear should be considered for the MTF patient who has a history of genital warts, particularly if the patient is immunocompromised.

Female-to-male. We recommend that clinicians follow the standard guidelines for natal females to screen for cervical cancer in FTMs. Cervical cancer screening guidelines vary from country to country, and between professional organizations. In North America, generally the recommendation is that natal females start screening within 3 years of sexual activity that

poses risk for HPV transmission, with Pap smears initially performed annually and then every 2-3 years if no significant abnormalities are noted after the first two Pap smears, until age 69-70 (Amy et al., 2005; Drouin et al., 1998; Smith, Cokkinides, & Eyre, 2006). Annual Pap smears are advised for immunosuppressed natal females. Following hysterectomy, regular Pap smears are not needed unless there is a prior history of high-grade cervical dysplasia or cervical cancer, in which case Pap smears of the vaginal cuff should be performed annually until three normal tests are documented, then performed every 2-3 years after that.

While we encourage regular Pap smears for FTM patients as part of primary care, Pap smears can be traumatic for some FTM patients and should be kept to a minimum for patients at low risk of HPV transmission (i.e., little sexual activity involving the genitals). Total hysterectomy should be considered if the patient is unable to tolerate Pap smears.

There is no evidence that testosterone increases or reduces the risk of cervical cancer. However, testosterone therapy can cause significant atrophy in the cervical epithelium, mimicking dysplasia on the Pap smear (Miller, Bedard, Cooter, & Shaul, 1986). The pathologist should therefore be informed of the patient's hormonal status. For patients otherwise at low risk of cervical cancer, ASCUS and low-grade SIL Pap smears are unlikely to represent pre-cancerous lesions. However, these changes are not well characterized in the literature, and colposcopy may be indicated in patients at increased risk. Total hysterectomy should be considered in the presence of high grade dysplasia.

In summary, Pap smear guidelines for natal females should be followed for the FTM patient who has not had total hysterectomy, with deferral in patients who are at low risk for HPV transmission. As testosterone can result in atrophic changes to the cervical epithelium mimicking dysplasia, the pathologist should be informed if the patient is on hormonal therapy. Total hysterectomy should be considered in the presence of high grade dysplasia or if the patient is unable to tolerate Pap smears.

Ovarian Cancer

Some studies suggest an increased risk of ovarian cancer among FTM patients on testosterone therapy (Hage, Dekker, Karim, Verheijen, & Bloemena, 2000; Pache et al., 1991) and non-transgender women with polycystic ovarian syndrome (Schildkraut, Schwingl, Bastos, Evanoff, & Hughes, 1996). Polycystic ovarian syndrome (PCOS) is a hormonal syndrome complex characterized by failure to ovulate, absent or infrequent menstrual cycles, multiple cysts on the ovaries, hyperandrogenism, hirsuitism, acne, hidradenitis suppurativa, acanthosis nigricans, obesity, and glucose intolerance or diabetes. We include discussion of PCOS in this article not to suggest that PCOS is related to the development of FTM identity, but rather because increased incidence of PCOS has been noted among FTMs even in the absence of testosterone use (Balen et al., 1993; Bosinski et al., 1997; Futterweit et al., 1985) and we believe this is relevant in considering primary health care needs in FTM patients.

No recommended screening tests for ovarian cancer exist for any population, and pelvic exams are currently the only screening modality utilized. As the risk of ovarian cancer increases with age, we recommend considering pelvic exams every 1 to 3 years in FTM patients over age 40 or with a family history of ovarian cancer, with annual pelvic exams recommended for patients with a history of signs and symptoms suggestive of PCOS. As pelvic exams may be distressing for FTM patients, a salpingo-oophorectomy should be considered if patients cannot tolerate ongoing pelvic exams.

In summary, we recommend screening for signs and symptoms of PCOS in all FTM patients, and conducting pelvic exams annually if PCOS is suspected. In the FTM without a history of PCOS, pelvic exams every 1-3 years are recommended in patients over age 40 or with a family history of ovarian cancer. Preventive salpingo-oophorectomy is recommended for FTMs who cannot tolerate pelvic exams.

Endometrial Cancer

No recommended screening tests for endometrial cancer exist for any population, as endometrial cancer is typically diagnosed early as a result of unexpected vaginal bleeding. While there does not appear to be an increased risk of endometrial carcinoma specifically among patients on masculinizing endocrine therapy, dysfunctional uterine bleeding is not uncommon. Dysfunctional uterine bleeding is usually related to missed doses or changes in a patient's testosterone therapy, but otherwise unexplained bleeding should be fully evaluated, especially in previously amenorrheic patients. If bleeding is prolonged, the endometrium should be evaluated with trans-vaginal ultrasound, pelvic ultrasound, and/or endometrial biopsy, particularly if the patient is above age 35. A preventive total hysterectomy should be considered if fertility is not an issue, the patient is under age 40, and the patient's health will not be adversely affected by surgery.

Prostate Cancer

Feminizing endocrine therapy appears to decrease the risk of prostate cancer, but the degree of reduction is unknown. Cases of prostate cancer have been reported in MTF patients taking feminizing hormones, both before and after genital surgery (Markland, 1975; Spritz, 2003; Thurston, 1994; van Haarst, Newling, Gooren, Asscheman, & Prenger, 1998; van Kesteren et al., 1997). In a study of non-transgender males with naturally acquired testosterone deficiency, prostate cancer was detected in 14% of participants prior to testosterone replacement (Morgentaler, Bruning, & DeWolf, 1996); it is unclear how this rate compares to MTFs who have reduced gonadal function as a result of exogenous estrogen.

The prostate is not removed in MTF genital surgery, and there is no evidence that genital surgery increases or decreases the risk for prostate cancer. Regardless of surgical status MTF patients should be educated regarding the small but possible risk of prostate cancer, and digital rectal exams should be performed at the same frequency as for natal males. In vaginoplasty the neovagina is positioned posterior to the prostate and digital palpation may be difficult, particularly if the prostate has atrophied as a result of feminizing endocrine therapy (Jin, Turner, Walters, & Handelsman, 1997; van Kesteren et al., 1996). However, digital rectal examination should still be used in the post-operative MTF patient, as there are not yet standardized protocols for prostate evaluation by digital vaginal exam.

Even in non-transgender individuals, PSA testing is of limited efficacy in screening for prostate cancer. In a sample (N = 2,950) of participants from the Prostate Cancer Prevention Trial, biopsy revealed prostate cancer in 15% of participants who had PSA levels within the normal range for the duration of the trial (Thompson et al., 2004). Androgen antagonists may decrease serum levels of PSA, further complicating interpretation of PSA results in the MTF patient who is taking feminizing endocrine agents (Guess, Heyse, & Gormley, 1993; Leo, Bilhartz, Bergstralh, & Oesterling, 1991). The risks and possible benefits of PSA screening should be discussed with all MTF patients, with screening considered in MTF patients over age 45 who have additional risks such as family history of prostate cancer.

In summary, digital rectal exam should be performed on MTFs at the same frequency as for natal males, regardless of hormonal or surgical status. Risks and possible benefits of PSA screening should be discussed with all MTF patients, and patients taking feminizing endocrine agents should be made aware that PSA levels may be falsely low in an androgen-deficient setting, even in the presence of prostate cancer. PSA screening should only be considered in patients over age 45 who have additional risks for prostate cancer.

Other Cancers

Currently, there is no evidence that transgender persons are at either increased or decreased risk of other cancers. Screening recommendations for other cancers–including colon cancer, lung cancer, and anal cancer–should be followed as with non-transgender patients.

Cardiovascular Disease

Assessing and treating cardiovascular risk factors is an essential primary care intervention for transgender patients. Regardless of hormone status, the transgender population as a whole has several risk factors for cardiovascular disease. Smoking (discussed in detail in a

subsequent section on substance use) is a concern for both FTM and MTF persons. MTF patients tend to present for transgender care at an older age (Blanchard, 1994), and with hypertension, diabetes, hyperlipidemia, and other conditions common in middle age male bodies. FTM patients who present with PCOS are at increased risk for hypertension, insulin resistance and hyperlipidemia. Finally, cardiovascular risk factors are often undiagnosed or undertreated among transgender patients due to their relative lack of primary care. Close monitoring for cardiac events or symptoms is recommended for transgender individuals with risk factors, especially during the first two years of transgender endocrine therapy.

Feminizing and masculinizing endocrine therapy further increases cardiovascular risks in an already high-risk population. We therefore recommend that cardiovascular risk factors be reasonably controlled before initiating feminizing or masculinizing endocrine therapy. As part of physical assessment prior to hormone prescription, stress testing should be considered for patients at very high risk of cardiovascular disease or with any cardiovascular symptoms (Dahl et al., 2006).

Early diagnosis and treatment of cardiovascular risk factors, ideally prior to the onset of cardiovascular disease, may decrease risks associated with transgender endocrine therapy in transgender patients. Modification of diet and exercise, with consultation with a dietician or nutritionist as needed, may be helpful initial steps in controlling risk factors such as hypertension, hyperlipidemia, and diabetes. Daily aspirin therapy should be considered for patients at high risk for coronary artery disease (CAD).

Coronary Artery Disease, Cerebrovascular Disease, and Hormones

Male-to-female. The effects of feminizing hormones on coronary artery disease and cerebrovascular disease in MTFs are not well characterized. There are several case reports of myocardial infarction and ischemic stroke among MTFs taking estrogen (Biller & Saver, 1995; deMarinis & Arnett, 1978; Fortin, Klein, Messmore, & O'Connell, 1984; van Kesteren et al., 1997). However, the retrospective 1997

Netherlands study found no increased incidence of CAD or cerebrovascular disease compared to rates in the general population (van Kesteren et al., 1997).

Increased risk of cardiovascular disease has been noted among non-transgender women taking oral contraceptives, and both the Heart and Estrogen/Progestin Replacement Study (HERS) and Women's Health Initiative (WHI) trials, prospective studies of hormone replacement among postmenopausal women, indicated no benefit and a probable increased risk for cardiovascular events with combined estrogen and progesterone therapy (Grady et al., 2002; Rossouw et al., 2002). The estrogen-only arm of the WHI trial demonstrated an increase in cerebrovascular events but not cardiac events. The HERS and WHI trials were conducted using oral conjugated estrogen; it is unclear whether these effects extend to other oral or transdermal estrogens, which show reduced risk of venous thromboembolic events (Scarabin, Oger, & Plu-Bureau, 2003). In both the HERS trial and the observational Nurses Health Study (Grodstein, Manson, & Stampfer, 2001), an increased number of cardiac events occurred in the first 1 to 2 years and decreased in subsequent years of hormone replacement.

Although the data on MTFs and cardiovascular disease are limited, based on evidence from studies of non-transgender women and hormone replacement therapy we consider MTFs with pre-existing CAD who are using estrogen and/or progestin to be at increased risk of future events. The extent of risk, resulting morbidity, and mortality is unclear; it may be substantial given that doses used for feminization in MTFs are typically much higher than post-menopausal hormone replacement therapy. It may be possible to reduce risks by using transdermal estrogen, reducing the estrogen dose, and omitting progestin from the regimen.

Female-to-male. The effect of testosterone on cardiovascular events in FTM patients is unclear. While both exogenous testosterone and hyperandrogen states (e.g., PCOS) are known to increase cardiac risk factors, current evidence of increase in cardiac morbidity or mortality with PCOS is limited (Cibula et al., 2000; Legro, 2003; Loverro, 2004; Pierpoint, McKeigue, Isaacs, Wild, & Jacobs, 1998; van Kesteren et al., 1997). Studies in non-trans-

gender men and women indicate that low endogenous androgens appear to increase the risk for men, while higher endogenous androgens increase the risk for women (Hak et al., 2002).

In FTMs with pre-existing CAD who are using testosterone, there may be increased risk of future events. The extent of risk, resulting morbidity, and mortality is unclear, given the contradictory effects of testosterone replacement in non-transgender men and increased androgens in non-transgender women. Close monitoring for cardiac events or symptoms is recommended for FTMs at moderate to high risk for CAD.

Hypertension

Hypertension increases the risk of cardiovascular events and strokes, in addition to the independent risks that may be posed by estrogen and testosterone (Rossouw et al., 2002). Studies suggest that these risks are reduced proportionately to the reduction in blood pressure (MacMahon & Rodgers, 1994). A systolic blood pressure goal of ≤ 130 mm Hg and a diastolic goal of ≤ 90 mm Hg is recommended for transgender individuals who are taking feminizing or masculinizing hormones. This is consistent with American recommendations for individuals with compelling indications such as diabetes (Chobanian et al., 2003).

Male-to-female. Standard protocols for screening and treatment of hypertension should be used with MTFs who are not taking feminizing hormones. A systolic blood pressure goal of ≤ 130 mm Hg and a diastolic goal of ≤ 90 mm Hg is recommended for MTFs planning to begin feminizing hormone therapy within 1 to 3 years.

Exogenous estrogen can increase blood pressure, and transgender patients at risk may develop overt hypertension. We recommend that clinicians check the blood pressure of MTF patients who are taking estrogen every 1 to 3 months to monitor for potential hypertension. While a significantly higher incidence compared to the non-transgender population was not noted in the Netherlands study (van Kesteren et al., 1997), the researchers defined hypertension as pressures greater than 160/95 mm Hg, considerably higher than current North American guidelines.

The anti-androgen spironolactone is a diuretic and can therefore lower blood pressure (Asscheman & Gooren, 1992; Feldman & Bockting, 2003, Futterweit, 1998, Steinbeck, 1997). Prior, Vigna, and Watson (1989) reported a significant reduction of systolic blood pressure when spironolactone was added to the regimen of patients who had been on high-estrogen doses, with a decrease from a baseline of 127.8 mm Hg (SD 13.6) to 120.5 mg Hg after one year ($p < 0.05$). Spironolactone should be considered as part of the feminizing endocrine regimen, both for its antihypertensive effect and to allow reduction in estrogen dose (Dahl et al., 2006).

In summary, MTFs who are not taking feminizing hormones should be monitored and treated for hypertension as per standard protocols for natal males. For the MTF patient taking estrogen, blood pressure should be monitored every 1 to 3 months. A systolic blood pressure goal of ≤ 130 mm Hg and a diastolic goal of ≤ 90 mm Hg is recommended for MTF patients who are planning to begin feminizing hormone therapy within 1 to 3 years or are currently taking estrogen. Spironolactone should be considered as part of an antihypertensive regimen.

Female-to-male. Standard protocols for screening and treatment of hypertension should be used with FTMs who are not taking masculinizing hormones. A systolic blood pressure goal of ≤ 130 mm Hg and a diastolic goal of ≤ 90 mm Hg is recommended for FTMs planning to begin masculinizing hormone therapy within 1 to 3 years.

The risk of hypertension in FTMs is unclear. Exogenous testosterone can increase blood pressure (Kirk & Rothblatt, 1995; Steinbeck, 1997), and natal females with PCOS, itself a hyperandrogen syndrome, are at increased risk of hypertension (Cibula et al., 2000). However, a prospective study (N = 28) found no significant change in blood pressure after an average of 18 months testosterone administration, even among participants taking double the normal dose of testosterone (Meyer et al., 1986). A retrospective chart review of 293 FTM patients reported hypertension in 4.1% of FTMs, slightly below norms for natal females and well below norms for natal males (van Kesteren et al., 1997); as noted earlier, this study defined hypertension as greater than 160/95 mm Hg,

which is considerably higher than current North American guidelines.

We recommend that FTMs taking testosterone have their blood pressure checked every 1 to 3 months, with a systolic blood pressure goal of ≤ 130 mm Hg and a diastolic goal of ≤ 90 mm Hg. Prevention, screening, and treatment of hypertension during hormone therapy is particularly important for FTM patients with PCOS or other risk factors for cardiovascular disease.

Lipids

Male-to-female. Studies in both non-transgender women (The Writing Group for the PEPI Trial, 1995) and MTFs (Damewood, Bellantoni, Bachorik, Kimball, & Rock, 1989; New et al., 1997; New, Duffy, Harper, & Meredith, 2000; Sosa et al., 2004) demonstrate increased HDL and decreased LDL cholesterol after initiation of estrogen therapy. However, both the HERS and WHI trials, prospective studies of hormone replacement among postmenopausal women, indicated no benefit and a probable increased risk for cardiovascular events with combined estrogen and progesterone therapy (Grady et al., 2002; Rossouw et al., 2002). Oral estrogen therapy, both in postmenopausal women and MTF patients, is known to increase triglycerides, and has precipitated pancreatitis in several cases (Glueck, Lang, Hamer, & Tracy, 1994).

We recommend that standard hyperlipidemia screening and treatment protocols used for non-transgender patients be used for MTFs who are not taking estrogen, with a LDL goal of < 3.5 mmol/L for patients planning to start feminizing endocrine therapy within 1 to 3 years. MTF patients taking estrogen should have high cholesterol treated to an LDL goal of < 3.5 mmol/L for low to moderate risk patients, and < 2.5 mmol/L for high risk patients. These targets are consistent with Canadian recommendations for the prevention of cardiovascular disease (Genest, Frohlich, Fodor, & McPherson, 2003).

An annual fasting lipid profile is recommended throughout feminizing endocrine therapy to monitor for hyperlipidemia. Transdermal estrogen is recommended for MTF patients with hyperlipidemia, particularly hypertriglyceridemia. Exercise is recommended in all groups to treat low HDL levels.

Female-to-male. Patients taking testosterone typically experience increases in LDL and decreases in HDL cholesterol, putting them at increased risk of atherosclerotic disease (Asscheman et al., 1994; Goh, Loke, & Ratnam, 1995; McCredie et al., 1998). However, no extra cardiovascular morbidity was found in the retrospective Dutch study (van Kesteren et al., 1997). Both FTM patients and non-transgender women with PCOS are at increased risk of dyslipidemias, although the effect on the risk of cardiac events is undetermined (Cibula et al., 2000; Legro, 2003; Loverro, 2004; Pierpoint et al., 1998).

We recommend that standard hyperlipidemia screening and treatment protocols used for non-transgender patients be used for FTMs who are not taking testosterone, with a LDL goal of < 3.5 mmol/L for patients planning to start testosterone therapy within 1 to 3 years. FTM patients taking testosterone should have high cholesterol treated to an LDL goal of < 3.5 mmol/L for low to moderate risk patients, and < 2.5 mmol/L for high risk patients. These targets are consistent with Canadian recommendations for the prevention of cardiovascular disease (Genest et al., 2003).

An annual fasting lipid profile is recommended throughout masculinizing endocrine therapy to monitor for hyperlipidemia. Supraphysiologic testosterone levels should be avoided in patients who have hyperlipidemia, with daily topical or weekly intramuscular injections preferred over bi-weekly injections. Exercise is recommended in all groups to treat low HDL levels.

Diabetes Mellitus

Male-to-Female

Estrogen is known to impair glucose tolerance (Espeland et al., 1998; Godsland et al., 1993; Troisi, Cowie, & Harris, 2000) and there have been case reports of new onset type 2 diabetes among male-to-female transgender patients on estrogen (Feldman, 2002). Studies of non-transgender women taking oral contraceptives or hormone replacement therapy have reported decreased glucose tolerance but no increased incidence of diabetes (Manson et al., 1992; Rimm et al., 1992; Russell-Briefel, Ezzati, Perlman, & Murphy, 1987). However, these findings may not apply to biologically male transgender patients who have other risk factors for Type 2 diabetes. A study of glucose tolerance among hyperandrogenic women on oral contraceptives demonstrated a significant reduction in glucose tolerance and the development of diabetes in two of the sixteen women (Nader, Riad-Gabriel, & Saad, 1997), suggesting that the presence of endogenous androgens plays a role in glucose metabolism. In addition, patients on feminizing hormones often gain weight and body fat, which may contribute to glucose intolerance.

Standard diabetes screening protocols used for the non-transgender population should be followed with MTF patients who are not taking estrogen. As MTFs who take estrogen may be at increased risk for Type 2 diabetes, an annual fasting glucose test is recommended in patients with family history of diabetes or weight gain exceeding 5 kilograms. Glucose tolerance testing (GTT)–or glycosylated hemoglobin (A1c) testing for patients unable to perform a GTT–should be considered in patients with evidence of impaired glucose tolerance without diabetes.

Regardless of hormone status, diabetes management is the same in the MTF patient as the non-transgender patient. In the MTF taking estrogen, given the underlying mechanism of insulin resistance, treatment with an insulin sensitizing agent may be warranted for treatment of glucose intolerance and Type 2 diabetes if dietary change is not sufficient. Decrease in estrogen dose may be recommended if glucose is difficult to control or the patient is unable to lose weight.

Female-to-Male

As noted previously, there is evidence of a higher incidence of PCOS among FTMs, which carries an increased risk of glucose intolerance. There is no current evidence of an altered risk of Type 2 diabetes in FTMs who are taking testosterone. Testosterone does increase visceral fat among FTM patients (Elbers, Asscheman, Seidell, Megens, & Gooren, 1997), and older non-transgender women with high testosterone levels are at increased risk of developing Type 2 diabetes as well (Oh, Barrett-Connor, Wedick, & Wingard, 2002). Further research is needed to clarify how these findings affect the risk of diabetes in the FTM population.

With FTM patients we recommend screening by patient history for PCOS, with subsequent diabetes screening if PCOS is suspected. Guidelines for managing diabetes mellitus are the same for FTMs as for the non-transgender population.

HIV and Hepatitis B/C

Because HIV and Hepatitis B/C are transmitted by blood as well as through sex, we consider prevention and screening of HIV and Hepatitis B/C separate from sexually transmitted infections (STIs). STIs are discussed in a later section of the article.

As a whole, the transgender population appears to have a disproportionately high rate of HIV/AIDS (Asscheman, Gooren, & Eklund, 1989; Boles & Elifson, 1994; Clements-Nolle, Katz, & Marx, 1999), although prevalence varies greatly across gender identity. Reported HIV rates from seroprevalence studies in the U.S. range from 20-35% among individuals in the MTF spectrum, with 2-3% incidence among FTMs (Clements-Nolle, Marx, Guzman, & Katz, 2001; Kellog, Clements-Nolle, Dilley, Katz, & McFarland, 2001; Kenagy, 2002; Kenagy & Bostwick, 2005; McGowan, 1999; Risser et al., 2005; Simon, Reback, & Bemis, 2000; Xavier & Simmons, 2000).

Although there is significant variation in sexual behaviours and risks among transgender individuals, American studies suggest that psychosocial cofactors relating to unsafe sex—such as poor self-esteem, lack of safety in a romantic relationship, substance use, compulsive sex to affirm identity—are common concerns among MTFs (Bockting, Robinson, & Rosser, 1998; Clements-Nolle et al., 2001; Keatley et al., 2002; Kenagy, 2002; Mathy, 2002; Nemoto, Sugano, Operario, & Keatley, 2004). The reported prevalence of HIV among FTMs is thus far low, but studies suggest three risk factors of particular concern for possible sexual transmission: (a) lack of knowledge relating to HIV transmission and prevention, (b) misperception that FTMs are intrinsically at low risk for HIV, and (c) failure to consistently use a latex barrier during receptive anal or vaginal intercourse (Kenagy, 2002; Namaste, 1999).

Although prevalence of Hepatitis B and C among transgender individuals is not known, the common co-infection of HIV and Hepatitis B and C among individuals who have contracted HIV through blood-borne transmission is cause for concern. Needle-sharing with injectable hormones or silicone is a trans-specific potential risk factor for transmission of HIV and Hepatitis B and C (Bockting et al., 1998; Nemoto, Luke, Mamo, Ching, & Patria, 1999), and patients need to be educated regarding the risks as well as safe handling of needles and syringes. The prevalence of needle-sharing for injection of street drugs is not known. One American study found that 20% of MTF participants had injected street drugs at least once in the past six months, and that nearly 50% of those reporting injection drug use had shared syringes (Clements-Nolle et al., 2001).

Prevention of HIV and Hepatitis B and C involves education and behavioral change specifically tailored to the economic, psychosocial and physical circumstances of transgender persons (Bockting et al., 2005; Clements-Nolle, Wilkinson, Kitano, & Marx, 1999; Kammerer, Mason, Connors, & Durkee, 2001; Nemoto et al., 2002; Sausa, 2003; Warren, 1999). Clinicians should treat all patients with STIs and their partners according to recommended guidelines for non-transgender patients, to reduce risk of HIV and Hepatitis B transmission.

HIV testing has been shown to be an effective element in reducing transmission and gaining access to life-extending treatment in all populations. Recent analysis suggests that at least one-time HIV screening for all patients, regardless of risk, is a cost-effective public health strategy (Sanders et al., 2005). If there is a history of prior STIs or ongoing risk behaviours for sexual or blood-borne transmission of HIV–including unprotected penile-vaginal or penile-anal intercourse and sharing needles for injection of hormones or illicit drugs–screening for HIV and Hepatitis B and C should be considered every 6 months.

Hepatitis C is primarily transmitted through blood contact, and patients at risk benefit from testing and treatment. Hepatitis B vaccination, recommended for all children and adolescents, is highly effective and should be offered to all adult transgender patients as well. Care should be taken to monitor liver enzymes in patients who have chronic hepatitis and are taking feminizing or masculinizing endocrine agents (Asscheman & Gooren, 1992; Futterweit, 1998; van Kesteren et al., 1997).

Some HIV medications increase or decrease serum estrogen levels (a list is available as an online supplement at http://www.vch.ca/transhealth/resources/library/tcpdocs/estrogen-interactions.pdf), but there is no evidence that transgender endocrine therapy interferes with the effectiveness of HIV medication or negatively affect the progression of HIV/AIDS. Protease inhibitors increase the risk of hyperglycemia and hyperlipidemia, and these patients may need to be monitored closely, especially if taking estrogen.

Little has been published regarding the risks of reassignment surgery among patients with HIV/AIDS. HIV-positive persons have an increased risk of infection with any major surgery, with the number and severity of complications related to CD4 count. SRS outcomes appear to be good with adequate patient selection and pre-operative preparation (Kirk, 1999; Wilson, 1999).

In summary, as with the non-transgender population, any transgender patients with ongoing risk behaviours for sexual or blood-borne transmission of HIV, Hepatitis B, and Hepatitis C should be counselled about risks and prevention. HIV and Hepatitis B and C screening should be considered every 6 months for those with ongoing transmission risks, with screening at least once during the lifetime for all other patients. To reduce risk of HIV and Hepatitis B transmission, transgender individuals with STIs and their sexual partners should be treated according to recommended guidelines for non-transgender patients. Hepatitis B vaccination should be offered to all patients who are not already immune.

Mental Health

Although studies are limited, there is no increased incidence of major psychopathology in individuals with gender dysphoria compared to the general population (Cole, O'Boyle, Emory, & Meyer, 1997). However, the impact of psychosocial stresses–including the transpho-bic harassment, discrimination, and violence experienced by many transgender individuals (Nemoto, Sugano, et al., 2004)–is cause for concern. Depression is not uncommon among transgender patients, with 30-40% of the respondents in a San Francisco study reporting having been prescribed medication for a mental health condition, and 32% reporting prior suicide attempts (Clements, Katz, et al., 1999). In a Canadian study, 42% of respondents reported needing mental health assistance in the past, with 39% stating a current need for mental health services (Goldberg et al., 2003).

The primary care provider should routinely screen for mental health concerns and refer to trans-competent mental health professionals as needed. Peer support resources may also be appropriate. Management of co-existing gender concerns and mental health concerns is discussed in greater detail elsewhere (Bockting et al., 2006).

Musculoskeletal Health

The effects of estrogen, anti-androgens, and testosterone on lean muscle mass are well established from both transgender studies (Elbers, Asscheman, Seidell, & Gooren, 1999; Gooren & Bunck, 2004) and non-transgender studies (Bhasin et al., 1996; Blackman et al., 2002; Dobs, Nguyen, Pace, & Roberts, 2002; Griggs et al., 1989; Katznelson et al., 1996). It is estimated that approximately 4 kilograms lean body mass is lost following initiation of androgen deprivation in MTFs, and approximately 4 kilograms gained following initiation of testosterone in FTMs (Gooren, 1999).

Exercise may help MTFs taking feminizing endocrine agents to maintain muscle tone. Case reports exist of tendon rupture in both FTM patients on testosterone and non-transgender men taking anabolic steroids (Morgenthaler & Weber, 2005; Strauss & Yesalis, 1991). To avoid tendon rupture, FTMs who are involved in strength training and are taking testosterone should be instructed to increase weight load gradually, with an emphasis on repetitions rather than weight.

Osteoporosis

There is no evidence of increased risk of osteoporosis for transgender patients who do not take feminizing or masculinizing endocrine agents and have not had orchiectomy or oophorectomy. For these patients, screening should follow protocols for natal males (MTF) and natal females (FTM).

The effects of feminizing and masculinizing endocrine agents on bone density are controversial. Research evidence and practice recommendations are discussed below.

Loss of bone density is most likely in transgender patients who are not fully adherent to endocrine therapy following gonadal removal, or who have other risk factors (e.g., Asian or European heritage, smoking, family history, high alcohol use, hyperthyroidism). Calcium and vitamin D supplementation and weight bearing exercise are indicated for all transgender patients taking hormones who are at risk for osteoporosis. Densitometry screening may be indicated for patients at increased risk of osteoporosis, although normative data for transgender patients have not been established. Regardless of hormonal or surgical status, if a transgender patient shows significant bone loss compared to natal sex norms, further intervention is warranted. Bisphosphonates have been demonstrated to increase bone density and decrease fracture risk in non-transgender men and women (Watts, 2001). There are no long-term studies in transgender patients examining the degree to which loss of bone density correlates to the risk of clinical fractures; however, data in non-transgender men and women strongly support this conclusion (De Laet, van Hout, Burger, Hofman, & Pols 1997).

Male-to-Female

Studies in MTF patients suggest that feminizing endocrine therapy does not result in loss of bone mineral density (Schlatterer, Auer, Yassouridis, von Werder, & Stalla, 1998; van Kesteren, Lips, Gooren, Asscheman, & Megens, 1998), but long-term prospective studies have not been done. Prior to orchiectomy, no screening is recommended for the MTF patient taking feminizing endocrine agents except as indicated by additional risk factors. Calcium and Vitamin D supplementation is recommended.

Estrogen therapy is advised following orchiectomy to reduce the risk of osteoporosis. It is unclear how much estrogen is needed following gonadal removal to protect against bone loss, but studies in postmenopausal non-transgender women suggest that very low doses such as 0.025 mg transdermal estradiol may be sufficient (Doeren & Samsioe, 2000; Evans & Davie, 1996). If there are contraindications to estrogen therapy, supplemental calcium (1200 mg daily) and Vitamin D (600 units daily) are recommended to limit bone loss. If there are additional risk factors for bone loss, consider weekly bisphosphonate (35-70 mg alendronate, 35 mg risedronate) for osteoporosis prevention. Bone density screening should be considered for patients over age 60 who have been off estrogen therapy for longer than 5 years.

Female-to-Male

The effect of masculinizing endocrine agents on bone density is controversial. Although studies have found that exogenous testosterone maintains bone density to some degree in FTMs (Goh & Ratnam, 1997; Schlatterer, Auer et al., 1998; Turner et al., 2004; van Kesteren et al., 1998) it may not be sufficient, especially after oophorectomy (Tangpricha, Turner, Malabanan, & Holick, 2001; van Kesteren et al., 1998). Some FTM patients may use depot medroxyprogesterone acetate to produce amenorrhea, which appears to result in bone density loss with long term use in non-transgender women (Scholes, LaCroix, Ichikawa, Barlow, & Ott, 2005). Regardless of surgical status, supplemental calcium (1200 mg daily) and Vitamin D (600 units daily) are recommended for FTMs taking testosterone, to help maintain bone density. Bone density screening should be considered in FTMs over age 50 who have been on testosterone therapy for longer than 5 years, with earlier screening for patients who have additional risk factors.

Following oophorectomy, it is unclear how much testosterone is needed to protect against bone loss. Dahl and colleagues (2006) recommend reducing the dosage of testosterone to the level needed to keep serum free testosterone within the lower-middle end of the male reference interval. If there are contraindications to testosterone therapy, consider weekly bisphosphonate (35-70 mg alendronate, 35 mg risedronate) for osteoporosis prevention.

Sexual Health

Sexually Transmitted Infections (STIs)

STI testing and diagnosis. The primary care provider's recommendation to test for STIs depends on prevailing epidemiology and assessment of individual risk (Laboratory Centre for Disease Control [LCDC] Expert Working Group on Canadian Guidelines for Sexually Transmitted Disease, 1998). Individual risk is considered to include signs and symptoms of a specific STI, history of sexual activity known to pose risk for STI transmission, and membership in a population known to be at heightened risk for STI transmission. If the category "men who have sex with men" (MSM) is extended to include transgender individuals of any gender who have sex with men (TSM), as discussed in the earlier section on vaccinations (Gay and Lesbian Medical Association, 2001), many transgender individuals would be considered in a population that is at increased risk for STIs–identified by LCDC (1998) as youth under 25, street-involved individuals, men who have sex with men, and commercial sex trade workers.

Data on the rates of STIs other than HIV among transgender populations is limited. In a 1999 San Francisco study, 53% of MTF participants and 31% of FTM participants reported a prior sexually transmitted infection (Clements-Nolle, Katz, et al., 1999), with 36% reported for both groups in a New York survey (McGowan, 1999). While from a population health perspective a significant percentage of the transgender community is at risk for STIs, sexual practices among transgender individuals vary greatly (Bockting et al., 2005; Coleman, Bockting, & Gooren, 1993; Devor, 1993; Lawrence, 2005), and assumptions should not be made about the gender of a patient's sexual partner(s), sexual activities, or individual risks.

Sexual activities vary depending on the patient's anatomy and preferences, as well as that of their partner(s). While some transgender individuals are strongly dysphoric about their genitals, others enjoy using them sexually. Both MTFs and FTMs may engage in receptive or insertive oral, vaginal, and anal intercourse. While digital-genital contact or use of dildos is considered low risk for transmission of HIV, Hepatitis B, syphillis, gonorrhea, and chlamydia,

other STIs (e.g., herpes, trichomonas, HPV) can be transmitted by sharing of sex toys or by unprotected genital touching.

Potentially high-risk sexual behaviours reported by transgender research participants include unprotected sex, sex while intoxicated, and sex with multiple partners (Avery, Cole, & Meyer, 1995; Clements-Nolle, Katz et al., 1999; Gross & Davis, 2004; Kenagy & Hsieh, 2005; Lindley, Nicholson, Kerby, & Lu, 2003; McGowan, 1999). Cofactors related to unsafe sex, such as depression, suicidal ideation, and physical or sexual abuse, are also increased among the transgender population (Clements-Nolle, Marx et al., 2001; Keatley et al., 2002; Kenagy, 2002; Mathy, 2002; Nemoto, Sugano et al., 2004). Studies indicate the need to affirm one's gender identity can drive high-risk sexual behaviors (Bockting et al., 1998; Clements-Nolle, Marx et al., 2001; Nemoto, Operario, Keatley, & Villegas, 2004).

Ideally, recommendations relating to STI testing are individualized, based on a thorough understanding of the specific sexual activities and behaviours a patient engages in. However, it is often awkward for both the clinician and patient to discuss explicit sexual details in the primary care setting (Boekeloo et al., 1991; Bull et al., 1999; Epstein et al., 1998; Haley, Maheux, Rivard, & Gervais, 1999; Verhoeven et al., 2003). As patient trust is particularly fragile in transgender care, discussion of genitals is sensitive for many transgender patients, and a paucity of clinical language exists to discuss sex in a way that is trans-inclusive and respectful, we feel it is more practical to recommend that any transgender patient who is sexually active be tested regularly for the STIs that are most common locally. For clinicians in North America, we recommend testing all sexually active transgender patients yearly for gonorrhea, chlamydia, and syphillis, with tests every 6 months if the patient reports recurrent STIs, unprotected sex with a partner who might be at risk for STIs, unprotected anal or vaginal sex with more than one partner, psychosocial cofactors relating to unsafe sex, or other risk factors. If there is strong clinician-patient rapport and the patient is comfortable talking about sexuality, more detailed discussion of sexual activities is preferable to facilitate individualized testing and prevention.

The variable anatomy of transgender patients affects how screening or diagnostic tests for gonorrhea and chlamydia are performed. A urine-based test of a non-clean catch specimen of the first 25 ml of urine (e.g., Gen-Probe™) can be used regardless of anatomy, making this the ideal testing method for most transgender patients. Alternatively, a urethral sample can be taken in patients with a natal penis (MTF pre-surgery), or a vaginal (MTF post-vaginoplasty, FTM pre-vaginectomy) or cervical sample (FTM pre-hysterectomy) may be appropriate. Rectal and pharyngeal samples can be used in patients with symptoms in these areas.

STI prevention. STI prevention should reflect the patient's anatomical and psychosocial needs. For example, non-penetrative sexual activities or penetration with a dildo can be recommended for MTF patients who are taking feminizing endocrine agents and therefore unable to sustain an erection sufficiently firm for condom use. To prevent condom breakage, supplemental lubrication should be made available to MTFs who have had vaginoplasty (as the neovagina is not self-lubricating) and to FTMs who take testosterone (as decreased estrogen can result in vaginal atrophy and dryness). The unique difficulties faced by transgender people in negotiating safe sex should be acknowledged and explored (Bockting et al., 1998; Bockting et al., 2005).

Sex trade workers are often mistakenly assumed to be at intrinsically higher risk for STIs due to failure to use condoms with clients. Like non-transgender women in the sex trade, MTFs in the sex trade report using condoms relatively consistently with clients, but far less consistently with romantic partners (Gras et al., 1997; Gwadz, Clatts, Goldamt, Lankenau, & Leonard, 2002; Nemoto, Operario, et al., 2004; Rodrigo Álvaro, Rodríguez-Arenas, Ramón, & Martín Martín, 2002; Scheer, Delgado, & Schwarcz, 2004). Counseling relating to STI prevention in romantic relationships should not be overlooked in primary care of transgender individuals involved in the sex trade.

STI treatment. Treatment of STIs should follow regional STI guidelines or recent updates by the Centre for Disease Control for treatment of non-transgender individuals. Transgender endocrine therapy does not affect treatment of STIs in the transgender individual.

Fertility Issues

Transgender endocrine therapy may reduce fertility and this may be permanent even if endocrine agents are discontinued. Potential reproductive impacts and options should be discussed with any transgender patient who is considering endocrine therapy (Meyer et al., 2001). Sperm banking is most useful prior to initiation of endocrine therapy, as feminizing endocrine agents can permanently impact fertility; ideally, several samples should be banked. With the patient's permission, an introductory letter should be sent by the primary care provider alerting the centre that the patient is transgender so the MTF who is already cross-living will be treated in a respectful manner. Oocyte cryopreservation is currently considered investigational, but should be discussed with FTMs as services develop.

Testosterone should not be considered a fail-safe contraceptive for FTM patients. FTMs may continue to ovulate on testosterone therapy, even if menses have stopped; the risk of pregnancy is reduced but not predictably. Additionally, testosterone can adversely affect a developing fetus. Depo-Provera®, barrier methods, and spermicides are possible contraceptive options for FTMs at risk of pregnancy who are on or considering testosterone therapy.

Sexual Function

Feminizing and masculinizing endocrine therapy may impact sexual function (Dahl et al., 2006). Testosterone therapy tends to increase libido among FTM patients, while feminizing endocrine agents tend to reduce libido, reduce erectile function, and decrease ejaculation among MTF patients. If an MTF patient is concerned about limiting erectile dysfunction while undergoing feminizing endocrine therapy, the prescribing clinician should first consider adjusting the dose of the feminizing agents, while addressing the patient's desires regarding the degree of feminization and level of erectile function. If this is unsuccessful, erection-enhancing drugs such as sildenafil may be considered.

Some clinicians have observed an increased incidence of acute prostatitis among MTF patients in the first few years of transition, which could be caused by cessation of ejaculation resulting in stagnant prostate secretions. There may also be increased risk for acute prostatitis or urinary tract infection after vaginoplasty, due to the shortened urethra.

Following genital surgery, overall sexual function, libido, arousal, orgasm, and pain during sex is variable. Outcomes depend on pre-operative sexual function, the type of surgery performed, and post-operative complications. Elsewhere, Bowman and Goldberg (2006) review research relating to sexual function following sex reassignment surgery.

Substance Use

Smoking

Little is known about smoking prevalence in the transgender population. In a study of transgender patients presenting to a Minnesota clinic for transgender endocrine therapy, 37% reported being current smokers compared to 20% for the Minnesota population overall (Feldman, Bockting, Allen, & Brintell, 2003). Among the transgender population there are commonly multiple identified risk factors for smoking, such as poverty, stressful living and work environments, and societal marginalization (Gilman, Abrams, & Buka, 2003; Gruskin, Hart, Gordon, & Ackerson, 2001; Tang et al., 2004). Accordingly, we recommend that all transgender patients be screened for past and present tobacco use.

Trans-specific risks associated with smoking include an increased risk of venous thromboembolic events with estrogen therapy and reassignment surgery, possible increased risk of cardiovascular disease with both feminizing and masculinizing endocrine therapy (especially over age 50), and delayed healing following surgery. Smoking cessation is strongly encouraged before initiating transgender endocrine therapy (Dahl et al., 2006) and is mandatory prior to phalloplasty or another free flap surgical procedure (Bowman & Goldberg, 2006). Smoking cessation interventions can be effective, particularly if they are incorporated into a comprehensive transgender care program. This approach involves consistent smoking cessation messages from all staff, frequent supportive follow-up of cessation efforts, and direct communication of the limitations and risks that smoking imposes on transgender endocrine therapy and sex reassignment surgery (Feldman & Bockting, 2003). Buproprion, nicotine replacement, and behavioral modification techniques may be appropriate.

Alcohol and Drug Use

Rates of alcohol and drug use among transgender individuals are not known, but may be increased due to self-medication for depression, as well as high rates of exposure to discrimination and abuse. A study of 209 MTFs in San Francisco found that 45% had used drugs or alcohol within the previous 30 days, and alcohol, marijuana, cocaine, and methamphetamines were the drugs most commonly used (Reback & Lombardi, 1999). Other trans-specific American studies reported substance use ranging from 20-30% (Bockting et al., 2005; Clements-Nolle, Katz et al., 1999; Cole et al., 1997; Valentine, 1998). Accordingly, we recommend that all transgender patients be asked about current and past alcohol and drug use, with referral to a trans-competent chemical dependency program as needed.

In all referrals, care should be taken to ensure the service is trans-competent prior to referral. In referral to residential addiction programs that have gender-specific programming or facilities, particular attention is needed to ensure the transgender person will be welcomed and that appropriate accommodations will be made in sleeping arrangements, shower use, bathroom use, and group activities. Other trans-specific issues in addiction treatment are discussed in further detail elsewhere (Bockting et al., 2006).

Venous Thrombosis, Thromboembolism, and Feminizing Hormones

As noted by Dahl and colleagues (2006), MTF patients taking any form of estrogen are at increased risk of venous thromboembolic events (VTE), with the risk potentially as high as a 20-fold increase (van Kesteren et al., 1997). These risks are greater for MTFs older than 40 years, those who smoke, and those who are sedentary. Risks may be reduced somewhat by use of transdermal estrogen in lower doses (Scarabin et al., 2003; van Kesteren et al., 1997). Patients should be warned regarding the risks of VTE, given information about the signs and symptoms, and counseled regarding preventive measures and lifestyle issues. Daily aspirin therapy should be considered in patients with risk factors for VTE who are taking estrogen. Estrogen therapy is contraindicated in MTF patients with a history of VTE or underlying thrombophilia such as anticardiolipin syndrome and Factor V Leiden.

THE PRIMARY CARE PROVIDER AND FEMINIZING OR MASCULINIZING MEDICAL INTERVENTIONS

Some transgender patients seek medical assistance to feminize or masculinize their bodies through endocrine therapy, surgery, or removal of hair through laser treatments or electrolysis. While specialists are often involved in this level of care, the primary care provider plays a vital role in coordinating care, providing referrals, co-managing endocrine treatment (including monitoring lab work and side effects, avoiding drug interactions, supporting smoking cessation, etc.), and providing post-surgical followup.

There is great variation in the extent to which hormonal or surgical changes are undertaken or desired. Not all transgender individuals feel a discrepancy between gender identity and the body. Among those who do, some seek maximum feminization or masculinization, while others experience relief with an androgynous presentation resulting from endocrinological or surgical minimization of sex characteristics.

Endocrinological and surgical treatment can profoundly increase quality of life for transgender individuals who desire to bring their bodies into greater congruence with their gender identity (Mate-Kole, Freschi, & Robin, 1990; Pfäfflin & Junge, 1998; Smith, Van Goozen, Kuiper, & Cohen-Kettenis, 2005). If medical concerns emerge regarding hormonal interventions or planned surgeries, efforts should be made to try to control them where possible through changes to behavior and lifestyle or through medication. Reduction or dis-

continuation of endocrine therapy or cancellation of planned surgery should be a last rather than first resort and is not to be undertaken lightly as there can be serious psychological consequences.

Transgender Endocrine Therapy in the Primary Care Setting

Transgender endocrine therapy–the provision of exogenous endocrine agents to induce feminizing or masculinizing changes–is a strongly desired medical intervention for many transgender individuals. In addition to inducing physical changes, the act of using cross-sex hormones is itself an affirmation of gender identity, which is a powerful incentive for this population (Gay and Lesbian Medical Association, 2001; Kammerer et al., 1999). Studies have shown improved psychological adjustment and quality of life with endocrine therapy (Kuiper & Cohen-Kettenis, 1988; Leavitt, Berger, Hoeppner, & Northrop, 1980).

Transgender patients desiring endocrine therapy may ask their primary care clinician to provide this treatment. In our experience, primary care providers tend to view transgender medicine as a specialty and often feel hesitant to initiate endocrine therapy, preferring instead to refer patients to endocrinologists for this care. However, we believe that with appropriate training and experience (Goldberg, 2006) primary care providers are well-suited to provide safe and effective masculinizing or feminizing endocrine therapy in the setting of comprehensive health care. As stated by Dahl and colleagues (2006), "medical visits relating to hormone maintenance provide an opportunity for broader care to a population that is often medically underserved, and many of the screening tasks involved in long-term hormone maintenance fall within the scope of primary care rather than specialist care" (p. 112). As the field of transgender medicine is continually evolving, primary care providers with patients undergoing endocrine therapy should become familiar and keep current with the medical literature, and discuss emerging issues with colleagues (through, for example, networks established by the World Professional Association for Transgender Health).

Primary care providers can increase their experience and comfort in providing transgender endocrine therapy through a variety of means. The primary care provider completely new to transgender medicine can begin by reading research reviews and practice guidelines (e.g., Dahl et al., 2006), and by co-managing care or consulting with a more experienced provider. Clinicians can further gain experience by providing maintenance of endocrine therapy to patients who started hormones in consultation with a specialist. Below we discuss the range of potential roles for the primary care clinician in transgender endocrine care.

Bridging. Transgender patients may present for care already taking feminizing or masculinizing endocrine agents, whether prescribed by a clinician or obtained through other means such as internet purchase. In these cases the primary care clinician who is uncomfortable providing long-term endocrine therapy can provide a 1 to 3 month "bridging" prescription for hormones while assisting the patient in finding a clinician who can provide access to long-term care. The patient's current regimen should be assessed for safety and drug interactions (using Dahl et al., 2006, or a similar protocol), with safer medications or doses suggested when indicated. If endocrine agents were previously prescribed, with the patient's permission, the previous medical records should be requested and the history of endocrine therapy documented in the current chart. Primary care providers who prescribe bridging hormones need to work with the patient to establish limits as to the time length of bridging therapy.

Endocrine therapy following gonad removal. Hormone replacement with estrogen or testosterone is usually continued lifelong after oophorectomy or orchiectomy, unless medical contraindications arise. Guidelines for post-operative endocrine therapy are discussed elsewhere (Dahl et al., 2006). Laboratory monitoring can be done yearly for otherwise healthy patients.

Hormone maintenance prior to gonad removal. Once patients have achieved maximal feminizing or masculinizing benefit from endocrine therapy–typically two or more years–they remain on a maintenance dose. Maintaining body changes generally requires lower doses of endocrine agents compared to initial induction. The maintenance dose is then adjusted for change in health conditions, aging, or lifestyle.

The patient presenting for maintenance endocrine therapy should have their current regimen assessed for safety and drug interactions, with safer medications or doses suggested when indicated. The patient should be monitored by physical exam and laboratory testing every six months (Dahl et al., 2006). For MTFs over age 40, transdermal rather than oral estrogen is recommended; over age 50, the clinician should consider decreasing the estrogen dose to 100 mcg twice per week or less, depending on the patient's health status and particularly cardiovascular risk. For FTMs, testosterone doses should be sufficient to maintain free testosterone levels in the low to normal male range.

Patients may occasionally need to reduce or temporarily stop their endocrine therapy in anticipation of upcoming medical procedures, such as surgery or sperm banking. MTF patients should discontinue estrogen 2 to 4 weeks prior to any major surgery to reduce the risk of thromboembolic events (Bowman & Goldberg, 2006). It is helpful to discuss any temporary interruption of endocrine therapy with the patient well in advance.

Initiating hormonal feminization or masculinization. Protocols for initiation of transgender endocrine therapy are discussed in detail elsewhere (Dahl et al., 2006). While the trans-experienced primary care provider can coordinate initiation of endocrine therapy in most cases, the patient should be referred to a trans-experienced endocrinologist if there is a pre-existing metabolic or endocrine disorder that may be affected by hormone therapy. Referral to other specialists may be appropriate if there are conditions that require further assessment prior to initiating transgender endocrine therapy (e.g., cardiovascular disease).

The WPATH *Standards of Care* advise that prior to initiation of transgender endocrine therapy patients should be assessed by a trans-experienced mental health professional to determine hormone eligibility and readiness (Meyer et al., 2001). As discussed by Bockting and colleagues (2006), physicians and nurse practitioners with appropriate training, expertise, and a practice structure that allows extended sessions may perform this assessment; alternatively, the patient may be referred to a mental health clinician who has the appropriate experience.

Whether the mental health assessment is performed by the prescribing clinician or by a third party, ideally the prescribing clinician and the patient will work with a therapist trained in treating gender identity issues as endocrine therapy begins. As stated in the WPATH *Standards of Care*, psychotherapy is not a requirement prior to initiation of transgender endocrine therapy (Meyer et al., 2001). However, the process of gender transition involves profound mental, social, emotional, economic, and legal changes in a patient's life. Endocrine therapy can be both an enriching and complicating element in this transition, and trans-competent mental health professionals can provide a wide variety of resources to assist the transgender patient (and prescribing clinician) in this complex process. If a therapist is involved, with the patient's consent regular communication is advised to ensure that the transition process is proceeding smoothly, both physically and psychosocially.

Primary Care of the Patient Undergoing Sex Reassignment Surgery

Sex reassignment surgery refers to a number of procedures that can be undertaken to surgically feminize or masculinize the face, neck, breasts or chest, genitals, and overall body contours; remove the gonads; stop menstrual periods (FTM); and raise voice pitch (MTF). Depending on the specific procedure sought, the patient may require referral to a plastic surgeon, urologist, gynecologist, reproductive endocrinologist, or otolaryngologist with expertise in SRS.

The Primary Care Clinician's Role Prior to SRS

The WPATH *Standards of Care* advise that patients seeking chest or breast surgery should be assessed by an appropriately trained mental health professional to determine SRS eligibility and readiness, with assessment by two mental health professionals required prior to genital surgery or gonadal removal (Meyer et al., 2001). Some surgeons provide these referrals;

in other cases the primary care provider may need to coordinate referral.

As with transgender endocrine therapy, psychotherapy is not an absolute requirement for SRS (Meyer et al., 2001). However, supportive professional and peer counseling can be helpful with preparation and adjustment, and should be accessible to all patients before and after surgery. The primary care provider can assist by discussing patient awareness of resources and, where needed, facilitating referrals to trans-experienced professionals.

Assessment of physical health and investigation of any medical conditions of concern are standard pre-operative procedures. Although the surgeon will do a full patient history and physical examination–usually several months prior to surgery–it is helpful if the primary care provider provides a letter reviewing the pertinent past medical history of the patient (Bowman & Goldberg, 2006). The primary care clinician also has an important role in helping the patient address any health concerns that will likely be of concern to the surgeon, such as smoking or uncontrolled diabetes. This is particularly important if the patient has to travel a great distance to the surgeon, as in these situations advance physical evaluation by the surgeon may be prohibitively expensive.

The Primary Care Clinician's Role Following SRS

As discussed by Bowman and Goldberg (2006), MTF breast augmentation and FTM chest surgery, hysterectomy, and oophorectomy involve relatively minor modification of surgical procedures routinely performed for the non-transgender population. While there are important trans-specific refinements to techniques used in these surgeries, post-operative care is the same as for the non-transgender population, and complications are usually minor and are typically managed by the primary care provider.

Genital reassignment surgery is a more complex procedure with multiple trans-specific considerations, and consultation with an experienced surgeon is advised for any postoperative concerns (Bowman & Goldberg, 2006). However, the primary care provider will likely be the first clinician the patient approaches if there are complications. At minimum, the primary care provider should expect to monitor wound healing following genital surgery. If there are complications, the expense and time involved in traveling back to the original surgeon may mean that the primary care provider must liaise between the patient, the original surgeon, and local specialists who are not expert in SRS to coordinate a care plan.

As the primary care provider will likely be the clinician providing ongoing preventive and health promotion care following sex reassignment surgery, the primary care provider should discuss with the patient any screening tests that will be needed on an ongoing basis and the types of procedures that will be involved. For example, the primary care clinician should ensure that MTFs are aware that prostate checks are still needed after genital surgery and discuss special mammogram procedures needed following breast implants, and should ensure that FTMs understand that even after chest surgery there is a risk of breast cancer. Following vaginoplasty, the primary care provider should check with the MTF patient periodically about dilation and provide recommendations relating to vaginal cuff Pap smears. For both MTFs and FTMs, STI prevention and sexual health should be discussed before and after genital surgery, as there is a paucity of trans-relevant information in consumer sexual health literature.

CONCLUDING REMARKS

Transgender persons represent an underserved community in need of sensitive, comprehensive health care. Primary medical care providers will likely encounter patients with gender identity issues at some point in their practice, whether or not they choose to provide transgender endocrine therapy. We hope this document helps primary care providers to feel more confident in clinical practice with the transgender community.

REFERENCES

Amy, R., Coldman, A., Ehlen, T., St. Germain, L., Hayes, M., Kan, L., Lo, J., Matisic, J., O'Connor, R., Chou, S., Sentell, J., Suen, K., Thomson, T., & van Niekerk, D. (2005). *Screening for cancer of the cer-*

vix: An office manual for health professionals (6th ed.). Vancouver, BC: BC Cancer Agency.

Asscheman, H., & Gooren, L. J. G. (1992). Hormone treatment in transsexuals. *Journal of Psychology & Human Sexuality, 5*(4), 39-54.

Asscheman, H., Gooren, L. J. G., & Eklund, P. L. (1989). Mortality and morbidity in transsexual patients with cross-gender hormone treatment. *Metabolism, 38,* 869-873.

Asscheman, H., Gooren, L. J. G., Megens, J. A. J., Nauta, J., Kloosterboer, H. J., & Eikelboom, F. (1994). Serum testosterone level is the major determinant of the male-female differences in serum levels of high-density lipoprotein (HDL) cholesterol and HDL2 cholesterol. *Metabolism, 43,* 935-939.

Avery, E. N., Cole, C. M., & Meyer, W. J., III (1995, September). *Transsexuals and HIV/AIDS risk behaviors.* Paper presented at the 14th Biennial Symposium of the Harry Benjamin International Gender Dysphoria Association, Kloster Irsee, Germany.

Bakker, A., van Kesteren, P. J., Gooren, L. J. G., & Bezemer, P. D. (1993). The prevalence of transsexualism in the Netherlands. *Acta Psychiatrica Scandinavica, 87,* 237-238.

Balen, A. H., Schacter, M. E., Montgomery, D., Reid, R. W., & Jacobs, H. S. (1993). Polycystic ovaries are a common finding in untreated female to male transsexuals. *Clinical Endocrinology, 38,* 325-9.

Baxter, N. (2001). Preventive health care, 2001 update: Should women be routinely taught breast self-examination to screen for breast cancer? *Canadian Medical Association Journal, 164,* 1837-46.

Bhasin, S., Storer, T. W., Berman, N., Callegari, C., Clevenger, B., Phillips, J., Bunnell, T. J., Tricker, R., Shirazi, A., Casaburi, R. (1996). The effects of supraphysiologic doses of testosterone on muscle size and strength in normal men. *New England Journal of Medicine, 335,* 1-7.

Blackman, M. R., Sorkin, J. D., Münzer, T., Bellantoni, M. F., Busby-Whitehead, J., Stevens, T. E., Jayme, J., O'Connor, K. G., Christmas, C., Tobin, J. D., Stewart, K J., Cottrell, E., St. Clair, C., Pabst, K. M., & Harman, S. M. (2002). Growth hormone and sex steroid administration in healthy aged women and men: A randomized controlled trial. *Journal of the American Medical Association, 288,* 2282-2292.

Biller, J., & Saver, J. L. (1995). Ischemic cerebrovascular disease and hormone therapy for infertility and transsexualism. *Neurology, 45,* 1611-3.

Blanchard, R. (1994). A structural equation model for age at clinical presentation in nonhomosexual male gender dysphorics. *Archives of Sexual Behavior, 23,* 311-320.

Bockting, W. O. (2003). *Transgender identity, sexuality, and coming out: Implications for HIV risk and prevention.* Proceedings of the NIDA-sponsored satellite sessions in association with the XIV International AIDS Conference, Barcelona, Spain, July 7-11, 2002 (pp. 163-172). U.S. Bethesda, MD: National

Institute on Drug Abuse, U.S. Department of Health and Human Services, National Institutes of Health.

Bockting, W. O., Knudson, G., & Goldberg, J. M. (2006). Counseling and mental health care for transgender adults and loved ones. *International Journal of Transgenderism, 9*(3/4), 35-82.

Bockting, W. O., Robinson, B. E., Forberg, J., & Scheltema, K. (2005). Evaluation of a sexual health approach to reducing HIV/STD risk in the transgender community. *AIDS Care, 17*, 289-303.

Bockting, W. O., Robinson, B. B. E., & Rosser, B. R. S. (1998). Transgender HIV prevention: A qualitative needs assessment. *AIDS Care, 10*, 505-526.

Boekeloo, B. O., Marx, E. S., Kral, A. H., Coughlin, S. C., Bowman, M., & Rabin, D. L. (1991). Frequency and thoroughness of STD/HIV risk assessment by physicians in a high-risk metropolitan area. *American Journal of Public Health, 81*, 1645-1648.

Boice, J. D. Jr., Friis, S., McLaughlin J. K., Mellemkjaer, L., Blot, W. J., Fraumeni, J. F. Jr., & Olsen, J. H. (1997). Cancer following breast reduction surgery in Denmark. *Cancer Causes and Control, 8*, 253-8.

Boice, J. D. Jr., Persson, I., Brinton, L. A., Hober, M., McLaughlin, J. K., Blot, W. J., Fraumeni, J. F. Jr., & Nyren, O. (2000). Breast cancer following breast reduction surgery in Sweden. *Plastic and Reconstructive Surgery, 106*, 755-62.

Boles, J., & Elifson, K. W. (1994). The social organization of transvestite prostitution and AIDS. *Social Science & Medicine, 39*, 85-93.

Bonin, E., Brehove, T., Kline, S., Misgen, M., Post, P., Strehlow, A. J., & Yungman, J. (2004). *Adapting your practice: General recommendations for the care of homeless patients.* Nashville: Health Care for the Homeless Clinicians' Network, National Health Care for the Homeless Council, Inc. Retrieved October 31, 2005, from http://www.nhchc.org/Publications/6.1.04GenHomelessRecsFINAL.pdf

Bosinski, H. A. G., Peter, M., Bonatz, G., Arndt, R., Heidenreich, M., Sippell, W. G., & Wille, R. (1997). A higher rate of hyperandrogenic disorders in female-to-male transsexuals. *Psychoneuroendocrinology, 22*, 361-80.

Bowman, C., & Goldberg, J. M. (2006). Care of the patient undergoing sex reassignment surgery. *International Journal of Transgenderism, 9*(3/4), 135-165.

Brinton, L., A., Lubin, J. H., Burich, M. C., Colton, T., Brown, S. L., & Hoover, R. N. (2000). Breast cancer following augmentation mammaplasty. *Cancer Causes Control, 11*, 819-827

Brinton, L. A., Persson, I., Boice, J. D. Jr., McLaughlin, J. K., & Fraumeni, J. F. Jr. (2001). Breast cancer risk in relation to amount of tissue removed during breast reduction operations in Sweden. *Cancer, 91*, 478-83.

Bryant, H., & Brasher, P. (1995). Breast implants and breast cancer: Reanalysis of a linkage study. *New England Journal of Medicine, 332*, 1535-9.

Bull, S. S., Rietmeijer, C., Fortenberry, J. D., Stoner, B., Malotte, K., Vandevanter, N., Middlestadt, S. E., &

Hook, E. W., III. (1999). Practice patterns for the elicitation of sexual history, education, and counseling among providers of STD services: Results from the Gonorrhea Community Action Project (GCAP). *Sexually Transmitted Diseases, 26*, 584-589.

Burcombe, R. J., Makris, A., Pittam, M., & Finer, N. (2003). Breast cancer after bilateral subcutaneous mastectomy in a female-to-male trans-sexual. *Breast, 12*, 290-3.

Chobanian, A. V., Bakris, G. L., Black, H. R., Cushman, W. C., Green, L. A., Izzo, J. L. Jr., Jones, D. W., Materson, B. J., Oparil, S., Wright, J. T. Jr., & Rocella, E. J. (2003). Seventh report of the Joint National Committee on Prevention, Detection, Evaluation, and Treatment of High Blood Pressure. *Hypertension, 42*, 1206-52.

Cibula, D., Cifkova, R., Fanta, M., Poledne, R., Zivny, J., & Skibova, J. (2000). Increased risk of non-insulin dependent diabetes mellitus, arterial hypertension and coronary artery disease in perimenopausal women with a history of the polycystic ovary syndrome. *Human Reproduction, 15*, 785-789.

Clements-Nolle, K., Katz, M. H., & Marx, R. (1999). *Transgender Community Health Project: Descriptive results.* San Francisco: San Francisco Department of Public Health.

Clements-Nolle, K., Marx, R., Guzman, R., & Katz, M. (2001). HIV prevalence, risk behaviors, health care use, and mental health status of transgender persons: Implications for public health intervention. *American Journal of Public Health, 91*, 915-921.

Clements-Nolle, K., Wilkinson, W., Kitano, K., & Marx, R. (1999). HIV prevention and health service needs of the transgender community in San Francisco. *International Journal of Transgenderism, 3*(1 + 2). Retrieved January 1, 2005, from http://www.symposion.com/ijt/hiv_risk/clements.htm

Colditz, G. A. (2005). Estrogen, estrogen plus progestin therapy, and risk of breast cancer. *Clinical Cancer Research, 11*, S909-S917.

Cole, C. M., O'Boyle, M., Emory, L. E., & Meyer, W. J., III (1997). Comorbidity of gender dysphoria and other major psychiatric diagnoses. *Archives of Sexual Behavior, 26*, 13-26.

Coleman, E., Bockting, W. O., & Gooren, L. J. G. (1993). Homosexual and bisexual identity in sex-reassigned female-to-male transsexuals. *Archives of Sexual Behavior, 22*, 37-50.

Dahl, M., Feldman, J., Goldberg, J. M., & Jaberi, A. (2006). Physical aspects of transgender endocrine therapy. *International Journal of Transgenderism, 9*(3/4), 111-134.

Damewood, M. D., Bellantoni, J. J., Bachorik, P. S., Kimball, A. W. Jr., & Rock, J. A. (1989). Exogenous estrogen effect on lipid/lipoprotein cholesterol in transsexual males. *Journal of Endocrinological Investigation, 12*, 449-454.

Davies, S., & Goldberg, J. M. (2006). Clinical aspects of transgender speech feminization and masculinization. *International Journal of Transgenderism, 9(3/4),* 167-196.

De Laet, C. E. D. H., van Hout, B. A., Burger, H., Hofman, A., & Pols, H. A. P. (1997). Bone density and risk of hip fracture in men and women: Cross sectional analysis. *British Medical Journal, 315,* 221-225.

de Vries, A. L. C., Cohen-Kettenis, P. T., & Delemarre-van de Waal, H. (2006). Clinical management of gender dysphoria in adolescents. *International Journal of Transgenderism, 9(3/4),* 83-94.

Deapen, D., Hamilton, A., Bernstein, L., & Brody, G. S. (2000). Breast cancer stage at diagnosis and survival among patients with prior breast implants. *Plastic and Reconstructive Surgery, 105,* 535-40.

deMarinis, M., & Arnett, E. N. (1978). Cerebrovascular occlusion in a transsexual man taking mestranol. *Archives of Internal Medicine, 138,* 1732-3.

Devor, H. (1993). Sexual orientation identities, attractions, and practices of female-to-male transsexuals. *Journal of Sex Research, 30,* 303-315.

Dobs, A. S., Nguyen, T., Pace, C., & Roberts, C. P. (2002). Differential effects of oral estrogen versus oral estrogen-androgen replacement therapy on body composition in postmenopausal women. *Journal of Clinical Endocrinology & Metabolism, 87,* 1509-1516.

Doeren, M., & Samsioe, G. (2000). Prevention of postmenopausal osteoporosis with oestrogen replacement therapy and associated compounds: Update on clinical trials since 1995. *Human Reproduction Update, 6,* 419-426.

Drouin, P., Fortier, M., Krepart, G., Inhaber, S., Paraskevas, M., Parboosingh, Riley, T., Roy, M., Sellors, J., Shaw, P., Stuart, G., & Wright, V. C., for the Quality Management Working Group of the Cervical Cancer Prevention Network (1998). *Programmatic guidelines for screening for cancer of the cervix in Canada.* Ottawa, ONT: Society of Gynecologic Oncologists of Canada.

Elbers, J. M. H., Asscheman, H., Seidell, J. C., & Gooren, L. J. G. (1999). Effects of sex steroid hormones on regional fat depots as assessed by magnetic resonance imaging in transsexuals. *American Journal of Physiology, 276,* E317-E325.

Elbers, J. M. H., Asscheman, H., Seidell, J. C., Megens, J. A. J., & Gooren, L. J. G. (1997). Long-term testosterone administration increases visceral fat in female to male transsexuals. *Journal of Clinical Endocrinology & Metabolism, 82,* 2044-2047.

Epstein, R. M., Morse, D. S., Frankel, R. M., Frarey, L., Anderson, K., & Beckman, H. B. (1998). Awkward moments in patient-physician communication about HIV risk. *Annals of Internal Medicine, 128,* 435-442.

Espeland, M. A., Hogan, P. E., Fineberg, S. E., Howard, G., Schrott, H., Waclawiw, M. A., & Bush, T. L. (1998). Effect of postmenopausal hormone therapy on glucose and insulin concentrations. *Diabetes Care, 21,* 1589-1595.

Evans, S. F., & Davie, M. W. (1996). Low and conventional dose transdermal oestradiol are equally effective at preventing bone loss in spine and femur at all post-menopausal ages. *Clinical Endocrinology, 44,* 79-84.

Eyler, A. E., & Whittle, S. (2001). FTM breast cancer: Community awareness and illustrative cases. Paper presented at the 17th Biennial Symposium of the Harry Benjamin International Gender Dysphoria Association, Galveston, TX. Abstract retrieved January 1, 2005, from http://www.symposion.com/ijt/hbigda/2001/41_eyler.htm

Feldman, J. (2002). New onset of type 2 diabetes mellitus with feminizing hormone therapy: Case series. *International Journal of Transgenderism, 6(2).* Retrieved January 1, 2005, from http://www.symposion.com/ijt/ijtvo06no02_01.htm

Feldman, J., & Bockting, W. O. (2003). Transgender health. *Minnesota Medicine, 86,* 25-32.

Feldman, J., Bockting, W. O., Allen, S., & Brintell, D. (2003, September). *Smoking cessation among transgender persons receiving hormone therapy.* Paper presented at the 18th Biennial Symposium of the Harry Benjamin International Gender Dysphoria Association, Gent, Belgium.

Fortin, C. J., Klein, T., Messmore, H. L., & O'Connell, J. B. (1984). Myocardial infarction and severe thromboembolic complications as seen in an estrogen-dependent transsexual. *Archives of Internal Medicine, 144,* 1082-3.

Futterweit, W. (1998). Endocrine therapy of transsexualism and potential complications of long-term treatment. *Archives of Sexual Behavior, 27,* 209-26.

Futterweit, W., Weiss, R. A., & Fagerstrom, R. M. (1986). Endocrine evaluation of forty female-to-male transsexuals: Increased frequency of polycystic ovarian disease in female transsexualism. *Archives of Sexual Behavior, 15,* 69-78.

Ganly, I., & Taylor, E. W. (1995). Breast cancer in a trans-sexual man receiving hormone replacement therapy. *British Journal of Surgery, 82,* 341.

Gay and Lesbian Medical Association (2001). *Healthy People 2010 companion document for lesbian, gay, bisexual, and transgender (LGBT) health.* San Francisco, CA: Author.

Genest, J., Frohlich, J., Fodor, G., & McPherson, R. (2003). Recommendations for the management of dyslipidemia and the prevention of cardiovascular disease: 2003 update. *Canadian Medical Association Journal, 168,* 921-924.

Gilman, S. E., Abrams, D. B., & Buka, S. L. (2003). Socioeconomic status over the life course and stages of cigarette use: Initiation, regular use, and cessation. *Journal of Epidemiology and Community Health, 57,* 802-808.

Glueck, C. J., Lang, J., Hamer, T., & Tracy, T. (1994). Severe hypertriglyceridemia and pancreatitis when estrogen replacement therapy is given to hypertriglyceridemic women. *Journal of Laboratory and Clinical Medicine, 123*, 59-64.

Godsland, I. F., Gangar, K., Walton, C., Cust, M. P., Whitehead, M. I., Wynn, V., & Stevenson, J. C. (1993). Insulin resistance, secretion, and elimination in postmenopausal women receiving oral or transdermal hormone replacement therapy. *Metabolism, 42*, 846-853.

Goffman, E. (1963). *Stigma: Notes on the management of spoiled identity.* Englewood Cliffs, NJ: Prentice-Hall.

Goh, H. H., Loke, D. F., & Ratnam, S. S. (1995). The impact of long-term testosterone replacement therapy on lipid and lipoprotein profiles in women. *Maturitas, 21*, 65-70.

Goh, H. H., & Ratnam, S. S. (1997). Effects of hormone deficiency, androgen therapy and calcium supplementation on bone mineral density in female transsexuals. *Maturitas, 26*, 45-52.

Goldberg, J. M. (2006). Training community-based clinicians in transgender care. *International Journal of Transgenderism, 9*(3/4), 219-231.

Goldberg, J. M., Matte, N., MacMillan, M., & Hudspith, M. (2003). *Community survey: Transition/cross-dressing services in BC–Final report.* Vancouver, BC: Vancouver Coastal Health and Transcend Transgender Support & Education Society.

Gooren, L. J. G. (1999). Hormonal sex reassignment. *International Journal of Transgenderism, 3.* Retrieved January 1, 2005, fromhttp://www.symposion.com/ijt/ijt990301.htm.

Gooren, L. J. G., & Bunck, M. C. (2004). Transsexuals and competitive sports. *European Journal of Endocrinology, 151*, 425-429.

Grady, D., Herrington, D., Bittner, V., Blumenthal, R., Davidson, M., Hlatky, M., Hsia, J., Hulley, S., Herd, A., Khan, S., Newby, L. K., Waters, D., Vittinghoff, E., & Wenger, N. (2002). Cardiovascular disease outcomes during 6.8 years of hormone therapy: Heart and Estrogen/Progestin Replacement Study follow-up (HERS II). *Journal of the American Medical Association, 288*, 49-57.

Gras, M. J., van der Helm, T., Schenk, R., van Doornum, G. J., Coutinho, R. A., & van den Hock, J. A. (1997). HIV infection and risk behaviour among prostitutes in the Amsterdam streetwalkers' district: Indications of raised prevalence of HIV among transvestites/transsexuals. *Nederlands Tijdschrift Voor Geneeskunde, 141*, 1238-1241.

Griggs, R. C., Kingston, W., Jozefowicz, R. F., Herr, B. E., Forbes, G., & Halliday, D. (1989). Effect of testosterone on muscle mass and muscle protein synthesis. *Journal of Applied Physiology, 66*, 498-503.

Grodstein, F., Manson, J. E., & Stampfer, M. J. (2001). Postmenopausal hormone use and secondary prevention of coronary events in the Nurses' Health Study: A prospective, observational study. *Annals of Internal Medicine, 135*, 1-8.

Gross, J., & Davis, M. (2004, July). *Female-to-male transgenders and HIV risk behaviors in Los Angeles, California.* Poster presented at the XV International AIDS Conference, Bangkok, Thailand.

Gruskin, E. P., Hart, S., Gordon, N., & Ackerson, L. (2001). Patterns of cigarette smoking and alcohol use among lesbians and bisexual women enrolled in a large health maintenance organization. *American Journal of Public Health, 91*, 976-9.

Guess, H. A., Heyse, J. F., & Gormley, G. J. (1993). The effect of finasteride on prostate-specific antigen in men with benign prostatic hyperplasia. *Prostate, 22*, 31-7.

Gumucio, C. A., Pin, P., Young, V. L., Destouet, J., Monsees, B., & Eichling, J. (1989). The effect of breast implants on the radiographic detection of microcalcification and soft-tissue masses. *Plastic and Reconstructive Surgery, 84*, 772-8.

Gwadz, M. V., Clatts, M. C., Goldsamt, L., Lankenau, S., & Leonard, N. (2002, July). *A behavioral profile of HIV risk behavior among a street-recruited sample of young men who have sex with men.* Presented at the XVI International AIDS Conference, Barcelona, Spain.

Hage, J. J., Dekker, J. J., Karim, R. B., Verheijen, R. H., & Bloemena E. (2000). Ovarian cancer in female-to-male transsexuals: report of two cases. *Gynecologic Oncology, 76*, 413-415.

Hak, A. E., Witteman, J. C., de Jong, F. H., Geerlings, M. I., Hofman, A., & Pols, H. A. (2002). Low levels of endogenous androgens increase the risk of atherosclerosis in elderly men: The Rotterdam study. *Journal of Clinical Endocrinology & Metabolism, 87*, 3632-9.

Haley, N., Maheux, B., Rivard, M., Gervais, A. (1999). Sexual health risk assessment and counseling in primary care: How involved are general practitioners and obstetrician-gynecologists? *American Journal of Public Health, 89*, 899-902.

Hayes, H. Jr., Vandergrift, J., & Diner, W. C. (1988). Mammography and breast implants. *Plastic and Reconstructive Surgery, 82*, 1-8.

Hultborn, R., Hanson, C., Kopf, I., Verbiene, I., Warnhammar, E., & Weimarck, A. (1997). Prevalence of Klinefelter's syndrome in male breast cancer patients. *Anticancer Research, 17*(6D), 4293-7.

Humphrey, L. L., Helfand, M., Chan, B. K., & Woolf, S. H. (2005). Breast cancer screening: A summary of the evidence for the U.S. Preventive Services Task Force. *Annals of Internal Medicine, 137*, 347-60.

Israel, G. E. & Tarver, D. E. I. (1997). *Transgender care: Recommended guidelines, practical information, and personal accounts.* Philadephia, PA: Temple University Press.

Jin, B., Turner, L., Walters, W. A., & Handelsman, D. J. (1997). The effects of chronic high dose androgen or estrogen treatment on the human prostate. *Journal of Clinical Endocrinology & Metabolism, 81*, 4290-4295.

Kammerer, N., Mason, T., Connors, M., & Durkee, R. (1999). Transgender health and social service needs in the context of HIV risk. *International Journal of Transgenderism, 3*(1 + 2). Retrieved January 1, 2005, from http://www.symposion.com/ijt/hiv_risk/kammerer.htm

Kammerer, N., Mason, T., Connors, M., & Durkee, R. (2001). Transgenders, HIV/AIDS, and substance abuse: From risk group to group prevention. In W. O Bockting & S. Kirk (Eds.), *Transgender and HIV: Risks, prevention, and care* (pp. 13-38). Binghamton, NY: The Haworth Press, Inc.

Katznelson, L., Finkelstein, J.S., Schoenfeld, D. A., Rosenthal, D. I., Anderson, E. J., & Klibanski, A. (1996). Increase in bone density and lean body mass during testosterone administration in men with acquired hypogonadism. *Journal of Clinical Endocrinology & Metabolism, 81*, 4358-4365.

Keatley, J., Nemoto, T., Operario, D., & Soma, T. (2002, July). *The impact of transphobia on HIV risk behaviors among male to female transgenders in San Francisco.* Poster presented at XVI International AIDS Conference, Barcelona, Spain.

Kellog, T. A., Clements-Nolle, K., Dilley, J., Katz, M. H., & McFarland, W. (2001). Incidence of human immunodeficiency virus among male-to-female transgendered persons in San Francisco. *Journal of Acquired Immune Deficiency Syndrome, 28*, 380-4.

Kenagy, G. P. (2002). HIV among transgendered people. *AIDS Care, 14*, 127-134.

Kenagy, G. P., & Bostwick, W. B. (2005). Health and social service needs of transgender people in Chicago. *International Journal of Transgenderism, 8*(2 + 3), 57-66.

Kenagy, G. P., & Hsieh, C. M. (2005). The risk less known: Female-to-male transgender persons' vulnerability to HIV infection. *AIDS Care, 17*, 195-207.

Kirk, S. (1999). Guidelines for selecting HIV positive patients for genital reconstructive surgery. *International Journal of Transgenderism, 3*(1 + 2). Retrieved January 1, 2005, fromhttp://www.symposion.com/ijt/hiv_risk/kirk.htm.

Kirk, S., & Rothblatt, M. (1995). *Medical, legal and workplace issues for the transsexual.* Watertown, MA: Together Lifeworks.

Kuiper, B., & Cohen-Kettenis, P. T. (1988). Sex reassignment surgery: A study of 141 Dutch transsexuals. *Archives of Sexual Behavior, 17*, 439-457.

Laboratory Centre for Disease Control (LCDC) Expert Working Group on Canadian Guidelines for Sexually Transmitted Disease (1998). *Canadian STD guidelines* (Report No.: H49-119/1998E). Ottawa: Health Canada.

Langström, N., & Zucker, K. J. (2005). Transvestic fetishism in the general population. *Journal of Sex & Marital Therapy, 31*, 87-95.

Lawrence, A. A. (2001). Vaginal neoplasia in a male-to-female transsexual: Case report, review of the literature, and recommendations for cytological screen-

ing. *International Journal of Transgenderism, 5*(1). Retrieved January 1, 2005, from http://www.symposion.com/ijt/ijtvo05no01_01.htm

Lawrence, A. A. (2005). Sexuality before and after male-to-female sex reassignment surgery. *Archives of Sexual Behavior, 34*, 147-166.

Leavitt, F., Berger, J. C., Hoeppner, J. A., & Northrop, G. (1980). Presurgical adjustment in male transsexuals with and without hormonal treatment. *Journal of Nervous and Mental Disease, 168*, 693-697.

Legro, R. S. (2003). Polycystic ovary syndrome and cardiovascular disease: A premature association? *Endocrine Reviews, 24*, 302-312.

Leo, M. E., Bilhartz, D. L., Bergstralh, E. J., & Oesterling, J. E. (1991). Prostate specific antigen in hormonally treated stage D2 prostate cancer: Is it always an accurate indicator of disease status? *Journal of Urology, 145*, 802-806.

Lindley, L. L., Nicholson, T. J., Kerby, M. B., & Lu, N. (2003). HIV/STI associated risk behaviors among self-identified lesbian, gay, bisexual, and transgender colleges students in the United States. *AIDS Education & Prevention, 15*, 413-429.

Lombardi, E. L., Wilchins, R. A., Priesing, D., & Malouf, D. (2001). Gender violence: Transgender experiences with violence and discrimination. *Journal of Homosexuality, 42*, 89-101.

Loverro, G. (2004). Polycystic ovary syndrome and cardiovascular disease. *Minerva Endocrinologica, 29*(3), 129-38.

MacMahon, S., & Rodgers, A. (1994). Blood pressure, antihypertensive treatment and stroke risk. *Journal of Hypertension–Supplement, 12*(10), S5-S14.

Manson, J. E., Rimm, E. B., Colditz, G. A., Willett, W. C., Nathan, D. M., Arky, R. A., Rosner, B., Hennekens, C. H., Speizer, F. E., & Stampfer, M. J. (1992). A prospective study of postmenopausal estrogen therapy and subsequent incidence of non-insulin-dependent diabetes mellitus. *Annals of Epidemiology, 2*, 665-673.

Markland, C. (1975). Transexual surgery. *Obstetrics & Gynecology Annual, 4*, 309-330.

Mate-Kole, C., Freschi, M., & Robin, A. (1990). A controlled study of psychological and social changes after surgical gender reassignment in selected male transsexuals. *British Journal of Psychiatry, 157*, 261-264.

Mathy, R. M. (2002). Transgender identity and suicidality in a nonclinical sample: Sexual orientation, psychiatric history, and compulsive behaviors. *Journal of Psychology & Human Sexuality, 14*, 47-65.

McCredie, R. J., McCrohon, J. A., Turner, L., Griffiths, K. A., Handelsman, D. J., & Celermajer, D. S. (1998). Vascular reactivity is impaired in genetic females taking high-dose androgens. *Journal of the American College of Cardiology, 32*, 1331-1335.

McGowan, C. K. (1999). *Transgender needs assessment.* New York City: Prevention Planning Unit, New York City Department of Health.

McPherson, K., Steel, C. M., & Dixon, J. M. (2000). ABC of breast diseases: Breast cancer–Epidemiology, risk factors, and genetics. *British Medical Journal, 321*(7261), 624-628.

Meyer, W. J., III, Bockting, W. O., Cohen-Kettenis, P. T., Coleman, E., Di Ceglie, D., Devor, H., Gooren, L., Hage, J. J., Kirk, S., Kuiper, B., Laub, D., Lawrence, A., Menard, Y., Monstrey, S., Patton, J., Schaefer, L., Webb, A., & Wheeler, C. C. (2001). *The standards of care for Gender Identity Disorders* (6th ed.). Minneapolis, MN: Harry Benjamin International Gender Dysphoria Association.

Meyer, W. J., III, Webb, A., Stuart, C. A., Finkelstein, J. W., Lawrence, B., & Walker, P. A. (1986). Physical and hormonal evaluation of transsexual patients: A longitudinal study. *Archives of Sexual Behavior, 15,* 121-138.

Miglioretti, D. L., Rutter, C. M., Geller, B. M., Cutter, G., Barlow, W. E., Rosenberg, R., Weaver, D. L., Taplin, S. H., Ballard-Barbash, R., Carney, P. A., Yankaskas, B. C., & Kerlikowske, K. (2004). Effect of breast augmentation on the accuracy of mammography and cancer characteristics. *Journal of the American Medical Association, 291,* 442-450.

Miller, N., Bedard, Y. C., Cooter, N. B., & Shaul, D. L. (1986). Histological changes in the genital tract in transsexual women following androgen therapy. *Histopathology, 10,* 661-669.

Morgentaler, A., Bruning, C. O., III, & DeWolf, W. C. (1996). Occult prostate cancer in men with low serum testosterone levels. *Journal of the American Medical Association, 276,* 1904-1906.

Morgenthaler, M., & Weber, M. (2005). Pathological rupture of the distal biceps tendon after long-term androgen substitution. *Zeitschrift für Orthopädie und Ihre Grenzgebiete, 137,* 368-370.

Mottet, L., & Ohle, J. M. (2003). *Transitioning our shelters: A guide to making homeless shelters safe for transgender people.* New York, NY: National Coalition for the Homeless & National Gay and Lesbian Task Force Policy Institute.

Nader, S., Riad-Gabriel, M. G., & Saad, M. F. (1997). The effect of a desogestrel-containing oral contraceptive on glucose tolerance and leptin concentrations in hyperandrogenic women. *Journal of Clinical Endocrinology & Metabolism, 82,* 3074-3077.

Namaste, V. K. (1999). HIV/AIDS and female-to-male transsexuals and transvestites: Results from a needs assessment in Quebec. *International Journal of Transgenderism, 3*(1 + 2). Retrieved January 1, 2005, from http://www.symposion.com/ijt/hiv_risk/namaste.htm

Nelson, H. D., Humphrey, L. L., Nygren, P., Teutsch, S. M., & Allan, J. D. (2002). Postmenopausal hormone replacement therapy: Scientific review. *Journal of the American Medical Association, 288,* 872-881.

Nemoto, T., Keatley, J., Operario, D., Soma, T., Fernandez, A., Adao, L., Eleneke, M., Arista, P., Soriano, C., & McCree, B. (2002, July). *Implementing HIV prevention, drug abuse treatment, and mental health services in the transgender community in San Francisco.* Poster presented at XVI International AIDS Conference, Barcelona, Spain.

Nemoto, T., Luke, D., Mamo, L., Ching, A., & Patria, J. (1999). HIV risk behaviours among male-to-female transgenders in comparison with homosexual or bisexual males and heterosexual females. *AIDS Care, 11,* 297-312.

Nemoto, T., Operario, D., Keatley, J., & Villegas, D. (2004). Social context of HIV risk behaviours among male-to-female transgenders of colour. *AIDS Care, 16,* 724-735.

Nemoto, T., Sugano, E., Operario, D., & Keatley, J. (2004, July). *Psychosocial factors influencing HIV risk among male-to-female transgenders in San Francisco.* Poster presented at XV International AIDS Conference, Bangkok, Thailand.

Netscher, D., Meade, R. A., Friedman, J. D., Malone, R. S., Brady, J. R., & Thornby, J. (1999). Mammography and reduction mammaplasty. *Aesthetic Surgery Journal, 19,* 445-451.

New, G., Duffy, S. J., Harper, R. W., & Meredith, I. T. (2000). Long-term oestrogen therapy is associated with improved endothelium-dependent vasodilation in the forearm resistance circulation of biological males. *Clinical and Experimental Pharmacology and Physiology, 27,* 25-33.

New, G., Timmins, K. L., Duffy, S. J., Tran, B. T., O'Brien, R. C., Harper, R. W., & Meredith, I. T. (1997). Long-term estrogen therapy improves vascular function in male to female transsexuals. *Journal of the American College of Cardiology, 29,* 1437-1444.

Nusbaum, M. R. H., & Hamilton, C. D. (2002). The proactive sexual health history. *American Family Physician, 66,* 1705-1712.

Oh, J. Y., Barrett-Connor, E., Wedick, N. M., & Wingard, D. L. (2002). Endogenous sex hormones and the development of type 2 diabetes in older men and women: The Rancho Bernardo Study. *Diabetes Care, 25,* 55-60.

Olsen, O., & Gotzsche, P. C. (2001). Screening for breast cancer with mammography. *Cochrane Database of Systematic Reviews, 4*(CD001877).

Oriel, K. A. (2000). Medical care of transsexual patients. *Journal of the Gay & Lesbian Medical Association, 4,* 185-194.

Pache, T. D., Chadha, S., Gooren, L. J. G., Hop, W. C., Jaarsma, K. W., Dommerholt, H. B., & Fauser, B. C. (1991). Ovarian morphology in long-term androgen-treated female to male transsexuals: A human model for the study of polycystic ovarian syndrome? *Histopathology, 19,* 445-452.

Pfäfflin, F. & Junge, A. (1998). *Sex reassignment–Thirty years of international follow-up studies; SRS: A comprehensive review, 1961-1991* (R. B. Jacobson & A. B. Meier, Trans.). Düsseldorf, Germany: Symposion Publishing. (Original work published 1992)

Pierpoint, T., McKeigue, P. M., Isaacs, A. J., Wild, S. H., & Jacobs HS. (1998). Mortality of women with polycystic ovary syndrome at long-term follow-up. *Journal of Clinical Epidemiology, 51,* 581-6.

Prior, J. C., Vigna, Y. M., & Watson, D. (1989). Spironolactone with physiological female steroids for presurgical therapy of male-to-female transsexualism. *Archives of Sexual Behavior, 18,* 49-57.

Pritchard, T. J., Pankowsky, D. A., Crowe J. P., & Abdul-Karim, F. W. (1988). Breast cancer in a male-to-female transsexual: A case report. *Journal of the American Medical Association, 259,* 2278-2280.

Reback, C. J., & Lombardi, E. L. (1999). A community-based harm reduction program for male-to-female transgenders at risk for HIV infection. *International Journal of Transgenderism, 3*(1 + 2). Retrieved January 1, 2005, from http://www.symposion.com/ijt/hiv_risk/reback.htm

Rimm, E. B., Manson, J. E., Stampfer, M. J., Colditz, G. A., Willett, W. C., Rosner, B., Hennekens, C. H., & Speizer, F. E. (1992). Oral contraceptive use and the risk of type 2 (non-insulin-dependent) diabetes mellitus in a large prospective study of women. *Diabetologia, 35,* 967-972.

Risser, J. M. H., Shelton, A., McCurdy, S. Atkinson, J., Padgett, P., Useche, B., Thomas, B., & Williams, M. (2005). Sex, drugs, violence, and HIV status among male-to-female transgender persons in Houston, Texas. *International Journal of Transgenderism, 8*(2 + 3), 67-74.

Rodrigo Álvaro, J., Rodríguez-Arenas, M. A., Ramón, P., & Martín Martín, S. (2002, July). *Risk factors for the HIV transmission in transgender sex workers.* Presented at the XVI International AIDS Conference, Barcelona, Spain.

Rossouw, J. E., Anderson, G. L., Prentice, R. L., LaCroix, A. Z., Kooperberg, C., Stefanick, M. L., Jackson, R. D., Beresford, S. A., Howard, B. V., Johnson, K. C., Kotchen, J. M., & Ockene, J. (2002). Risks and benefits of estrogen plus progestin in healthy postmenopausal women: Principal results from the Women's Health Initiative randomized controlled trial. *Journal of the American Medical Association, 288,* 321-333.

Russell-Briefel, R., Ezzati, T. M., Perlman, J. A., & Murphy, R. S. (1987). Impaired glucose tolerance in women using oral contraceptives: United States, 1976-1980. *Journal of Chronic Diseases, 40,* 3-11.

Sanders, G. D., Bayoumi, A. M., Sundaram, V., Bilir, S. P., Neukermans, C. P., Rydzak, C. E., Douglass, L. R., Lazzeroni, L. C., Holodniy, M., & Owens, D. K. (2005). Cost-effectiveness of screening for HIV in the era of highly active antiretroviral therapy. *New England Journal of Medicine, 352,* 570-585.

Saslow, D., Runowicz, C. D., Solomon, D., Moscicki, A., Smith, R. A., Eyre, H. J., & Cohen, C. (2002). American Cancer Society guideline for the early detection of cervical neoplasia and cancer. *CA: A Cancer Journal for Clinicians, 52,* 342-362.

Sausa, L. A. (2003). The HIV prevention and educational needs of trans youth: A qualitative study [Ph.D.] University of Pennsylvania. *Dissertation Abstracts International, 64*(4A), 1186. (University Microfilms No. AAT 3087465)

Scarabin, P. Y., Oger, E., & Plu-Bureau, G. (2003). Differential association of oral and transdermal oestrogen-replacement therapy with venous thromboembolism risk. *Lancet, 362,* 428-432.

Schairer, C., Lubin, J., Troisi, R., Sturgeon, S., Brinton, L., & Hoover, R. (2000). Menopausal estrogen and estrogen-progestin replacement therapy and breast cancer risk. *Journal of the American Medical Association, 283,* 485-491.

Scheer, S., Delgado, V., & Schwarcz, S. (2004, July). *Use of HIV prevention services and HIV risk reduction strategies among male-to-female transgenders in San Francisco (USA).* Presented at the XV International AIDS Conference, Bangkok, Thailand.

Schildkraut, J. M., Schwingl, P. J., Bastos, E., Evanoff, A., & Hughes, C. (1996). Epithelial ovarian cancer risk among women with polycystic ovary syndrome. *Obstetrics & Gynecology, 88,* 554-559.

Schlatterer, K., Auer, D. P., Yassouridis, A., von Werder, K., & Stalla, G. K. (1998). Transsexualism and osteoporosis. *Experimental and Clinical Endocrinology and Diabetes, 106,* 365-368.

Schlatterer, K., Yassouridis, A., von Werder, K., Poland, D., Kemper, J., & Stalla, G. K. (1998). A follow-up study for estimating the effectiveness of a cross-gender hormone substitution therapy on transsexual patients. *Archives of Sexual Behavior, 27,* 475-492.

Scholes, D., LaCroix, A. Z., Ichikawa, L. E., Barlow, W. E., & Ott, S. M. (2005). Injectable hormone contraception and bone density: Results from a prospective study. *Epidemiology, 13,* 581-587.

Sember, R., Lawrence, A. A., & Xavier, J. (2000). Transgender health concerns. *Journal of the Gay & Lesbian Medical Association, 4,* 125-134.

Simon, P. A., Reback, C. J., & Bemis, C. C. (2000). HIV prevalence and incidence among male-to-female transsexuals receiving HIV prevention services in Los Angeles County. *AIDS, 14,* 2953-2955.

Smith, R. A., Cokkinides, V., & Eyre, H. J. (2006). American Cancer Society guidelines for the early detection of cancer, 2006. *CA: A Cancer Journal for Clinicians, 56,* 11-25.

Smith, R. A., Saslow, D., Sawyer, K. A., Burke, W., Costanza, M. E., Evans, W. P., III, Foster, R. S. Jr., Hendrick, E., Eyre, H. J., & Sener, S. (2003). American Cancer Society guidelines for breast cancer screening: Update 2003. *CA: A Cancer Journal for Clinicians, 53,* 141-169.

Smith, Y. L. S., Van Goozen, S. H. M., Kuiper, A. J., & Cohen-Kettenis, P. T. (2005). Sex reassignment: Outcomes and predictors of treatment for adolescent and adult transsexuals. *Psychological Medicine, 35,* 89-99.

Sosa, M., Jodar, E., Arbelo, E., Dominguez, C., Saavedra, P., Torres, A., Salido, E., Liminana, J. M., Gomez De Tejada, M. J., & Hernandez, D. (2004). Serum lipids and estrogen receptor gene polymorphisms in male-to-female transsexuals: Effects of estrogen treatment. *European Journal of Internal Medicine, 15*, 231-237.

Sperber, J., Landers, S., & Lawrence, S. (2005). Access to health care for transgendered persons: Results of a needs assessment in Boston. *International Journal of Transgenderism, 8*, 75-91.

Spritz, M. (2003). *Effects of cross gender hormonal therapy on prostates of 20 male-to-female postoperative patients.* Paper presented at the 18th Biennial Symposium of the Harry Benjamin International Gender Dysphoria Association, Gent, Belgium.

Steinbeck, A. (1997). Hormonal medication for transsexuals. *Venereology: Interdisciplinary, International Journal of Sexual Health, 10*, 175-177.

Strauss, R. H., & Yesalis, C. E. (1991). Anabolic steroids in the athlete. *Annual Review of Medicine, 42*, 449-457.

Symmers, W. S. (1968). Carcinoma of breast in transsexual individuals after surgical and hormonal interference with the primary and secondary sex characteristics. *British Medical Journal, 2*(597), 82-85.

Takata, L. L., & Meltzer, T. R. (2000). Procedures, postoperative care, and potential complications of gender reassignment surgery for the primary care physician. *Primary Psychiatry, 7*, 74-78.

Tang, H., Greenwood, G. L., Cowling, D. W., Lloyd, J. C., Roeseler, A. G., & Bal, D. G. (2004). Cigarette smoking among lesbians, gays, and bisexuals: How serious a problem? *Cancer Causes Control, 15*, 797-803.

Tangpricha, V., Turner, A., Malabanan, A., & Holick, M. (2001). *Effects of testosterone therapy on bone mineral density in the FTM patient.* Paper presented at the 17th Biennial Symposium of the Harry Benjamin International Gender Dysphoria Association, Galveston, TX. Abstract retrieved January 1, 2005, from http://www.symposion.com/ijt/hbigda/2001/39_tangpricha.htm

The Writing Group for the PEPI Trial (1995). Effects of estrogen or estrogen/progestin regimens on heart disease risk factors in postmenopausal women: The Postmenopausal Estrogen/Progestin Interventions (PEPI) Trial. *Journal of the American Medical Association, 273*, 199-208.

Thompson, I. M., Pauler, D. K., Goodman, P. J., Tangen, C. M., Lucia, M. S., Parnes, H. L., Minasian, L. M., Ford, L. G., Lippman, S. M., Crawford, E. D., Crowley, J. J., & Coltman, C. A. Jr. (2004). Prevalence of prostate cancer among men with a prostate-specific antigen level < or = 4.0 ng per milliliter. *New England Journal of Medicine, 350*, 2239-2246.

Thurston, A. V. (1994). Carcinoma of the prostate in a transsexual. *British Journal of Urology, 73*, 217.

Troisi, R., Cowie, C. C., & Harris, M. I. (2000). Hormone replacement therapy and glucose metabolism. *Obstetrics & Gynecology, 96*, 665-670.

Turner, A., Chen, T. C., Barber, T. W., Malabanan, A. O., Holick, M. F., & Tangpricha, V. (2004). Testosterone increases bone mineral density in female-to-male transsexuals: A case series of 15 subjects. *Clinical Endocrinology, 61*, 560-566.

Valentine, D. (1998). *Gender Identity Project report on intake statistics.* New York: Lesbian and Gay Community Services Center of New York.

van Haarst, E. P., Newling, D. W., Gooren, L. J. G., Asscheman, H., & Prenger, D. M. (1998). Metastatic prostatic carcinoma in a male-to-female transsexual. *British Journal of Urology, 81*, 776.

van Kesteren, P. J. M., Asscheman, H., Megens, J. A. J., & Gooren, L. J. G. (1997). Mortality and morbidity in transsexual subjects treated with cross-sex hormones. *Clinical Endocrinology, 47*, 337-342.

van Kesteren, P. J. M., Lips, P., Gooren, L. J. G., Asscheman, H., & Megens, J. A. J. (1998). Long-term follow-up of bone mineral density and bone metabolism in transsexuals treated with cross-sex hormones. *Clinical Endocrinology, 48*, 347-354.

van Kesteren, P. J. M., Meinhardt, W., van der Valk, P., Geldof, A. A., Megens, J. A. J., & Gooren, L. J. G. (1996). Effects of estrogens only on the prostates of aging men. *Journal of Urology, 156*, 1349-1353.

Verhoeven, V., Bovijn, K., Helder, A., Peremans, L., Hermann, I., Van Royen, P., Denekens, J., & Avonts, D. (2003). Discussing STIs: Doctors are from Mars, patients from Venus. *Family Practice, 20*, 11-15.

Warren, B. E. (1999). Sex, truth and videotape: HIV prevention at the Gender Identity Project in New York City. *International Journal of Transgenderism, 3*(1 + 2). Retrieved January 1, 2005, from http://www.symposion.com/ijt/hiv_risk/warren.htm

Watts, N. B. (2001). Treatment of osteoporosis with bisphosphonates. *Rheumatic Disease Clinics of North America, 27*, 197-214.

White Holman, C., & Goldberg, J. M. (2006a). Ethical, legal, and psychosocial issues in care of transgender adolescents. *International Journal of Transgenderism, 9*(3/4), 95-110.

White Holman, C., & Goldberg, J. M. (2006b). Social and medical transgender case advocacy. *International Journal of Transgenderism, 9*(3/4), 197-217.

Wilson, A. N. (1999). Sex reassignment surgery in HIV positive transsexuals. *International Journal of Transgenderism, 3*(1 + 2). Retrieved January 1, 2005, from http://www.symposion.com/ijt/hiv_risk/wilson.htm.

World Health Organization (1978). *Alma-Ata 1978: Primary health care.* Report of the International Conference on Primary Health Care, Alma-Ata, USSR, 6-12 September 1978. WHO "Health for All" series, No. 1. Geneva: Author.

Xavier, J., & Simmons, R. (2000). *Final report of the Washington Transgender Needs Assessment Survey.* Washington, DC: Administration for HIV and AIDS, District of Columbia Department of Health.

doi:10.1300/J485v09n03_02

Counseling and Mental Health Care
for Transgender Adults and Loved Ones

Walter O. Bockting, PhD
Gail Knudson, MD, MPE, FRCPC
Joshua M. Goldberg

SUMMARY. Increasingly, transgender individuals and loved ones (partners, family, and friends) are seeking assistance from mental health professionals working in the community rather than in university or hospital-based gender identity clinics. Drawing on published literature specific to transgender mental health, interviews with expert clinicians, the authors' clinical experience, and three key guiding principles (a transgender-affirmative approach, client-centered care, and a commitment to harm reduction), we suggest protocols for the clinician providing mental health services in the community setting. Practice areas discussed include assessment and treatment of gender concerns, trans-specific mental health issues, and trans-specific elements in general counseling of transgender individuals and their loved ones. doi:10.1300/J485v09n03_01 *[Article copies available for a fee from The Haworth Document Delivery Service: 1-800-HAWORTH. E-mail address: <docdelivery@ haworthpress.com> Website: <http://www.HaworthPress.com> © 2006 by The Haworth Press, Inc. All rights reserved.]*

KEYWORDS. Transgender, mental health, counseling, gender dysphoria

INTRODUCTION

Transgender individuals and loved ones (partners, family, and friends) may seek assistance from mental health professionals for trans-specific or more general health concerns. Transgender mental health practice may include: (a) Evaluation, care planning, and treatment of gender identity concerns; (b) evaluation, care planning, and treatment of mental

Walter O. Bockting, PhD, is Associate Professor and Coordinator of Transgender Health Services, Program in Human Sexuality, Department of Family Medicine and Community Health, University of Minnesota Medical School, Minneapolis, MN, USA. Gail Knudson, MD, MPE, FRCPC, is affiliated with the Department of Sexual Medicine, University of British Columbia and Vancouver Hospital, Vancouver, BC, Canada. Joshua M. Goldberg is Education Consultant of the Transgender Health Program, Vancouver, BC, Canada.

Address correspondence to: Dr. Walter O. Bockting, Program in Human Sexuality, University of Minnesota, 1300 South Second Street, Suite 180, Minneapolis, MN, USA, 55454 (E-mail: bockt001@umn.edu).

This manuscript was created for the Trans Care Project, a joint initiative of Transcend Transgender Support & Education Society and Vancouver Coastal Health's Transgender Health Program, with funding from the Canadian Rainbow Health Coalition. The authors thank Lin Fraser, Melady Preece, Rupert Raj, Oliver Robinow, Hershel Russell, Sandra Samons, and Julian Young for their comments on an earlier draft, and Donna Lindenberg, Olivia Ashbee, A. J. Simpson, and Rodney Hunt for research assistance.

[Haworth co-indexing entry note]: "Counseling and Mental Health Care for Transgender Adults and Loved Ones." Bockting, Walter O., Gail Knudson, and Joshua M. Goldberg. Co-published simultaneously in *International Journal of Transgenderism* (The Haworth Medical Press, an imprint of The Haworth Press, Inc.) Vol. 9, No. 3/4, 2006, pp. 35-82; and: *Guidelines for Transgender Care* (ed: Walter O. Bockting, and Joshua M. Goldberg) The Haworth Medical Press, an imprint of The Haworth Press, Inc., 2006, pp. 35-82. Single or multiple copies of this article are available for a fee from The Haworth Document Delivery Service [1-800-HAWORTH, 9:00 a.m. - 5:00 p.m. (EST). E-mail address: docdelivery@haworthpress.com].

health concerns; (c) psychotherapy for individuals, couples, families, and groups; (d) short-term consultation (typically 1-3 sessions)–including information, resources, and referral assistance for a transgender individual or loved one, or peer consultation for another clinician; (e) psychoeducational workshops and groups offering information and facilitated discussion on specific topics (e.g., sexual health, feminizing or masculinizing hormone therapy, gender role transition), as well as training for employers, schools, and other interested members of the public; (f) case and global advocacy (see article in this volume by White Holman and Goldberg, 2006b); (g) clinical support or supervision for facilitators of peer-led support group; and (h) training of other clinicians.

This article addresses *trans-specific* elements of mental health practice, including assessment, care planning, and treatment. It is intended to assist clinicians providing mental health services in the community setting–counselors, family physicians, nurses, psychologists, psychiatrists, psychiatric nurses, and social workers–who are already familiar with basic terms and concepts in transgender care and are seeking more advanced clinical guidance in work with transgender adults. Mental health practice with transgender adolescents is discussed elsewhere in this volume (de Vries, Cohen-Kettenis, & Delemarre-van de Waal, 2006; White Holman & Goldberg, 2006a).

Mental health is intrinsically connected to cultural, physical, sexual, psychosocial, and spiritual aspects of health. Complete mental health care for the transgender community must similarly be considered in the context of a holistic approach to transgender health that includes comprehensive primary care as well as psychosocial care (Keatley, Nemoto, Sevelius, & Ventura, 2004; Raj, 2002). Close coordination between mental health and other services is essential for optimal practice (Bockting & Fung, 2005; Feldman & Bockting, 2003).

This article should not be perceived as a rigid set of guidelines or standards for care. In any clinical practice it is paramount that protocols be tailored to the specific needs of each client, and mental health practice is particularly dynamic in this regard. Research in transgender health is still in its infancy, and there are widely diverging clinical and consumer opinions about

"best" practice. In this article we offer suggestions based on published literature specific to transgender mental health, interviews with expert clinicians, the authors' clinical experience, and the guiding principles of the co-sponsoring organizations–a transgender-affirmative approach, client-centered care, and a commitment to harm reduction (Kopala, 2003). Ongoing interdisciplinary research and collegial meetings are important in further developing practice protocols. Clinicians are encouraged to adapt and modify our suggested protocols to address changing conditions and emerging issues in practice.

CLINICAL PICTURE

As a heterogeneous population, there is great diversity among transgender individuals and their needs relating to mental health services. In a 2002 survey of individuals in British Columbia requiring transgender health services (N = 179), 53% of respondents reported a current need for counseling relating to gender issues, with 32% requiring mental health assessment relating to pursuit of feminizing or masculinizing hormones or surgery and 39% stating a current need for mental health care for issues not relating to gender identity concerns (Goldberg, Matte, MacMillan, & Hudspith, 2003). Clients may present seeking assistance with mental health issues, concerns relating to gender identity or expression, or non-transgender-specific psychosocial issues. For some clients all three concerns may be relevant, and the focus of treatment may need to shift over time to address the most pressing concerns.

Regardless of the presenting concern, the clinician must be able to evaluate the impact of transgender-specific issues on mental health (e.g., transphobia, impact of gender issues on psychosocial and identity development, psychological effects of feminizing or masculinizing hormones) and the implications for treatment. For individuals seeking help relating to gender identity concerns, the clinician must be knowledgeable about gender and sexual identity development, transgender "coming out," crossdressing, gender dysphoria, gender transition, and the common concerns and reactions of loved ones.

Figure 1 outlines the basic assessment, treatment, and evaluation process in mental health care for transgender individuals. The initial evaluation (A) involves determination of the client's reasons for seeking service and a general client history. If the client has current gender identity concerns, the next step may be a gender assessment (B) to provide more detailed information about the client's gender identity issues and to determine any co-existing conditions, or it may be to provide supportive counseling until the client feels ready to engage in such a process. If the client does not have gender concerns but is instead presenting with mental health concerns, a more detailed mental health assessment (C) is performed. Based on the assessments, a clinical impression is generated, including a multi-axial diagnosis and assessment formulation where appropriate. The next step, care planning (D), involves recommendations for treatment and discussion of treatment options. If the client wishes to pursue hormonal or surgical feminization or masculinization, a specialized assessment (E) must be done to evaluate eligibility and readiness (Meyer et al., 2001). Each of these tasks is discussed in detail below.

INITIAL EVALUATION

Initial evaluation typically consists of one to three 50-minute clinical interview sessions with a new client. The goals of the initial evaluation are to build therapeutic rapport, discuss client and assessor goals and expectations, record client history and objectives, evaluate current psychological concerns and capacity to consent to care, and form an initial clinical impression. Each task is discussed below.

After the rules of confidentiality and other information required at any mental health consultation have been discussed, the next question should be an open question as to what leads the client to seek assistance at this time. Once the client has been able to describe the presenting complaint, the interviewer should decide which assessment tasks are most appropriate for the initial visit and which should be postponed to subsequent sessions. For clients in acute crisis, stabilization is the immediate priority; assessment will, by necessity, be more brief and focused on content directly related to the current situation, rather than a detailed life history.

Trans-Specific Issues in Building Therapeutic Rapport

Many transgender individuals and loved ones have had negative experiences with health and social service professionals, and may be wary about entering unreservedly into a relationship with the clinician. This is particularly true when the interaction is mandated–for example, as part of obtaining access to hormone therapy or surgery–rather than voluntarily sought (Bockting, Robinson, Benner, & Scheltema, 2004; Brown & Rounsley, 1996). Issues relating to hormone and surgery assessment are discussed in detail in a later section of the article.

In addition to the regular techniques used to build therapeutic rapport, it can be helpful to actively demonstrate transgender-specific sensitivity by discussing privacy issues in setting appointment times (e.g., whether a message can be left at the client's home or workplace) and the client's preferred name and pronouns. Visible transgender brochures, books, and posters signal to clients that you are aware of transgender concerns and are supportive of the transgender community. Similarly, intake forms should be transgender-inclusive.

Discussing Client and Clinician Goals and Expectations

Every client has goals and expectations, and often fears, about working with a mental health professional. Transgender clients may have a particular idea about what to expect based on previous experience with health professionals or the experiences of transgender peers. Clinicians also come to this work with particular goals and expectations, as well as a framework for how the initial evaluation and subsequent care planning and treatment will proceed. It is recommended that the protocols and approach used by the clinician be explained in detail so the client knows what to expect.

FIGURE 1. Clinical Pathways and Task in Mental health Practice with Transgender Individuals

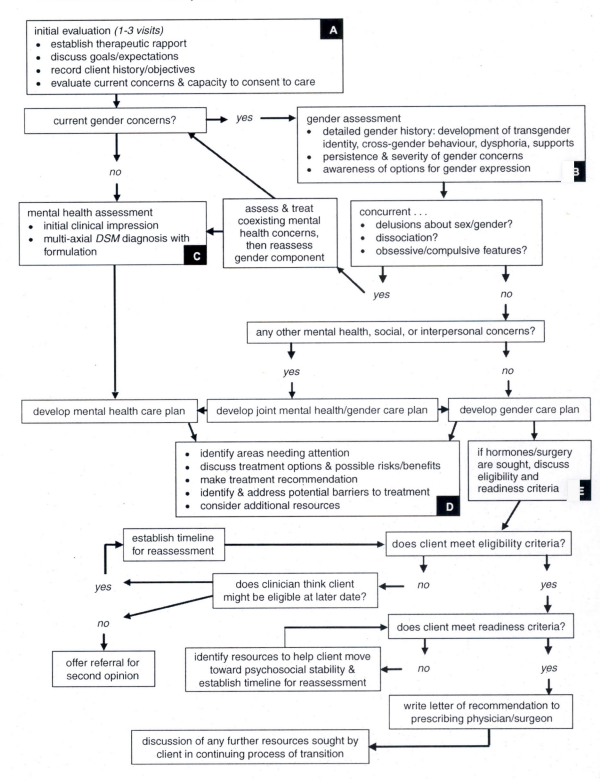

In particular, if the client is presenting with a desire to be assessed for hormones or surgery, it is important to ensure the client understands the process the clinician will use to conduct the evaluation, the specific eligibility and readiness criteria to be evaluated, and the way the clinician will handle possible outcomes of the evaluation process. Whether pursuing hormone therapy or surgery is the main issue or not, it is helpful to make it clear that you are not judging the client's gender presentation or passability. Instead, the assessment will focus on core gender identity, authentic self, and psychosocial adjustment.

Documenting Client History and Current Concerns

Documentation of client history–including relevant medical, gender, and psychosocial information–is addressed in the evaluation interview by asking the type of questions listed in Table 1. Initial evaluation and documentation should be paced to facilitate therapeutic rapport. For some clients, in-depth discussion of potentially sensitive topics at an early stage helps reassure the client that the therapist is knowledgeable, sensitive, and non-judgmental; for other clients it can be anxiety-provoking

TABLE 1. Potential Areas of Inquiry in Initial Evaluation

Topic	Questions
Medical history	Does anyone in your family have a history of chronic physical or mental health concerns? Do you have any chronic physical or mental health conditions, and if so, what are they? Have you ever been diagnosed with a physical or mental health condition, and if so, when and what was the diagnosis? Have you ever been hospitalized, and if so, when and what for? Are you currently taking any medication (including illicitly obtained hormones) or herbal supplements, and if so, what is the name, dose, and length of time you have been taking it? Have you ever had any injuries or surgeries?
Substance use	Do you smoke, and if so how much per day? Have you ever had any concerns relating to drugs or alcohol? Has anyone else ever expressed concern about, or objected to, your use of alcohol or drugs? Have there been any unpleasant incidents where alcohol or drugs were involved? Do you have any concerns about drugs or alcohol now?
Family	People define 'family' in many ways; who do you define as being in your family? How would you characterize your relationships with your family members when you were a child, and now? Do you have any concerns relating to your family?
Sexuality	How do you identify in terms of your sexual orientation? Are you sexually attracted to men, women, or both? Are you sexually attracted to transgender people? Are you currently involved with anyone romantically, and if so, how do you feel about your relationship? Have you had any concerns about relationships or sexuality in the past? Do you have any current concerns about relationships or sexuality today? Have you ever had any concerns about sexual abuse or sexual assault?
Social	What are your social supports? When you are under stress, who do you turn to for help? Are you currently working, in school, or volunteering? Do you have any concerns relating to work, school, or community involvement? Do you feel connected to any particular communities– e.g., transgender community, ethnic or cultural community, lesbian/gay/bisexual community, youth groups, seniors' groups, Deaf community? What are your hobbies or social interests?
Economic	What is your primary source of income? Do you have any current financial stress? Are you worried about future financial stress? Are you satisfied with your current housing? Do you have any concerns about housing? Do you have any concerns about work?
Gender concerns	Have you ever had any concerns relating to your gender? Do you currently have concerns or questions relating to your gender? How do you feel about being transgender? Are there any cultural or religious conflicts for you as a transgender person? Have you ever pursued any changes to your appearance or body to bring it closer to your sense of self? Have you ever sought to change your body through hormones or surgery, or thought about pursuing this in the future? Do you have any concerns about your appearance or body now? Are there any kinds of supports you feel might be helpful as a transgender person?

to be asked questions about drug and alcohol use, sexual concerns, history of sex work, etc.

Standardized psychological testing and paper-and-pencil questionnaires are helpful tools to screen for a range of health and psychosocial adjustment issues and to assess the client's identity in greater depth. Using these instruments as an adjunct to the clinical interview can make the interview more efficient by reducing the areas and questions to be explored verbally, and allows cross-referencing of verbal and written responses (as clients vary in their comfort to reveal certain personal information verbally or in writing). In addition to instruments used to evaluate general mental and physical health, Table 2 presents an overview of commonly used tests and questionnaires relevant to transgender-specific concerns. The instruments chosen depend on the client's presenting complaint.

While it is important to gain an accurate sense of areas of concern, evaluation should also include discernment of client strengths. Determining personal strengths and positive supports is necessary not only to give a complete picture of the client's life and psychosocial adjustment, but also to bolster a client's sense of competency and agency. The care plan that will be developed based on the evaluation will build on these strengths to promote resilience.

In some cases, evaluation by another professional may be useful. For example, if the initial interview is conducted by someone other than a psychiatrist, a separate psychiatric evaluation may be indicated to assess psychiatric symptomatology and, if there are co-existing mental health issues, explore options for pharmacological or other treatment. Depending on answers to screening questions about drug and alcohol use, a formal chemical dependency evaluation may be recommended. The stigma associated with substance use may lead clients to be hesitant to frankly discuss details of drug and alcohol use during an initial evaluation. However, given the relatively high prevalence of drug and alcohol use among transgender individuals (Hughes & Eliason, 2002; Lombardi & van Servellen, 2000; Nemoto, Operario, Keatley, Nguyen, & Sugano, 2005; Pasillas, Anderson, & Fraser, 2000) and the difficulties faced by transgender individuals in accessing substance abuse treatment that is transgender-sensitive and competent, we believe it is important to enquire about drug and alcohol use as part of the intake process. Visible pamphlets about substance abuse treatment and harm reduction can be helpful in providing clients with reassurance that it is safe to discuss these concerns.

Evaluating Capacity to Make Care Decisions

Decision-making capacity is the ability to understand relevant information and to appreciate the reasonable foreseeable consequences of a decision (Appelbaum & Grisso, 1988). As in the non-transgender population, most transgender clients will not present any challenge in terms of ability to consent to care, and the evaluation is usually a spontaneous and straightforward judgment based on routine interactions between a clinician and client (Tunzi, 2001). Sometimes determination of the capacity to make medical decisions is more challenging because a client has limited cognitive capacity due to neurological illness, developmental disability, head injury, or intoxication. In these cases, formal capacity assessment such as the Aid to Capacity Evaluation (ACE) may be used by the mental health clinician or the patient's primary care provider (Etchells et al., 1999). ACE is a semi-structured decisional tool that prompts inquiry into the seven relevant areas outlined in Table 3.

TABLE 2. Testing and Questionnaire Instruments

Assessment area	Possible instruments
Transgender identity	Gender Identity Questionnaire (Docter & Fleming, 2001)
Internalized transphobia	Transgender Identity Survey (Bockting, Miner, Robinson, Rosser, & Coleman, 2005)
Components of sexual identity	Assessment of Sexual Orientation (Coleman, 1987)
Psychosexual functioning	Derogatis Sexual Functioning Inventory (Derogatis & Melisaratos, 1979), Compulsive Sexual Behavior Inventory (Coleman, Miner, Ohlerking, & Raymond, 2001)

TABLE 3. Aid to Capacity Evaluation[1]

Area of capacity to assess	Interview questions
Ability to understand the medical problem	What problem are you having now?
Ability to understand the proposed treatment	What is the treatment for your problem? What can we do to help you?
Ability to understand the alternatives to the proposed treatment (if any)	Are there any other treatments? What other options do you have?
Ability to understand the option of refusing treatment (including treatment withdrawal)	Can you refuse the treatment? Can we stop the treatment?
Ability to accept the reasonably foreseeable consequences of accepting treatment	What could happen to you if you have the treatment? How could the treatment help you? Could the treatment cause problems and side effects?
Ability to accept the reasonably foreseeable consequences of refusing proposed treatment	What could happen to you if you don't have the treatment? Could you get sicker or die without the treatment?
Ability to make a decision that is not substantially based on hallucinations, delusions, or cognitive signs of depression	Why have you decided to accept or refuse the treatment? Do you think we are trying to hurt or harm you? Do you deserve to be treated? Do you feel that you are being punished? Do you feel that you are a bad person?

[1]An ACE scoring form is available online at the University of Toronto Joint Centre for Bioethics website, http://www.utoronto.ca/jcb/disclaimers/ace_form.htm
Adapted from Etchells, E. (n.d.). Aid to Capacity Evaluation (ACE). Toronto, ONT: University of Toronto Joint Centre for Bioethics. Retrieved January 1, 2005, from http://www.utoronto.ca/jcb/disclaimers/ace.pdf

In complex cases, additional evaluation should be sought from a psychologist or other clinician who specializes in medical competency evaluation. It may also be appropriate to seek collateral information from loved ones or caregivers (see case studies of Jamie and Patricia in Appendix A).

Initial Clinical Impression

After the interview is complete and any testing is scored, the assessor should review the completed questionnaires, the interview notes and test results, supplemental evaluations (e.g., psychiatric assessment, chemical dependency evaluation, competency testing) and collateral evidence, and integrate the information gathered into an overall assessment of the client's presenting complaint, goals and expectations, background, and biopsychosocial adjustment. In complex cases the clinical impression may be tentative at this point, and will need to be confirmed during the course of treatment.

ASSESSMENT AND TREATMENT OF GENDER CONCERNS

The prevalence of gender concerns is unknown. There are no data about the number of persons who have concerns or questions about gender identity or crossdressing, only some limited data on those who have sought surgical sex reassignment. The prevalence of transsexuals pursuing sex reassignment surgery is estimated at 1 in 11,900 for male-to-female transsexuals and 1 in 30,400 for female-to-male transsexuals (Bakker, van Kesteren, Gooren, & Bezemer, 1993) and annual incidence rates are estimated to range from 0.15-1.58 per 100,000 (Kesteren, Gooren, & Megens, 1996; Olsson & Möller, 2003).

Gender identity concerns can affect individuals of all ages. Male-to-female (MTF) transsexuals may not seek psychological or medical intervention until middle age (Blanchard, 1994), while female-to-male (FTM) transsexuals typically present somewhat younger. However, gender issues can affect all age groups, including children and adolescents. Seniors may also present with previously unarticulated or untreated gender concerns.

Gender issues can arise in a variety of ways in mental health practice. Some clients disclose at the first session that they are seeking help for gender issues, and may specifically ask about the clinician's experience in working with the transgender community as part of the initial meeting. Others are unsure how to articulate their concerns or are more cautious about divulging gender issues, presenting with generalized depression or anxiety, seeking help "coping with stress," or other general concerns. As gender-variance is often assumed to be evidence of homosexuality, individuals who are questioning their gender or are confused about gender identity issues may describe their feelings in terms of confusion about sexual orientation. In some cases gender issues emerge over time as part of the clinical picture for clients who initially seek help relating to substance use, self-harming behavior, disordered eating, or other issues.

The language used by transgender individuals is continually changing, as transgender people become more visible and are better able to articulate similarities and differences in identities and experiences. To facilitate communication, it is helpful for the clinician and client to reach a common understanding of terms and concepts key in discussion of gender concerns, including those relating to gender, sex, and sexual orientation.

Gender Assessment

Assessment of gender concerns involves a detailed history of transgender identity development and gender expression. In addition to the interview questions outlined in Table 4, paper-and-pencil instruments listed earlier in Table 2 (e.g., Gender Identity Questionnaire, Transgender Identity Survey) may be utilized. If the client presents with gender confusion or is in the early stages of exploring identity, it may be too soon in their identity development to allow an in-depth gender assessment. In these cases, further exploration of identity and experimentation with the various options to manage or express one's transgender identity in the context of psychotherapeutic treatment is advised before completion of a full gender assessment. For clients in later stages of incorporating transgender identity into daily life, a more detailed interview will be possible.

There is controversy within the transgender community and among mental health professionals about the *DSM-IV-TR* (American Psychiatric Association, 2000) diagnoses of *Gender Identity Disorder* (GID) and *Transvestic*

Fetishism (TF) as part of evaluation and treatment planning (Bockting & Ehrbar, 2006). Some clinicians feel that a diagnosis of GID or TF is fundamentally important to guiding clinical consideration of options for treatment and helps promote client access to health care, including access to hormone therapy and sex reassignment surgery (Brown & Rounsley, 1996). Others believe that these diagnoses pathologize transgenderism, normalize dominant Western gender binary norms as culturally universal, and conflate distress relating to societal marginalization with distress relating to a condition that may require medical intervention (Davis, 1998; Hill, Rozanski, Carfaginni, & Willoughby, 2003; Israel & Tarver, 1997; Moser & Kleinplatz, 2003; Wilson & Lev, 2003). Although a diagnosis of GID is not explicitly required to gain access to hormones or surgery in the World Professional Association for Transgender Health (WPATH) *Standards of Care* (Meyer et al., 2001), the diagnosis is required by many individual clinicians as a prerequisite to hormonal or surgical treatment.

Regardless of approach and beliefs relating to GID and TF diagnosis, or a history of GID or TF diagnosis, we consider it essential to evaluate specific parameters in assessment of clients who present with gender identity concerns. These include the specific nature of the gender concerns, their persistence and severity, any associated mental health concerns (e.g., obsessive or compulsive features, delusions relating to sex and gender, dissociation, personality disorders), any associated concerns about sexual identity (e.g., sexual orientation), and any co-existing conditions such as anxiety and mood disorders (Bockting, Coleman, Huang, & Ding, 2006; Clements-Nolle, Marx, Guzman, & Katz, 2001) or Asperger's Disorder (Robinow & Knudson, 2005). Appendix B provides two sample letters summarizing the gender assessment findings of a MTF and FTM transgender client.

Nature of the Gender Concerns

Not all transgender individuals struggle with gender issues; among those who do, there are varying concerns. Some individuals seek help because they are confused about their identity; others are struggling with despair, shame, or

TABLE 4. Potential Areas of Inquiry in Gender Evaluation: Transgender Person

Topic	Questions
Gender identity	How would your describe your gender identity? How did you come to recognize that your experience of gender is different than most individuals? Were there any life events that you feel were significant in influencing your gender identity? Have there been changes to your gender identity over time? What do you remember feeling about your gender as a child, during puberty, and as an adolescent? How do you feel about your gender now? Do you have any questions or concerns about your gender? How does your gender identity impact how you feel about work, relationships, family, or other aspects of your life?
Gender expression	Are there any activities you did as a child or that you do now as an adult that you think of as being cross- or trans-gendered, and if so, how have these been viewed by your family and others in your life? Did you prefer to be around individuals of any particular gender as a child, and if so, is this different than your preferences now? Have you ever crossdressed; if so, what was that experience like for you, and if not, what do you imagine it would be like? If you could change your external appearance in any way you wanted to more closely match your sense of who you are, what would this look like in terms of your gender? Have you ever taken feminizing or masculinizing hormones or had sex reassignment surgery, and if so, what was that like for you?
Perceptions of others	How do you think others perceived your gender when you were a child, and how do you think others perceive your gender now? How do you want to be perceived in terms of your gender? How important is it to you that there be a fit between how you feel about your gender and how others perceive you?
Sexuality	How does gender play out in your sexual desires or fantasies? Does gender impact the kinds of sexual activities you do (on your own or with others) or wish you could do? What is a typical sexual fantasy for you? Do your sexual fantasies involve other men, women, or transgender people, or do you mainly fantasize about yourself? If you are in your fantasies, do you imagine yourself to be female, male, or transgender? What are your feelings about the parts of your body that are often associated with sexuality (e.g., genitals, chest/breasts)?
Support resources	Do the people in your life know that you are transgender; if so, what was it like to tell them, and if not, how do you feel about them not knowing? Have you had any contact with other transgender individuals, and if so, what was that like for you? What do you see your relationship being to the transgender community now, and what would you like it to be in the future? Have you used the Internet to access support and information about being transgender; if so, what have you learned, and in what ways was it helpful or not helpful for you?

guilt relating to crossdressing or transgender feelings; others are dysphoric about physical characteristics associated with their sex, the perceptions of others relating to gender, and/or the social roles associated with their sex and gender assigned at birth.

Persistence and Severity of Gender Concerns

For some individuals, gender concerns are mild and/or transient; for others they are persistent and severe enough to cause "clinically significant distress or impairment in social, occupational, or other important areas of functioning"–considered the minimum clinical threshold necessary for diagnosis of Gender Identity Disorder or Transvestic Fetishism (American Psychiatric Association, 2000). Clients who are gender-variant but not preoccupied with gender concerns to the degree that it is negatively affecting their quality of life should not be diagnosed with GID or TF. Distress relating to others' transphobia is not GID; if it is so severe that the transphobia of others is negatively affecting quality of life, a diagnosis of Adjustment Disorder may be appropriate (Israel & Tarver, 1997).

Associated Obsessive or Compulsive Features

Compulsive crossdressing, obsessive pursuit of validation of transgender identity through sexual pursuits, or other obsessive or compulsive behaviors should be evaluated. If there is sexual compulsivity, a diagnosis of Sexual Disorder NOS or Transvestic Fetishism may be appropriate (American Psychiatric Association, 2000). If the client is not seeking hormones or surgery, compulsivity can be treated concurrent with addressing transgender issues. If the client is seeking hormones or surgery, the obsessive or compulsive features should first be addressed, with subsequent reassessment to determine whether gender identity concerns persist (Bockting, 1997).

Delusions About Sex or Gender

In rare cases, schizophrenia or other thought disorders manifest as gender- or sex-based delusions (Campo, Nijman, Evers, Merckelbach, & Decker, 2001; Manderson & Kumar, 2001). For example, the client may believe that their body has spontaneously transformed from one sex to another, or that internal organs of the other sex are present even after laboratory examination confirms there is no evidence of intersexuality. In some cases the delusion may be expressed as "really being of another gender." This can be distinguished from gender dysphoria, the latter usually being more persistent and longstanding, and present also when the client is not actively delusional.

Dissociation

For some individuals, growing up transgender is experienced as traumatic. Others have experienced additional trauma such as physical or sexual abuse. Coping strategies with such trauma may include dissociation of the self, and this may involve a split of identity into a separate male and female self (Bockting & Coleman, in press). By addressing this trauma in therapy, an integrated self can be achieved (Bockting & Coleman, in press; Brown & Rounsley, 1996). A diagnosis of Dissociative Identity Disorder as defined in the *DSM-IV-TR* is not a contraindication to sex reassignment surgery (Brown, 2001) but should be very carefully evaluated as part of the overall care plan. A diagnosis of Dissociative Identity Disorder is not appropriate for individuals who have a bi-gender identity but no dissociation, even if they describe their gender as having different "personalities"

or "selves." As stated by Israel and Tarver (1997), "The transition from one gender to another occurs across psychological and physical planes and is experienced as self-fulfilling and stress-relieving for the transgender individual, in contrast to the increased confusion and insecurity felt by the person with a dissociative condition" (pp. 29-30).

Personality Disorders

It can be challenging to evaluate gender identity concerns in clients with personality disorders such as borderline personality disorder. Sometimes it is difficult to determine whether symptoms of gender dysphoria are solely due to the personality disorder or were pre-existing, with the personality disorder evolving as a way of coping with the dysphoria. In other cases, gender dysphoria and a personality disorder may be unrelated and simply co-exist.

Internalized Homophobia

Clients who have difficulty accepting same-sex or same-gender sexual feelings or attractions may fantasize about or describe themselves as being of the other gender (Brown & Rounsley, 1996). Assessment of gender concerns should include a thorough sexual history, and appropriate counseling offered for any concerns about sexual orientation. Gender identity concerns should be reassessed after sexual orientation has been clarified and comfort with sexual orientation has been achieved.

Asperger's Disorder

Asperger's Disorder is classified in the *DSM-IV-TR* as a qualitative impairment in social functioning with restricted repetitive and stereotypical patterns of behavior, interests, and activities (American Psychiatric Association, 2000). There is no clinically significant delay in language and cognitive development. This disorder is typically diagnosed in childhood.

For reasons that are not understood, gender dysphoria is present in clients with Asperger's Disorder at a greater rate than those in the unaffected population (Robinow & Knudson, 2005). The gender dysphoria is usually present quite early in life but may not become apparent until later. Because of the obsessive and compulsive nature of Asperger's Disorder, clients will usually be very persistent in obtaining sex reassignment surgery, but do not appear to be as concerned about social adjustment as their observance of social cues is impaired (see case of Patricia in Appendix A). Diagnosis of previously unrecognized Asperger's Disorder can facilitate any needed social, education, or pharmacotherapeutic interventions (Volkmar, Cook, Pomeroy, Realmuto, & Tanguay, 1999), as well as ensuring that treatment of co-existing gender concerns accommodates the communication patterns typical of Asperger's. It may also be relevant in determining competency in making care decisions.

Care Plan for Gender Identity Concerns

Treatment of gender concerns depends on numerous factors, including the client's stage of transgender identity development, the client's knowledge of and pre-existing pursuit of gender identity management options, and co-existing mental health or psychosocial concerns. Prior to treatment of gender issues, co-existing conditions that are more emergent or that present a barrier to treatment must be addressed, and if other concerns become more emergent during treatment of gender issues the focus of care should shift accordingly. Mental health or psychosocial concerns identified during the initial evaluation or during treatment of gender identity concerns should be evaluated and incorporated into the overall care plan. Axis IV psychosocial stressors are best addressed through coordination with social, housing, legal, and vocational services (White Holman & Goldberg, 2006b).

Care planning should include consideration of socioeconomic factors that influence clients' ability to access or engage in treatment. Seventy-two percent of participants in a survey in British Columbia (N = 179) reported difficulty accessing services relating to crossdressing or gender transition; the most common barriers reported were cost (40%), lack of services in the client's home region (31%), and waitlists for services (26%) (Goldberg et al., 2003). As private psychotherapy is often not covered by public health insurance, psychotherapy may not be economically accessible even when the client is highly motivated to engage in treatment. Global advocacy is needed to ensure that transgender individuals in need of professional assistance are able to access psychotherapeutic services.

Psychotherapy for Gender Identity Concerns

Some individuals explore gender identity issues through peer support, use of the internet, or self-directed reading, writing, and reflection. Others voluntarily seek professional psychotherapeutic assistance, or have psychotherapy recommended as a prerequisite to consideration for feminizing or masculinizing hormone therapy or sex reassignment surgery.

Mental health professionals may, depending on their theoretical orientation and training, apply a number of different therapeutic approaches to the treatment of gender identity concerns (Fraser, 2005). What is most important is that the treating clinician has developed specific competence in transgender care, which often includes a re-examination of theory on gender and sexual identity development within their own discipline and training under supervision of an established gender specialist (Israel & Tarver, 1997). A trusting, authentic relationship with the client is paramount to the success of any psychotherapeutic approach. Because working with transgender clients can involve challenging transference and countertransference issues (Koetting, 2004; Milrod, 2000), ongoing clinical supervision and peer consultation are essential.

Addressing Co-Existing Mental Health or Psychosocial Concerns

Unless treatment of gender identity concerns and concurrent mental health concerns are embedded in safeguarding or improving the client's social adjustment, it is unlikely that the goal of achieving better mental health and well-being will be achieved. Treatment of concurrent mental health concerns is necessary both to relieve the distress associated with these concerns and also to help the client engage in psychotherapy to address the gender identity issues. It takes courage and persistence on the client's part to confront gender identity concerns that have often been surrounded with fear, shame, hopelessness, and despair. Addressing the overall mental health of the client will improve the client's ability to work toward resolution of gender confusion or distress and, if desired, to pursue gender transition.

Many clients are appreciative of an integrated approach, but others see the discussion of psychosocial or mental health concerns as a "distraction" from working on gender issues. To promote active client engagement in treatment, it can be helpful to explain to the client how addressing co-existing concerns will be of benefit not only in terms of improved mental health, but also in terms of achieving and sustaining resilience in living life as a transgender person in the face of social stigma. Moreover, the client's strengths and resilience displayed so far should be acknowledged and validated, and treatment should build on these strengths.

Exploring Gender History and Development of Transgender Identity

The emphasis of this aspect of therapy is on internal reflection and on the meaning the client assigns to past and present experiences (Bockting, 1997). The goal is not to theorize or speculate about causative factors relating to transgender identity, but rather to explore the client's understanding of their own identity development and the impact of life events.

Exploration of gender history, development of transgender identity, and related concerns begins with an in-depth review of the client's personal history. This review of personal history provides the opportunity to cognitively restructure significant events and experiences, facilitate grief and healing, and foster a stronger sense of self and identity. It can also aid in identifying and changing patterns of compulsivity, understanding the development of Axis I and II disorders, and illuminating and changing present maladaptive thoughts and behaviors. The telling of one's history to a willing listener is also validating and, by speaking of it, helps to clarify and consolidate the client's self-understanding. It may be helpful to discuss these experiences in a framework of developmental stages of transgender coming out or emergence (Bockting & Coleman, in press; Lev, 2004).

Journaling has been shown to lessen the impact of trauma and improve health (Esterling, L'Abate, Murray, & Pennebaker, 1999). Clients who are literate can write their life stories chronologically as homework between therapy sessions, and bring this journal to share in individual or group therapy. Those who struggle with writing can create genograms, photo montages or collages, or other visual depictions of life story.

During therapy, issues may arise relating to family-of-origin intimacy dysfunction, abuse, or neglect. Consultation or referral to specialized services may be useful if clients need assistance for childhood sexual abuse. In some cases, transgender clients may seek to involve family members in therapy to explore and resolve childhood issues, and use this as an opportunity to improve these relationships. Support from family and friends has been associated with resilience of transgender individuals facing gender-related stigma and discrimination (Bockting, Coleman, Huang et al., 2006).

Another area of focus may be internalized transphobia. Clients who have internalized societal stigma (Goffman, 1963) typically struggle with profound shame, guilt, and self-loathing. This may manifest in a hope that psychotherapy will stop transgender feelings or, more typically, in an over-emphasis on passing as a non-transgender woman or man and a discomfort associating with other transgender individuals onto whom feelings of guilt and self-hatred are projected. Exploring these issues may help the client move toward self-acceptance (Bockting & Coleman, in press). For some clients, psychotherapy to alleviate internalized transphobia is a long-term process.

After personal history has been reviewed and gender identity concerns have been clarified, it is appropriate to shift to actively exploring options for expression and management of gender identity. However, such exploration may trigger a need to revisit issues in the past, resulting in new insights and further resolution. To maintain a trusting therapeutic relationship, it is helpful to continue to clarify expectations of the degree and value of reflecting on the past, or "soul-searching," to facilitate the client in making a fully informed decision about the various options for expression and management of gender identity.

Exploration of Options for Gender Expression

The WPATH *Standards of Care* (Meyer et al., 2001) list a range of possible options for transgender identity exploration and expression, including (a) participation in peer support/self-help groups or in the transgender community, (b) counseling to explore gender identity and to deal with pressures relating to work or family (c) learning about transgenderism from the Internet, guidelines for care, or literature relating to legal rights, (d) disclosing transgender identity to family, friends, and other loved ones ("coming out"), (e) integration of gender awareness into daily living, (f) temporary and potentially reversible changes to appearance, such as changes in hairstyle or makeup; shaving, plucking, or waxing facial or body hair; applying facial hair; wearing prosthetic breasts or penile prosthesis; tucking or binding the chest or genitals; and crossdressing, (g) change in vocal expression, pitch/tone, inflection, and other aspects of speech, (h) episodic cross-living, (i) change in gender pronoun or name, in common usage or legal change, (j) semi-permanent changes to appearance such as masculinizing or feminizing hormones (some changes are reversible, while others are not), and (k) permanent changes to appearance, such as surgical reconstruction of the face, chest, or genitals, or electrolysis or laser removal of facial and body hair. This list is not meant to be exhaustive, but simply to illustrate that there are multiple options that may be pursued, and that there is no right or wrong way to manage one's identity. Frequently, a client's expression of transgender identity evolves over time, requiring re-evaluation of possible options. The role of the mental health professional is to assist the client to consider all of the options and make an informed decision regarding identity management. Whatever options the client considers, there should be thought as to how the client will realistically integrate changes into daily life.

Discussion of options should take into account previous treatment and identity exploration. For example, if the client is already living full-time in the desired gender role and is satisfied with this, exploring options such as integrating crossgender feelings into the gender role assigned at birth or "episodic crossliving" would not be appropriate; ensuring the client is cognizant that there is not one way to be transgender will suffice.

Gender role transition, hormone therapy, and each surgical procedure may be considered separately. A gender role transition could be undertaken with or without hormone therapy or surgery; similarly, hormone therapy does not need to be followed by surgery, and chest or breast surgery is not necessarily accompanied by hormone therapy or followed by genital surgery. Feminizing or masculinizing hormones have systemic effects and it is not possible to pick and choose specific changes, but endocrine agents that cause menstrual cessation (FTM) or mild feminization without breast development (MTF) may be appropriate for clients who identify as androgynous, bi- or non-gendered and wish only to minimize sex and gender characteristics (Dahl et al., 2006).

Contact with peers who are expressing their gender identity in various ways can help clients appreciate the multiplicity of options for gender expression, understand what is involved in the various possible change processes that may be pursued, and anticipate potential challenges. Peer contact may include group therapy, self-help groups, participation in Internet discussions, social contact, or one-to-one peer support available through transgender community organizations. Peers can help with information about ways other than medical intervention to feminize or masculinize appearance, such as clothing, hairstyle, breast prostheses, chest binders, and genital prostheses.

Many transgender individuals initially immerse themselves in a specific transgender social network or group as part of their desire to find community. While strong transgender identification and community affiliation can be a helpful path to self-discovery, peer opinion can at times also be a negative force if there is pressure to conform to group norms or to pursue a particular identity or course of action. For example, some transgender individuals emphasize physical change and transition, whereas others reject the idea of transition to pass as a member of the other sex as "selling out" to fit mainstream norms. The mental health clinician can assist with referral to peer groups that explicitly support diversity of gender identity and expression, and individual choice in decisions relating to identity management.

Implementation of Identity Management Decisions

Once the client has come to a decision for gender identity expression and management, therapy focuses on supporting the individual to implement this decision. Some clients may choose strategies that do not require disclosure of transgender identity to others, keeping transgender identity and expression private. For others, disclosing transgender identity to family and friends, co-workers, teachers, or students, community, and others in the transgender person's life is an important step.

Disclosure of transgender identity is often considered analogous to disclosure and coming out for lesbian women, gay men, and bisexual individuals. However, the two processes are not identical (Brown & Rounsley, 1996). While both processes involve disclosure of a personal secret that may evoke a negative response by others, the existence of homosexuality and bisexuality is generally recognized; in contrast, transgenderism is not widely recognized or understood, and challenges societal beliefs about sex, gender, and sexuality in a way that is disorienting to many non-transgender individuals. For those undergoing gender transition, coming out involves not only the disclosure of a secret, but also subsequent visible changes in social role and physical appearance; for loved ones the consequences are also different as physical changes cannot be concealed and gender-based definitions of relationships may change. (e.g., the loss of a "father" who changed gender roles).

Despite the differences, the tools for disclosure of transgender identity are the same as those used in other circumstances where a client wants to discuss a potentially emotionally charged issue (Israel & Tarver, 1997). Clients are encouraged to take calculated risks in disclosure (Bockting & Coleman, in press; Horton, 2001), starting with people who are most likely to be accepting. This builds a base of support for the client and possibly for other individuals in the transgender person's life who may have difficulty following disclosure. Although some loved ones are not surprised by disclosure

of transgender identity and are strongly supportive, in most cases immediate acceptance is not a realistic expectation. Loved ones often go through stages of adjustment involving feelings of shock, disbelief, denial, fear, anger, and betrayal, followed by sadness and eventual acceptance (Ellis & Eriksen, 2002; Emerson & Rosenfeld, 1996). Peer support can be vital to help clients put reactions of loved ones in perspective. Family therapy or counseling for loved ones of a transgender person can be helpful as well.

The importance of social support cannot be underestimated. Research has shown that transgender individuals often have low levels of social support and that support from family and peers buffers the negative effects of social stigma and discrimination on transgender individuals' mental health (Bockting, Coleman, Huang et al., 2006; Nemoto, Operario, Sevelius et al., 2004). One study found that lack of familial support was predictive of regret following sex reassignment surgery (Landen, Walinder, Hambert, & Lundstrom, 1998).

Clients going through a gender role transition–with or without hormones or surgery–face many challenges. These include the adjustment of learning a new gender role and also the discrimination and harassment that is frequently experienced by someone who is visibly gender-variant, as many clients are–especially in the early stages of transition. During this time the counselor can be an important support, helping the client to cope with stress and to reflect on how the changes are affecting gender identity and overall comfort. The mental health professional can play an important role in assisting with planning and pacing such a transition.

For any of the feminizing or masculinizing medical interventions–including hormones, surgery, speech change, and permanent hair removal–the counselor can assist the client in obtaining information about the procedures; understanding the possible impact of these interventions on mental, physical, and sexual health; and, if surgery is needed, planning for pre-operative and post-operative care and support. As discussed in a later section, the clinician may also be asked to evaluate the client's eligibility and readiness to begin hormones or undergo surgery. If the clinician providing therapy will be assessing hormone or surgery eligibility and readiness, it is important for the client and therapist to mutually agree on psychotherapeutic tasks, goals, or milestones relating to eligibility and readiness criteria to be reached before the recommendation can be made. Doing so helps prepare the client for this assessment and emphasizes that this is a shared process. The weight and implications of identity management decisions, and the associated fears, may lead the client to look to the therapist to affirm that making a gender role transition is the right course to take; it is important that the responsibility for the actual decision as to how to express or manage gender identity be consistently directed back to the client.

Ongoing Management of Gender Issues Throughout the Client's Life

Coming out does not end with realizing one's option of choice for identity management. Rather, transgender coming out is a lifelong process. Identities may continue to evolve, and psychosocial challenges will continue to arise. Disclosure issues continue throughout life with the establishment of new relationships with friends, co-workers, partners, and others. The client may seek ongoing counseling or return to counseling in the future to further improve or maintain mental health, address concerns about gender identity and aging, deal with grief and loss, and/or address relationship issues. Even after years of living in the preferred gender role, clients may seek support relating to social stigma, such as coping with discrimination and harassment or internalized transphobia.

Some transgender individuals have an unchanging gender identity, while others have a more fluid identity that evolves over time. For example, a client may initially identify as bi-gender and spend time in both gender roles, but after doing so for many years pursue a more full-time gender role transition. Conversely, a client who initially transitions and strongly identifies as one gender may later feel more comfortable with a blended or androgynous presentation. Some clients initially focus on passing as a non-transgender woman or man, but in time express a consciously transgendered identity; others who initially dismissed passing-

ability later come to value it more. Identity shifts may happen spontaneously over the course of one's life, or may be in response to new situations, experiences, and challenges relating to aging or relationships with others (e.g., retirement, children leaving home, divorce).

Developmental tasks that were previously disrupted or halted because of gender dysphoria are often taken up once comfort with one's gender identity has been achieved. For many, this includes dating and relationships. The working relationship that the client has established with the therapist can be an important resource to assist with such issues as questions about sexual orientation, disclosure of transgender identity within dating and sexual relationships, safer sex, and sexual functioning. Hormones can affect sexual desire and responsiveness. Increased comfort with one's role and body may result in a sexual renaissance, including possible high risk behavior (Bockting, Robinson, & Rosser, 1998).

For those who have surgery, adequate postsurgical care is crucial. In addition to physical care following surgery, clients may need counseling to deal with physical discomfort or pain, altered physical sensation or sexual function, complications that may be transient or persistent, and psychosocial adjustment. Hormones will also need to be changed following removal of the ovaries/testicles, and fluctuations in hormone levels may cause psychological changes requiring therapeutic intervention.

The vast majority of clients are satisfied and report further reduction in gender dysphoria following surgery (Green & Fleming, 1990; Pfäfflin & Junge, 1998). However, clients may also experience grief over lost time or mourning for the idealized fantasy of self prior to change (Hansbury, 2005). Clients who have been very focused on surgery to the exclusion of other life goals may need support to explore other directions in their lives once the long sought after surgery has been achieved.

Hormonal and Surgical Treatment of Gender Dysphoria

Some individuals with gender dysphoria seek hormonal and/or surgical feminization or masculinization to reduce a discrepancy between their sense of self and their primary or secondary sex characteristics. The clinicians involved in the care of the individual presenting with gender dysphoria have a shared responsibility to determine the client's eligibility and readiness for hormone therapy or sex reassignment surgery. Ultimately, the prescribing clinician or the surgeon must decide whether to prescribe or perform the surgical procedure.

Most clinicians follow the WPATH *Standards of Care* (Meyer et al., 2001), which outline guidelines for clinical evaluation of eligibility and readiness in both adults and adolescents. The WPATH guidelines for transgender adults are summarized in Table 5; guidelines for adolescents are discussed elsewhere in this volume (de Vries, Cohen-Kettenis, & Delemarre-van de Waal, 2006). *Eligibility* refers to the minimum criteria that anyone seeking these medical interventions must meet, and *readiness* refers

to the client being mentally ready for the procedure. Readiness does not imply that the client can no longer have any mental health concerns to be ready for reassignment services; rather, sufficient stability needs to be in place to both make an informed decision and to be adequately prepared to deal with the physical, emotional, and social consequences of the decision.

Although psychotherapy is not an absolute requirement in the WPATH *Standards of Care*, the *Standards* do require mental health assessment by one qualified professional prior to hormone therapy or breast/chest surgery, and assessments by two mental health clinicians–including one with a doctorate degree–prior to hysterectomy or genital reconstructive surgery (Meyer et al., 2001). As with other types of psychological assessment, evaluation of hormone or surgery eligibility and readiness may take

TABLE 5. Summary of the World Professional Association for Transgender Health's *Standards of Care: Hormone and Surgery Eligibility and Readiness Criteria for Adults* (Meyer et al., 2001)

Hormones	
Eligibility	Readiness
1. Able to give informed consent 2. Informed of anticipated effects and risks 3. Completion of 3 months of "real life experience" OR have been in psychotherapy for duration specified by a mental health professional (usually minimum of 3 months)[1]	1. Consolidation of gender identity 2. Improved or continuing mental stability 3. Likely to take hormones in a responsible manner

Chest or Breast Surgery	
Eligibility	Readiness
1. Able to give informed consent 2. Informed of anticipated effects and risks 3. Completion of 3 months of "real life experience" OR have been in psychotherapy for duration specified by a mental health professional (usually minimum of 3 months) 4. FTM chest surgery may be done as first step, alone or with hormones; MTF breast augmentation may be done after 18 months on hormones (to allow time for hormonal breast development)	1. Consolidation of gender identity 2. Improved or continuing mental stability

Genital Surgery, Hysterectomy, and Oophorectomy	
Eligibility	Readiness
1. Able to give informed consent 2. Taking hormones for at least 12 months (if needing and medically able to take hormones) 3. At least 1 year "real life experience" 4. Completion of any psychotherapy required by the mental health professional 5. Informed of cost, hospitalization, complications, aftercare, and surgeon options	1. Consolidation of gender identity 2. Improved or continuing mental stability

[1]The WPATH *Standards* note that "in selected circumstances, it can be acceptable to provide hormones to patients who have not fulfilled criterion 3–for example, to facilitate the provision of monitored therapy using hormones of known quality, as an alternative to black-market or unsupervised hormone use" (Meyer et al., 2001, p. 13).

place in the context of a pre-existing therapeutic relationship, or the evaluation may be performed as a circumscribed process by a clinician who has not previously worked with the client.

A client-centered approach generally emphasizes care as a collaborative process involving the clinician, the client, and other clinicians or loved ones that the client wants to be included in decision-making. While evaluation of hormone or surgery eligibility and readiness technically does not involve a fully collaborative process as the client does not have latitude to negotiate the eligibility or readiness criteria, it is important to be flexible enough during the assessment to consider areas that may be open to negotiation and to discuss these with the client. For example, interpretation of what constitutes "real life experience" or "mental stability" may be negotiated and mutually agreed upon.

Qualifications of Hormone and Surgery Assessors

Most prescribing clinicians and surgeons require that the evaluation for hormone therapy or sex reassignment surgery be performed by an assessor who meets the competency requirements outlined in the WPATH *Standards of Care* (Meyer et al., 2001), including completion of specialized training and demonstrated competence in the assessment of sexual and gender identity disorders (e.g., certification by the American Association of Sex Therapists, Counselors and Therapists).

Prescribing clinicians with a practice structure that allows extended appointments and appropriate training in transgender medicine–including training in behavioral health and in the mental health aspects of gender dysphoria–may choose to take sole responsibility for initiating hormone therapy. In this situation, the prescribing clinician will conduct both physical screening (Dahl et al., 2006) and psychological screening to determine whether hormone therapy is appropriate. A mental health clinician may be asked to conduct an additional psychological assessment if a more detailed assessment or second opinion is desired.

Some insurance plans that provide coverage for sex reassignment surgery set requirements for evaluation beyond those in the WPATH

Standards of Care. If the client is considering surgery, determination of assessor credentials required by the third party payer is recommended as early in the process as possible. It can be devastating for clients who have completed a gender role transition, with or without hormone therapy, to be told years into the process that they do not qualify for coverage of surgery.

The "Gatekeeper" Role and Its Impact on Therapeutic Rapport

Clinicians conducting the assessment to determine eligibility and readiness of hormone therapy or surgery are in a "gatekeeper" role that involves a power dynamic which can significantly affect therapeutic rapport (Bockting et al., 2004; Rachlin, 2002). The client often perceives the evaluation not as a desired tool to help them therapeutically determine a plan of action, but rather as a hoop that must be jumped through to reach desired goals, a frightening loss of autonomy over one's body and life, or a type of institutionalized oppression or discrimination, as a mental health evaluation is not required for non-transgender individuals requesting hormones, breast augmentation, or hysterectomy (Brown & Rounsley, 1996).

The approach to building rapport during hormone and surgery assessment depends on the nature of the clinical relationship. Some clients come for evaluation having already made a clear decision supported by self-directed research about treatment options, substantial internal reflection, and in some cases peer or professional counseling; having already disclosed their transgender identity to loved ones, co-workers, or others; and having relatively good supports and overall stability. In these cases a relatively short evaluation may be feasible, and the strategies to build rapport will be different than in circumstances where a more prolonged relationship is required to determine whether hormonal or surgical treatment is appropriate.

If tension arises related to the assessor's role of gatekeeper to the desired medical interventions, it may be helpful to openly discuss this. Strategies used to manage client anxiety and anger and promote a collaborative relationship in mandated treatment settings can be useful (de Jong & Berg, 2001). Normalizing emotional reactions and behaviors clients commonly display–such as anger, anxiety, and fear; being belligerent, uncooperative, or manipulative; or telling the assessor what the client thinks they want to hear (Bolin, 1988)–helps frame this as a systems issue rather than a personal power struggle. Discussion about what the assessment process involves is imperative as the client's anxiety or anger is often heightened by inaccurate understanding of the process.

When the gatekeeper issue is posing a serious barrier to rapport in an ongoing psychotherapeutic relationship, it may be advisable to separate assessment from psychotherapy so two different clinicians are working with the same client (Anderson, 1997). The psychotherapist's role would then be to work with the client towards their stated goal of meeting hormone or surgery eligibility or readiness criteria, making it clear that there can be no guarantee of a particular outcome. The combined advocate-therapist role (Lev, 2004) can be particularly appropriate if a client needs to work on issues such as substance use, borderline personality disorder, or self harm, as there is often anxiety that a history of these concerns will be considered evidence that the client is not stable enough to proceed with hormones or surgery. Separating psychotherapeutic treatment of present issues from a future assessment can help reassure the client that assessment will focus on the adaptation they have achieved rather than on a history of instability or mental health concerns.

In our experience, clients who feel prepared for hormone or surgery evaluation are more willing to share information than clients who are highly anxious or fearful about the process. At minimum we recommend a letter explaining the assessment process (Appendices C and D) be sent well in advance of the appointment to the client and their primary care provider, both to ensure the parameters of assessment are understood and also to ensure that the client is aware of required supporting documentation.

Clinicians not involved in the assessment can assist by engaging in therapeutic discussion relating to any previous experience, such as anxiety related to having been denied support for hormone therapy or surgery in the past, and open discussion about the topics the client is most worried about. Some clinicians may feel hesitant to discuss terms of the hormone or surgery evaluation for fear they are "coaching" the client; however, asking the client how they might respond if they are asked questions about specific topics is different than coaching the client on how to answer questions about those topics.

Evaluating Eligibility

Informed consent. Informed consent requires the capacity to make decisions relating to medical care and an understanding of the specific treatment options that are proposed. Mental health clinicians are not expected to have detailed knowledge of the medical risks and benefits of specific hormones or surgical feminization or masculinization procedures–these will be discussed with the client by the prescribing physician or surgeon–but should be sufficiently knowledgeable to be able to assess whether the client has a generally accurate understanding of medical options, risks, and benefits. Clinician-reviewed consumer education materials developed by the Trans Care Project are available online (Ashbee & Goldberg, 2006a, 2006b; Simpson & Goldberg, 2006a, 2006b). Key issues are the irreversibility of some changes even if hormone therapy is discontinued and an appreciation that the long-term impact of hormone therapy on one's physical health is not fully known.

The mental health clinician should explore the client's awareness of possible psychosocial risks and benefits, including the possible impact of visible physical changes on existing relationships. In some cases hormone therapy or sex reassignment surgery improves the ability to pass as a non-transgender woman or man, reducing the risk of harassment and discrimination; in other cases the changes increase visibility as a transgender person, thus adding to the social risks. Awareness of these risks relates to informed consent; capacity to anticipate, withstand, and cope with the challenges posed is relevant in evaluating readiness.

"Real-life experience." The WPATH *Standards of Care* define the "real life experience" as the act of "fully adopting a new or evolving gender role or gender presentation in everyday life" (Meyer et al., 2001, p. 17), with the inten-

tion of achieving an experiential understanding of the familial, interpersonal, socioeconomic, and legal consequences of gender transition. The "real life experience" is a way for the transgender person who wishes to permanently change gender roles to move from an imagined experience to a lived experience. For some individuals this experience is liberating and exhilarating; for others there is disappointment that the real experience does not live up to a fantasized ideal.

A fundamental premise of the "real life experience" is that the person should experience life in the desired role before making irreversible physical changes. The WPATH *Standards of Care* do not require a "real life experience" prior to hormone therapy, breast surgery, or chest surgery, but do include a minimum of one year of "real life experience" as an eligibility criterion for genital reconstructive surgery or gonadal removal (Meyer et al., 2001). The WPATH *Standards* explicitly state that the "real life experience" is not a diagnostic test to evaluate the severity or nature of the gender identity concerns, but that the process tests "the person's resolve, the capacity to function in the preferred gender, and the adequacy of social, economic, and psychological supports" (Meyer et al., 2001, p. 18). For FTM transsexuals it is often difficult to live in the desired role without first undergoing chest surgery, hence a real life experience is not required for such surgery.

It is important to note that the "real life experience" is not defined by adherence to stereotypical ideas of masculinity or femininity. Just as there is a range of gender expression among non-transgender women–with many choosing not to wear makeup, dresses, or otherwise displaying attributes conventionally considered feminine–transgender women also have a range of gender expression. Similarly, not all transgender men are masculine in appearance or behavior. The real life experience is not defined by ability to pass as a non-transgender woman or man. Rather, it is defined by actualizing and continuously expressing one's unique gender identity.

Too often the "real life experience" is perceived by the client only in terms of an eligibility criterion that must be met to gain access to surgery, with the client feeling pressure to demonstrate uncritical adoption of a stereotypical

feminine or masculine role. From a therapeutic perspective, the "real life experience" is a time of adjustment, exploration, and experimentation, learning how to relate to oneself and to others as the previously hidden self emerges. Psychotherapy is not an absolute requirement during this process, but it can be a valuable support during a time of profound internal and external change. Some assessors prefer to see the client periodically throughout the "real life experience" to try to get a sense of how the client is progressing and to offer support to those who are having difficulty. If the clinician or client feels that the assessor's role as gatekeeper prevents frank discussion of challenges, disappointments, and surprises during the "real life experience," involvement of a peer or external professional counselor may be useful in providing a space for the client to discuss problems or concerns without fear that access to surgery will be delayed or blocked.

In evaluating completion of the required "real life experience," the WPATH *Standards of Care* suggest a review of involvement in the community via work, volunteering, student activity, or a combination of all three; the acquisition of a name that conforms to a person's gender identity; and evidence that individuals other than the mental health professional know the patient in the desired gender role (Meyer et al., 2001). Flexibility in interpreting the "real life experience" is needed for clients who are housebound, living in a prison or residential long-term care facility, or who are otherwise unable to work, volunteer, or attend school. Additionally, we encourage a broad understanding of "work" that validates the life experience of those who are caregivers or parents, sex trade workers, and others who may not be able to provide documentation of employment. Ideally, the means of validating this aspect of transition will be at the discretion of the clinician who is performing the evaluation. Some insurance plans that cover the cost of surgery require specific documentation and may have "real life experience" criteria beyond the WPATH *Standards*.

Assessing Readiness

As discussed earlier, *readiness* relates to stability of gender identity and also the psychological stability needed to cope with the physical, emotional, and social consequences of the decision to undergo hormone therapy and/or sex reassignment surgery. To assess readiness it is important to determine what the consequences of the treatment will likely be based on the individual circumstances of the client, including awareness and preparedness to cope with the potential challenges.

While some degree of ambivalence and uncertainty is to be expected with any life-changing process, the client should have a clear sense of the gendered self prior to initiating hormones or surgery. Physical change is not appropriate for clients who are just beginning to explore their identity or options for gender expression. While it is not necessary for transgender feelings or gender dysphoria to have existed since childhood, a longer period of assessment is required if the dysphoria is newly discovered, episodic, or possibly transient.

As per Figure 1, delusions about sex or gender, dissociative disorders, thought disorders, or obsessive or compulsive features should be evaluated and treated prior to proceeding with hormone therapy or surgery. Thought disorders, dissociative disorders, and obsessive-compulsive disorders can, rarely, cause a transient wish for sex reassignment which disappears or significantly lessens when the underlying mental health condition is treated. It is important to treat these disorders before proceeding with hormones or surgery to ensure that the desire for alteration of primary or secondary sex characteristics is not a temporary desire.

Other mental health concerns, psychosocial concerns, or substance use are not absolute contraindications to sex reassignment. Sometimes these issues are a direct result of the gender dysphoria or suppressed transgender feelings and alleviate or remit entirely as the gender identity concerns are addressed. However, the clinician should be confident that supports are adequate and that any co-existing conditions are under control to the degree that (a) the introduction of a new stressor will not seriously destabilize the client, and (b) the client has sufficiently clear thinking to be competent to consent to treatment (Brown & Rounsley, 1996). If there are any questions about competency or substance use, a formal evaluation may be required.

If the client returns for hormone or surgery assessment long after the initial evaluation, it may be necessary to repeat some of the standardized psychological testing administered during the initial evaluation to determine progress. Improvement in mental health and psychosocial adjustment should be documented and the care plan for addressing these concerns updated.

Evaluation of hormone or surgery readiness should include the gender assessment described earlier to explore issues relating to stability of gender identity and appropriateness of hormones or surgery. Table 6 lists additional areas of inquiry specific to evaluating readiness to start hormone therapy or undergo sex reassignment surgery.

Recommendation Regarding Treatment

If the assessor judges the client to be an appropriate candidate for hormone therapy or sex reassignment surgery, a letter of recommendation should be written to the prescribing clinician or surgeon confirming eligibility and readiness as per the WPATH *Standards of Care* (Meyer et al., 2001). Sample letters are included as Appendices E and F. As outlined in the WPATH *Standards*, these letters should include (a) the client's general identifying characteristics, (b) explanation of the duration of professional relationship, including type of evaluation and/or therapy, (c) initial diagnoses relating to gender identity issues or any other concerns, (d) the rationale for hormones or surgery (why it is appropriate treatment), (e) evaluation of the client's eligibility and readiness for hormones or surgery, (f) the degree to which the client and mental health professional have followed the WPATH *Standards of Care*, and the likelihood that this will continue, (g) explanation of the clinician's relationship to others involved in the client's care, and (h) a statement that the clinician welcomes a phone call to verify any of the information in the letter.

If the assessor feels the treatment is generally appropriate but the client does not meet eligibility or readiness criteria, the reasons for this should be explained to the client and a timeline established for reassessment. If the client is consistently cross-living and just needs more time to complete the required "real life experi-

TABLE 6. Potential Areas of Inquiry: Hormonal or Surgical Evaluation

Topic	Questions
General readiness	What leads you to come for hormonal or surgical assessment at this time in your life? What are your hopes and dreams relating to hormones or surgery? What do you expect hormones or surgery to change, and what do you think is not likely to change? How do you think hormones or surgery may affect your relationships with loved ones, and how do you think they will impact you at work, at school, or in the broader community? What will you do if the hormonal or surgical change process doesn't turn out as you had hoped? Have you taken any other steps to change your outward appearance, and if so, what was that like for you? Are there any issues in your life that you think might complicate a decision to take hormones or have surgery, or that might increase stress during this time? What kinds of supports do you feel might be helpful before or during hormonal therapy, or before and after surgery?
Hormones	Which changes are you most looking forward to from hormone therapy? Are there any changes from hormone therapy that you are not sure about? What medical care do you need to monitor for side effects, and who will provide this? If you experience side effects as a result of hormone therapy, what will you do? Are there any side effects of hormones that you are particularly concerned about? How do you feel about the permanence of some effects of hormone therapy, including the possibility of permanent sterility? The long-term effects of cross-sex hormones are not yet clear; how do you feel about taking this risk?
Sex reassignment surgery	What medical care might you need following surgery, and how will you obtain this care? Where will you rest and heal after surgery? Are there people who can help look after you as you recover following surgery? How do you feel about the permanence of surgery? How do you feel about the possibility of scarring? How do you feel about the risk of possible change in sensation, including the possibility of loss of sexual sensation or ability to achieve orgasm? Even when surgery is wanted there is sometimes a sense of loss, as with any big change; how do you feel about the changes to your body, and how have you dealt with other losses in your life? What additional issues or adjustments do you anticipate after surgery?

ence," the reassessment plan is straightforward; if the client is not consistently cross-living, psychotherapeutic interventions may be necessary to explore reasons for this and to assist the client to gain the support needed to be able to live full-time in the desired role. In some cases, referral to a transgender-sensitive financial planner or advocate may be helpful in identifying economic resources for the costs of transition. If there are psychosocial readiness concerns, resources should be identified to help the client move toward psychological and social stability, with specific and measurable goals established. Denial of access to desired treatment can be highly disappointing and it is important to emphasize that reassessment is believed to be appropriate, and to ensure that clients are aware of peer and professional supports in the interim.

In some cases, the assessor may feel that hormonal or surgical feminization or masculinization is not an appropriate treatment and that future reassessment of eligibility and readiness is not indicated. This may be the case if a client is seeking hormones or surgery for reasons other than gender dysphoria, where another type of assessment is more appropriate (e.g., a male without gender dysphoria seeking hormonal or surgical castration to reduce sexual urges). If the prescribing physician or surgeon has informed the client that their physical health is too fragile to ever proceed, or a client is judged to be incompetent to make medical decisions and the cause for diminished competency is not likely to change, the client should be supported to come to terms with this and to explore alternative forms of transgender expression rather than false hope being held out of eventual reassignment.

Counseling of Loved Ones

Significant others, family members, friends, or allies of transgender persons (SOFFAs) typically come to therapy to address their own concerns relating to a loved one's disclosure of being transgender or the impact of transgender issues on their relationships over time. Alternatively, SOFFAs may participate in family or relationship therapy as part of a transgender person's therapeutic process.

As with the transgender population, SOFFAs are a heterogeneous group. Some SOFFAs are encouraging and supportive, and may take a strong stand in helping counter the shame and embarrassment that many transgender individuals feel. For others, transgender issues are a source of conflict. Evaluation of the SOFFA who presents for individual counseling includes discussion of the nature of their relationship to the transgender person, the impact of gender issues on this relationship and on the relationships with others, and awareness of available support resources (see Table 7).

Some SOFFAs may have always known or suspected that their loved one is transgender. More typically, SOFFAs are shocked and surprised. Responses upon disclosure range from acceptance to disgust, depending on the individual's frame of reference, their relationship with the transgender person, cultural beliefs about gender variance, and the timing and means of disclosure. When transgender issues have been a secret and are disclosed late in a relationship, there can be feelings of betrayal and questioning of intimacy, as with the disclosure of any large secret (Reynolds & Caron, 2000). Adjustment also varies depending on the degree of change requested in a specific aspect of the relationship. For example, disclosure relating to the hope that a partner will participate in erotic crossdressing is different than disclosure that will affect the entire relationship, such as a gender transition.

Ellis and Eriksen (2002) describe an emotional process for SOFFAs similar to stages of bereavement (Kübler-Ross, 1969). Stage 1 may include denial, shock (Lantz, 1999), post-traumatic reactions (Cole, Denny, Eyler, & Samons, 2000), and trying to bargain with the transgender person or a higher power for the gender issues to disappear (Covin, 1999). Stage 2 may include anger at the transgender person (Lantz, 1999), fear of others' reactions (Bullough & Weinberg, 1988; Reynolds & Caron, 2000), and fear about how the transgender person will be treated (Samson, 1999). Parents may blame themselves, assuming their child is transgender because of a failure in parenting (Lantz, 1999). At this stage sexual dysfunction may occur in the relationship between the transgender client and their partner (Cole et al., 2000). Counseling may be helpful at this stage to help restore intimacy and reduce isolation. During Stage 3, family and loved ones are able to start to grieve the losses on many levels, and may seek support from others who are in similar situations. Peer support or social contact with other SOFFAs can be helpful at this stage (Weinberg & Bullough, 1988). Stage 4 involves self-discovery and change. SOFFAs may not agree on the

TABLE 7. Potential Areas of Inquiry in Gender Evaluation: Loved One of a Transgender Person

Topic	Questions
Disclosure	When did you learn that your (partner, child, sibling, etc.) was transgender? How did you find out that your (partner, child, sibling, etc.) was transgender? What was your initial reaction to finding out about your loved one's feelings, and how do you feel about it now? Do individuals in your life know that your (partner, child, sibling, etc.) is transgender, and how do you feel about them knowing/not knowing?
Impact on relationships	It is common for loved ones to have fears and questions about gender issues, and question their relationship to the transgender person or their own identity (including sexual orientation); are any of these concerns for you? Have you ever seen your (partner, child, sibling, etc.) crossdressed, and if so, how was that for you? Has your (partner, child, sibling, etc.) ever taken hormones or had surgery to bring their body closer to their sense of self, or is this something they are considering; if so, how do you feel about this? How have transgender issues affected your relationships with others (e.g., other family members, friends)? Do you worry about how others might react when they learn that your loved one is transgender?
Support resources	Have you had any contact with other (partners, parents, siblings, children, etc.) of transgender people, and if so, what was that like for you? What do you see your relationship being to the transgender community now, and what would you like it to be in the future?

changes the transgender individual is making and counselors can be helpful in conflict resolution. At this stage, couples may decide whether to stay together. Stage 5 is a time for acceptance and welcoming the transgender person into daily life. At this point, the SOFFA often joins the journey of the transgender person, including the adjustments that must be made. Counselors may help by providing a place to process the anger and frustration that arises as a result of discrimination and harassment directly experienced or witnessed by the SOFFA. Finally, the goal of stage 6 is pride in their loved one's courage. This pride may take the form of advocating for transgender people and educating others about them (Lantz, 1999).

TRANSGENDER-SPECIFIC ASSESSMENT AND TREATMENT OF MENTAL HEALTH ISSUES

Although studies are limited, one team of researchers found that a large group of transgender individuals (N = 435) who sought services from a gender clinic did not appear to have increased rates of major psychiatric illness (operationally defined as disruption in mood or personality that affected life, work, and relationships in identifiable ways) compared to the general population (Cole, O'Boyle, Emory, & Meyer, III, 1997). However, the impact of psychosocial stressors, including harassment, discrimination, and violence experienced by many transgender individuals (Lombardi, Wilchins, Priesing, & Malouf, 2001), as well as the high incidence of poverty resulting from employment discrimination (Nemoto, Operario, Keatley, & Villegas, 2004), are cause for concern. In a study of 515 transgender individuals in San Francisco, 62% of MTF and 55% of FTM respondents met clinical criteria for depression, 22% of MTFs and 20% of FTMs reported a history of mental health hospitalization, and 32% of MTFs and 32% of FTMs reported prior suicide attempts (Clements-Nolle, Katz, & Marx, 1999). As a medically underserved population (Feldman & Bockting, 2003), transgender individuals with mental health concerns are at risk for late diagnosis and treatment. Those undergoing a gender transition may avoid disclosing symptoms of mental illness for fear that this will jeopardize access to hormone therapy or surgery, further delaying treatment.

The presence of apparent mental health symptoms in initial sessions does not necessarily indicate chronic mental health issues. Transgender people who are seeking help for gender identity concerns are often anxious or defensive about seeing a mental health professional. Moreover, establishment of a trusting relationship with a trans-positive, supportive clinician can result in release of longstanding suppressed emotions and feelings of powerlessness related to past experiences of neglect or mistreatment, with the potential for transference of anger. Lack of language to articulate gender identity concerns can lead the transgender individual to appear confused, disoriented, temporarily unable to communicate, profoundly frustrated, or labile. Nevertheless, evidence of mental health symptoms should not be ignored. Even when mental health symptoms are the sequelae of social stigma or oppression, relief of these symptoms may help give the client the stability and resilience needed to engage in psychotherapeutic healing. Careful evaluation is required. Regardless of the reason for the mental distress, the transgender client deserves appropriate mental health care to alleviate these symptoms and treat any existing mental disorders.

In our experience, in the overwhelming majority of cases mental health symptoms have psychosocial causes. Rarely, there may be a physiological component. As per the standard diagnostic process outlined in the *DSM-IV-TR*, there should be consideration of possible pharmacologic or medical factors as part of the standardized mental health interview for any client with acute mental health symptoms. There are rare case reports of psychosis in transsexual women related to sudden cessation of estrogen therapy (Faulk, 1990; Mallett, Marshall, & Blacker, 1989), and observations of depressive mood changes related to initiation of estrogen or progesterone therapy (Asscheman, Gooren, & Eklund, 1989; Feldman & Bockting, 2003; Flaherty et al., 2001; Israel & Tarver, 1997; Steinbeck, 1997). Psychiatric decompensation has been observed in some FTM clients with pre-existing Schizoaffective Disorder, Bipolar Disorder, and Schizophrenia upon initiation of testosterone therapy (Feldman, 2005). Additionally, as a medically underserved population, transgender individuals can present with untreated physical conditions that may have psychological symptoms, including HIV and syphilis.

After a thorough evaluation and history, the clinician should offer a diagnostic opinion based on the multi-axial system of the *DSM-IV-TR* (American Psychiatric Association, 2000) and a diagnostic formulation. During initial evaluation any psychiatric diagnosis should be considered tentative, to be confirmed during the course of treatment. This is particularly true for personality disorders or other complex conditions that usually take more time to assess than the initial diagnostic evaluation allows.

Treatment options may include psychotherapeutic techniques such as cognitive-behavioral therapy, dialectical behavior therapy, and eye movement desensitization and reprocessing; pharmacotherapy; and social or advocacy interventions. If the client intends to start or stop hormones while undergoing pharmacologic treatment for mental health concerns, medication may need to be re-evaluated as part of this process. Potential interactions between hormones and psychoactive medications should be carefully evaluated by the prescribing physician, and regular visits scheduled to monitor the risk of psychological decompensation (Dahl et al., 2006).

In some cases, referral to other clinicians may be needed for pharmacologic treatment or to overcome socioeconomic barriers to treatment. When multiple clinicians are involved, close communication is required to ensure coordinated care. Ideally, all clinicians involved in care of a transgender client will have transgender-specific training. If no practitioners with transgender health expertise are available, the client should be informed of this. In some cases clients may feel they or an advocate can sufficiently educate the practitioner about transgender issues, while in other cases a clinician with transgender-specific training will be needed to effectively treat the client's concerns.

In determining a care plan, the presenting complaint of the client is the starting point. When there are multiple co-existing mental health concerns, a staged approach is recommended that begins with the issues that most negatively impact the client's quality of life and/or ability to engage in treatment. The client should be meaningfully involved in creating the treatment plan, and goals and expectations of treatment should be clear. While the client is ultimately responsible for deciding among the available treatment options, the clinician is expected to provide an informed clinical opinion and recommendations as part of care planning. Recommendations may include type of treatment, anticipated duration of treatment, timeline and criteria for re-evaluation, and involvement of peer or additional professional resources. Ideally, mental health care plans will be developed in coordination with the client's primary care provider and any other clinicians involved in the client's care. The timeline of the overall treatment plan should be explicitly discussed, jointly agreed upon, and reviewed on a regular basis. For some clients, it is better to discuss goals in terms of tasks rather than time, or at least the timeframe should be tentative. Progress in meeting the goals of the care plan should be reviewed regularly during the course of treatment; adjustments may have to be made.

Some transgender individuals have sophisticated knowledge about mental health treatment options, and have a clear direction they wish to pursue. Others have no knowledge and expect guidance from a professional. As part of care planning it is important to assess the individual's knowledge and the accuracy of their information, and to offer consumer education materials discussing treatment options if needed. In all cases, the clinician is responsible to ensure that clients understand what is involved in specific types of treatment.

Depression, Anxiety, and Suicidality

Depression and suicidality are not uncommon among transgender individuals. Among 181 transgender seminar participants at the University of Minnesota, 52% reported depression and 47% had considered or attempted suicide in the last three years (Bockting, Huang, Ding, Robinson, & Rosser, 2005). A comparison of psychosocially matched transgender and non-transgender individuals found that transgender individuals reported significantly more suicidal ideation and attempts (Mathy, 2002).

Depression and anxiety may be directly related to gender issues. For example, a long history of suppression of transgender feelings may have resulted in isolation, loneliness, and feelings of hopelessness; the fear of disclosing this secret to partners, family, friends, and coworkers–risking rejection and employment discrimination–can provoke a great deal of anxiety. In other cases, however, depression and anxiety may be unrelated to gender issues and may simply be a result of a predisposition to these symptoms or a result of other life experiences such as childhood neglect, death of a loved one, or relationship violence. Whatever the etiology, the goal is to alleviate the symptoms, address situational issues that create or contribute to the depression or anxiety, and build resilience (Israel & Tarver, 1997). Such resilience is particularly important as life as a transgender person may be highly stressful due to the prevailing social stigma. If psychoactive medication is part of the treatment plan, continued use should be re-evaluated as psychotherapeutic or other treatment progresses.

Self-Harm

Self-harm refers to intentional head-banging, cutting, burning, self-poisoning, car crash, or other behavior likely to cause injury, and may or may not be accompanied by suicidality. Self-harm may be a ritualized, chronic behavior used to self-regulate hyperarousal, dissociative states, or otherwise uncontrollable stress (Sachsse, Von der Heyde, & Huether, 2002), or an attempt to channel emotional futility, despair, and hopelessness into visible physical form (Israel & Tarver, 1997).

The prevalence of self-harm among transgender individuals is not known. A therapist who specializes in transgender care at a health centre in Toronto described seeing numerous transgender clients seeking care for self-injurious behaviors (Gapka & Raj, 2003). Deliberate damage to the testicles or penis by gender dysphoric MTF transsexuals has been described in a number of published case reports (Martin & Gattaz, 1991; McGovern, 1995; Mellon, Barlow, Cook, & Clark, 1989; Murphy, Murphy, & Grainger, 2001), and may reflect despair, lack of awareness of options for medical intervention, lack of access to transgender-specific and competent care, or ineligibility for desired surgery. Impulsively attempted auto-castration, auto-penectomy, or auto-mastectomy may be

followed by contrition, shame, and fear of ridicule or institutionalization for having committed a self-destructive act (Israel & Tarver, 1997).

No-harm agreements are commonly used in clinical practice where there are concerns about the risk for self-injurious behavior. A verbal or written no-harm agreement should not be considered a substitute for careful clinical assessment, and should not be relied upon as the sole tool for prevention of further attempts (American Psychiatric Association, 2003). In any instance of self-harm, medical treatment of injuries should take priority. Mental health treatment focuses on reducing further harm by detecting and treating underlying mental health problems (e.g., underlying Axis I or II disorder), reducing distress–including distress about having engaged in self-injurious behavior–and strengthening coping skills and resources (Boyce, Carter, Penrose-Wall, Wilhelm, & Goldney, 2003). There is no evidence regarding optimal treatment for transgender individuals who are chronically self-harming, but in our clinical experience, dialectical behavior therapy has been helpful. This treatment modality has been shown to reduce self-harm in chronically suicidal non-transgender women diagnosed with Borderline Personality Disorder (Linehan, Armstrong, Suarez, Allmon, & Heard, 1991).

Compulsivity

Compulsive crossdressing or obsessive/compulsive features of gender dysphoria–whether secondary to an anxiety or mood disorder or, as is more commonly the case, simply associated with suppression, shame, and anxiety about transgender feelings–can often be alleviated through psychotherapy. If necessary, pharmacotherapy (e.g., Selective Serotonin Re-uptake Inhibitors) may also be employed in conjunction with psychotherapy.

Psychotherapy focuses on identifying the pattern of obsessive/compulsive behaviors that developed over time and on changing this pattern through defining and adhering to boundaries that prevent self-destructive behaviors (see case vignette of Carlos in Appendix A). In addition, therapy aims to decrease isolation, alleviate shame and self-hatred, and confront internalized transphobia. Alternative, more constructive ways of expressing or validating one's transgender feelings are explored.

Thought Disorders

Schizophrenia, Schizo-affective Disorder, and other thought disorders should be treated as per standard protocols. For clients with co-existing gender dysphoria and delusional disorders, it is critical to manage the thought disorder through medications and support, monitor the client's identity over time, encourage experience in the preferred gender role, and require an extended period of stability prior to initiating medical interventions. Coordination with all the other health providers that work with the client—and, with the client's consent, inclusion of caregivers, family, and friends in therapy—can create a strong support system to facilitate an eventual gender transition if that is the direction chosen by the client. If well controlled, a thought disorder is not necessarily a contraindication for sex reassignment. Addressing gender dysphoria as part of a comprehensive care plan has the potential of rehabilitating a client with schizophrenia to a level that previously seemed out of reach (see case vignette of Jamie in Appendix A).

Personality Disorders

Personality disorders may be found among transgender clients (Bodlund, Kullgren, Sundbom, & Höjerback, 1993) and can be challenging to treat. Personality disorders may be unrelated to gender issues, or may seem to be linked to transgender concerns. Little is known about a possible relationship between the development of personality disorders and gender identity concerns; we offer the following speculative theoretical formulation derived from clinical observation.

Growing up transgender in a society that does not understand or accept gender-variance can be a challenge to the development of a coherent and confident sense of self. In children with transgender feelings who are also visibly gender-role-nonconforming, an early transgender "coming out" involves learning to cope with social stigma; possible rejection, harassment, ridicule, and abuse by age-peers and/or family; and an ensuing sense of shame and low

self esteem—all of which could potentially contribute to the development of a personality disorder. In children with transgender feelings who are not visibly gender-variant, the response to social stigma and pressure to conform is more likely to lead to suppression of crossgender feelings and dissociation. This can lead to a "split" identity of a "false" self presented to the world that overcompensates or conforms to the expectations associated with the sex assigned at birth, and a hidden "true" self that is compartmentalized and may be expressed in imagination, fantasy, and emerging sexuality that may be of a paraphilic or compulsive nature. In this scenario, mirroring by the social environment of the "false" instead of the "true" self may play a role in the development of psychological difficulties in identity and attachment (Fraser, 2005).

Whatever the etiology, management of personality disorders needs to be part of the treatment plan. A variety of psychotherapeutic techniques such as rational emotive therapy, cognitive behavior therapy, or dialectical behavior therapy can be applied, possibly in combination with pharmacotherapy. Selective Serotonin Reuptake Inhibitors have been used to treat clients with compulsive behaviors, and atypical antipsychotics have been used with success for clients with impulse control problems. If gender identity concerns co-exist, treatment of the gender concerns, potentially including a gender role transition, often aids in lessening symptoms of personality disorders.

If well managed, personality disorders are not a contraindication for a gender role transition, hormones, or surgery. However, any issues of concern should be discussed with the client, with clear goals for treatment and stabilization.

TRANSGENDER-SPECIFIC ELEMENTS IN GENERAL COUNSELING

Transgender individuals experience the same general life problems as everyone else, and may seek counseling for assistance with general life stressors. Although gender identity concerns may not be a factor, social stigma, internalized transphobia, and untreated gender dysphoria can have a significant impact on a transgender client's general psychosocial development, resilience, and functioning. Common transgender psychosocial concerns outlined below include body image problems, multiple losses resulting in cumulative grief, sexual concerns, social isolation and resultant social skill deficits, spiritual or religious concerns, substance use issues, and difficulty coping with historical or current violence or abuse. While employment dissatisfaction, discrimination, and loss of employment are also common, vocational counseling is a specialized area outside the scope of this article; issues relating to employment discrimination and transition planning in the workplace are discussed elsewhere in this volume (White Holman & Goldberg, 2006b).

For transgender individuals who seek general counseling, areas to explore in the initial evaluation may include any of the questions outlined in the previous sections. Questions depend in large part on the client's chief presenting concern. For example, if the presenting concern is grief relating to the recent death of a loved one, it is not appropriate to include detailed questions about gender history in the initial interview. If the client does not indicate whether transgender issues are relevant to the presenting concern, the clinician can ask about transgender issues with appropriate framing (e.g., "For some transgender people, being transgender affects their relationships–is this an issue for you?").

Body Image

The cultural norms of femininity and masculinity include strong cultural messages about what "real" men and "real" women should look like as well as norms relating to attractiveness. Some transgender individuals have difficulty accepting their bodies regardless of gender dysphoria, although gender dysphoria obviously complicates this picture. Weight gain associated with estrogen or testosterone can be distressing and can be a health risk in some cases.

Eating disorders can appear in both MTF and FTM transgender individuals (Fernández-Aranda et al., 2000; Hepp & Milos, 2002; Surgenor & Fear, 1998; Winston, Acharya, Chaudhuri, & Fellowes, 2004). Eating disor-

ders may originate in attempts to conform with societal conventions relating to thinness, may relate to a feeling of estrangement from the body (Gapka & Raj, 2003), or may be unrelated to body image per se (but rather may develop as a type of compulsive behavior to provide relief from stress). The published case reports cited above suggest that MTF transgender individuals typically struggle with anorexia, bulimia, or other disordered eating more typically seen in girls and women, while FTM transsexuals more often struggle with a drive to be muscular as typically seen in men with body image problems. However, FTM transgender individuals may also seek to minimize hips and breasts by excess exercising or disordered eating, or prevent menstruation by staying underweight. FTM transgender individuals who are attracted to other men may be particularly vulnerable to struggles with body image in an attempt to conform to the overemphasis on norms of appearance, weight, and muscularity in some gay communities (Williamson & Hartley, 1998; Yelland & Tiggemann, 2003).

Surgical procedures intended to alter primary or secondary sex characteristics can reduce gender dysphoria and are not intrinsically problematic; indeed, they are an important part of medical treatment for some transgender individuals. However, other transgender individuals desperately pursue cosmetic procedures in an attempt to erase any perceived sign of their birth sex or of being transgender (see case study of Anne in Appendix A) or to alleviate body image concerns. The clinician should focus on the underlying internalized transphobia or other psychological issues (e.g., anxiety and fears, isolation and loneliness, low self esteem, body image distortions or Body Dysmorphic Disorder, possible personality disorder) rather than focus on the cosmetic procedures themselves.

Following sex reassignment surgery, there may be body image concerns related to visible scarring or surgical results that do not fit the client's hopes and expectations in terms of aesthetic outcome. The clinician should distinguish between surgical complications, normal adjustment, and excessive preoccupation with the physical results.

Grief and Loss

Grief and loss can appear at many levels. Transgender individuals may experience multiple losses when they disclose that they are transgender, including loss of work as well as rejection by family, friends, and ethnocultural or faith community. This may be especially painful for transgender individuals who have high value for familial and cultural continuity.

On a developmental level, there can be a feeling of loss associated with aspects of physical and social experiences associated with sex or gender that are not possible even with transition. For example, some MTF transsexuals grieve the inability to menstruate, become pregnant and give birth (De Sutter, Kira, Verschoor, & Hotimsky, 2002); some FTM transsexuals grieve their inability to impregnate a partner. Some transgender individuals seek to create gendered rites of passage typically associated with adolescence to mark emergence as women or men (Cameron, 1996), or approach aspects of gender transition as a rite of passage into womanhood or manhood (Bolin, 1988; Fleming & Feinbloom, 1984).

Hormonal and surgical sex reassignment procedures can reduce fertility and lead to permanent sterility. Regrets and grief relating to sterility were noted in one study of transsexual women who had already undergone hormonal treatment (De Sutter et al., 2002). Discussion of reproductive impacts and options such as sperm banking for MtF transsexuals is advised in the WPATH *Standards of Care* as part of the informed consent process prior to hormonal or surgical intervention (Meyer et al., 2001). In some cases reproductive counseling may be advised.

As discussed earlier, even when surgical feminization or masculinization is highly desired there can be grief following surgery. Doubt, dissatisfaction, or regret immediately after surgery may relate to physical issues such as post-operative pain, surgical complications, or changes to sexual function; disappointment with the results; or stress caused by disclosure to loved ones (Lawrence, 2003; Michel, Ansseau, Legros, Pitchot, & Mormont, 2002). These type of regrets are typically temporary and resolve spontaneously or with psychotherapeutic assistance (Pfäfflin, 1992), and do not necessarily

signify regret about having made the transition. A review of 82 outcome studies published between 1961 and 1991 found that gender dysphoria in the new gender role accompanied by attempts at reversal of surgery or role change was less than 1% among FTM transsexuals and less than 1.0-1.5% among MTF transsexuals (Pfäfflin & Junge, 1992/1998). In most cases, regret resulted from improper differential diagnosis and treatment of co-existing mental health concerns, failure to complete the "real life experience," and unsatisfactory surgical results.

Sexual Concerns

As in the general population, there is a range of sexual identification, practices, and concerns among transgender individuals (Bockting, Robinson, Forberg, & Scheltema, 2005; Coleman, Bockting, & Gooren, 1993; Devor, 1993; Lawrence, 2005). Trans-specific sexual concerns may include managing gender dysphoria in a sexual relationship; concerns relating to erotic crossdressing; shifts in sexual orientation or sexual preferences as part of gender exploration or gender transition; and the impact of hormonal or surgical feminization or masculinization on sexual desire, sexual functioning, and safer sex negotiation.

Frank discussion of sexuality is comfortable for some transgender individuals, and not for others. Transgender individuals are often asked invasive and inappropriate questions by strangers or health professionals relating to genitals or sexual practices (O'Brien, 2003), and may be wary of the therapist's motivations if explicit questions are asked. Discomfort discussing sexuality in a therapeutic relationship may or may not extend to discomfort communicating about sex in an intimate relationship. In addition to feelings of embarrassment and shame commonly associated with sexuality, transgender individuals may have extra difficulty discussing sexual issues because of the dysphoria associated with their genitals and body, and with sexual roles associated with gender. Therefore, many transgender clients can benefit from exploring strategies for disclosure of identity, sexual negotiation, and setting boundaries regarding touch and sexual activity. Psychotherapeutic strategies proven effective for victims of sexual abuse may be useful in addressing anxiety or dissociation that some transgender clients may experience during sex.

In a therapeutic relationship and in intimate relationships, communication about transgender sexuality is made more difficult by the paucity of sexual language that is respectful and inclusive of the sexual experiences of transgender individuals and their partners. O'Brien (2003) describes this as "assumptions about bodies, genders, and genitals that simply do not speak to the real bodies that some transgender people live with, or the specific ways a transgender person might understand and describe their body" (p. 2). For example, an MTF transsexual who is married to a woman, transitioned late in life, and who has had little contact with the lesbian community may or may not describe her relationship as a lesbian one. Transgender individuals may also conceptualize their genitals in ways that fit their sense of self, with FtM transgender individuals using language such as a phantom penis, dicklit, or phalloclit rather than clitoris to refer to their genitals (Bockting, 2003; Kotula, 2002; O'Brien, 2003). For some transgender clients, discomfort discussing sexual issues in the therapy environment is due to difficulty finding appropriate language to refer to body parts that do not match their gender identity. In these cases, it may be helpful to normalize the discomfort and to spend time exploring language that feels comfortable to the client (Bockting, Robinson, et al., 2005).

Assumptions should not be made about sexual activities. While some transgender individuals are strongly dysphoric about their genitals and do not like them to be touched or looked at, others are comfortable using their genitals. For example, some FTM transsexuals may engage in receptive vaginal intercourse with other men (Coleman et al., 1993). Like non-transgender people, both MTF and FTM transgender individuals may engage in a wide variety of sexual behaviors, including erotic touch; receptive or insertive oral, vaginal, and anal penetration; and role-playing. Some transgender individuals identify as asexual and/or choose to be celibate.

Despite the challenges in talking about sex and the great need for sensitivity in approach, it is important for therapists to inquire about sexual issues in working with transgender clients.

Unaddressed sexual concerns can significantly impact quality of life. This is most obvious in case of sexual trauma or sexually transmitted infections, but more generally, sexual concerns can negatively impact self esteem and identity development. For example, an FTM transsexual who likes vaginal penetration may doubt his masculinity, as might a man who likes to have sex while crossdressed. Conversely, gender identity concerns can negatively impact sexual health. For example, attempts to affirm one's gender identity can drive drive high-risk sexual behaviors (Bockting, Robinson, & Rosser, 1998; Clements-Nolle et al., 1999; Nemoto, Operario, Keatley et al., 2004; Nuttbrock, Rosenblum, & Blumenstein, 2002).

No surveillance data are available to accurately enumerate the prevalence of HIV and other sexually transmitted infections (STI) among transgender people. However, needs assessment studies indicate that HIV/STI prevalence is high, particularly among transgender individuals who have sex with men (Bockting & Avery, 2005). For example, in a study of 392 MTF and 123 FTM transgender individuals in San Francisco, 35% of MTFs and 2% of FTMs tested positive for HIV, and 53% of MTFs and 31% of FTMs had been diagnosed with an STI (Clements-Nolle et al., 1999); among respondents in a New York survey, 36% of MTFs and 36% of FTMs indicated having had an STI (McGowan, 1999). Cofactors related to unsafe sex, such as low self-esteem, depression, suicidal ideation, substance use before sex, and physical or sexual abuse, are increased among the transgender population (Clements-Nolle et al., 2001; Keatley, Nemoto, Operario, & Soma, 2002; Kenagy, 2002; Mathy, 2002; Nemoto, Sugano, Operario, & Keatley, 2004). To promote safer sex, transgender individuals are in need of psychoeducational interventions to promote sexual health (Bockting et al., 2005; Nemoto, Sugano, Operario, & Keatley, 2004).

As discussed previously, changes relating to gender transition commonly impact sexuality, and psychotherapeutic assistance may be required to adjust to changes in sexual desire and function resulting from feminizing or masculinizing hormones or surgery. Additionally, gender transition can be accompanied by shifts in sexual orientation (Daskalos, 1998; Lawrence, 2005). For example, an MTF transgender person who has been primarily attracted to women prior to transition may experience attraction and pursue relationships with men following transition. Adjustment to these changes often involves developmental tasks similar to those in adolescence (Bockting & Coleman, in press). In other cases, the client's attractions remain consistent throughout transition but the gender role transition may involve change in sexual orientation identity (e.g., an FTM transgender person who loses a previously held lesbian identity).

Crossdressing for sexual excitement is a relatively common phenomenon. In a random sample of 18- to 60-year-olds in the general population of Sweden (N = 2,450), 2.8% of men and 0.4% of women reported at least one experience of crossdressing for erotic purposes (Langström & Zucker, 2005). Erotic crossdressing is not intrinsically problematic, and is a celebrated aspect of sexuality in some relationships (Vitale, 2004). However, as erotic crossdressing is a stigmatized act that is often considered sexually deviant, it is not uncommon for erotic crossdressers to need psychotherapeutic assistance to cope with shame, guilt, and conflict with partners (Dzelme & Jones, 2001). The stigma can lead to secretive and increasingly compulsive behavior which may need to be addressed.

Social Isolation

Visibly gender-variant individuals often have difficulty with public spaces, experiencing stares, harassment, and threats or actual violence. This can lead to increasing difficulty navigating public life, social seclusion, and anxiety. Anxiety disorders such as Social Anxiety Disorder, Agoraphobia, and Panic Disorder can be extreme and debilitating. If the individual presents with an anxiety disorder such as these, a combination of pharmacological treatment and cognitive-behavioral therapy is recommended.

Individuals who are not open about being transgender may find that concealment of identity and history causes decreased intimacy or feelings of disconnection and social alienation. This can be particularly difficult for transsexuals after transition, as much of life prior to transition cannot be discussed without disclosing transsexuality. Crossdressers may similarly experience isolation if there is rigid separation between social life, work life, and home life. For those who are fully open about being transgender or are comfortable talking about life prior to transition, there can still be a feeling of social disconnection based on differences in history and life experience compared to non-transgender peers.

Transgender people who feel socially disconnected may look to other transgender people for companionship, support, and a sense of belonging or community. While peer contact can be a significant positive element in many transgender individuals' lives (Grimaldi & Jacobs, 1996; Odo, 2002; Schrock, Holden, & Reid, 2004), as in any oppressed group there are complex social dynamics within transgender communities that may result in disappointments when expectations of safety, acceptance, and support are not met; when internalized transphobia results in hostility toward peers; or when a shared transgender identity is insufficient common ground for close and supportive relationships.

Some transgender individuals shun connection with the transgender community in an effort to normalize and mainstream their lives in conformity with prevailing social norms. While fear of others' reactions can be a driving force behind attempts to live life away from the transgender community, avoidance of transgender people suggests a degree of internalized transphobia that may negatively affect health and well being.

Spiritual and Religious Concerns

There is a diverse range of attitudes toward gender-variance, crossdressing, and transsexuality across spiritual traditions (Ramet, 1996; Sheridan, 2002). Transgender individuals from spiritual or religious traditions that prohibit cross-dressing and other transgender behavior often struggle with shame and guilt, feeling torn between self and community beliefs. Even those who are not actively involved in religious practice may have concerns about transgenderism rooted in the religion of upbringing or religious norms reflected in society. It can be helpful to assist the client to explore the impact that religious beliefs have on reactions of family members and society at large toward their transgender identity and behavior. However, reactions and attitudes of individuals are not always consistent with the doctrine promulgated by their religious institutions. Within many communities of faith acceptance can be found.

As with gay, lesbian, and bisexual persons hoping for religious salvation from same-sex desire, transgender individuals who are deeply religious and pray for help to overcome transgender feelings may feel betrayed if no answers are forthcoming. In addition, experiences of rejection, discrimination, and violence by members of a religious community can also impair faith.

Supportive spiritual counseling can be helpful in resolving dilemmas of faith and in finding acceptance. Consultation with progressive spiritual leaders can be helpful in determining ways for transgender individuals to be accommodated and included in gender-specific ceremonies and rituals.

Substance Use

Studies across North American suggest that alcohol and drug use (including nicotine use) is common among transgender individuals (Bockting, Huang, et al., 2005; Clements-Nolle et al., 1999; Hughes & Eliason, 2002; Macfarlane, 2003; Mason, Connors, & Kammerer, 1995; McGowan, 1999; Reback, Simon, Bemis, & Gatson, 2001; Risser & Shelton, 2002; Xavier, 2000). As with the general population, reasons for substance use vary widely among transgender individuals. Some use alcohol or drugs in an attempt to cope with transgender feelings, mental health issues, painful emotions relating to socioeconomic concerns, memories of physical or sexual abuse or assault, work-related stress and fatigue, or physical pain. Others start using alcohol or drugs to facilitate social interactions or to meet peer expectations.

As in the non-transgender population, there is great diversity in patterns of substance use; not all individuals who use drugs experience a negative impact in overall function. A chemical dependency evaluation by a trained evaluator may be necessary to determine to what extent the substance use is problematic. In a survey of transgender individuals (N = 179) conducted in British Columbia, 12% reported a current need for substance abuse or addiction services; 16% reported a past need and 8% anticipated the need for services in the future (Goldberg et al., 2003).

As with other areas of care, in substance abuse treatment we encourage a client-centered approach that supports the individual's choice of treatment goals and treatment modalities. Possible goals range from reduction of risky patterns of use to total cessation of drug or alcohol consumption. Treatment options depend on the drugs being used; for some substances both psychotherapeutic and pharmacologic treatment options are available.

Clients with co-existing mental health issues may require a dual diagnosis program where substance use and mental illness are treated in an integrated fashion (Osher & Drake, 1996). Similarly, an integrated approach is needed in working with clients whose substance use is affected by their gender identity concerns. While substance use can negatively impact psychotherapy and potentially affect the client's capacity to make medical decisions, a client who is struggling with substance use should not be excluded from treatment for gender identity concerns, and substance abuse treatment should not require that clients have resolved their gender identity concerns first. Rather, the clinician should focus on helping the client to address substance use as an integral part of the care plan toward resolution of the gender identity concerns.

Although transgender individuals may be highly motivated to engage in substance abuse treatment, particularly if they feel that substance use is interfering with their ability to transition, it can be difficult to find transgender-sensitive and competent treatment providers. Many drug and alcohol programs are gender-specific (i.e., for men or for women), posing a problem for individuals who are in the middle of transition, who do not identify as either man or woman, or who are visibly transgender. Residential treatment facilities must consider transgender-specific accommodations in sleeping, bathing, and group activities (White Holman & Goldberg, 2006b).

As with all other areas of transgender care, it is not enough for substance abuse treatment programs to be accessible and welcoming. Successful treatment requires understanding of the multiple issues that commonly drive transgender individuals' substance use and make recovery difficult. These issues may include coping with gender dysphoria, social stigma, experiences of abuse or violence, and mental health concerns. Specific strategies beyond those discussed in this article are needed to build capacity for transgender-competent substance abuse prevention and treatment services (Barbara & Doctor, 2004; Leslie, Perina, & Maqueda, 2001; Lombardi & van Servellen, 2000; Oggins & Eichenbaum, 2002).

Violence and Abuse

It is difficult to estimate the extent of violence against transgender people as the vast majority of violence is not reported. Tracking mechanisms typically do not differentiate between lesbian, gay, bisexual, and transgender individuals (Goldberg & White, 2004), and there are no mechanisms to track transgender-related violence against non-transgender loved ones. Transgender-specific studies suggest high prevalence of sexual abuse, sexual assault, relationship violence, and hate-motivated assault (Courvant & Cook-Daniels, 1998; Devor, 1994; Kenagy, 2005; Lombardi et al., 2001). Data relating to transgender-specific hate crimes indicate that 98% of incidents were perpetrated against MtF transgender individuals (Currah & Minter, 2000). Non-transgender SOFFAs are also vulnerable to hate-motivated violence, as evidenced by the murders of Philip DeVine, Lisa Lambert, Willie Houston, and Barry Winchell (Cook-Daniels, 2001; Goldberg, 2006).

Vulnerability related to being transgender may be exploited in an abusive relationship. For example, abuse may include hurtful statements that invalidate gender identity (e.g., "You'll never be a real woman") or threats to "out" the transgender person to family members or co-workers. Violence may also include attempts to harm gendered aspects of the body or destruction of clothing, make-up, wigs, or prosthetic devices used for gender expression (Goldberg, 2006). Fears of being exposed as a transgender person and the possibility of additional abuse or ridicule upon disclosure pose a barrier to reporting violence and to accessing support services.

Transgender issues can also affect SOFFAs who are experiencing abuse in a relationship (Cook-Daniels, 2003). For example, a SOFFA who is being abused by a transgender person may be reluctant to seek assistance for fear of further isolating their transgender loved one, having to disclose transgender issues to friends and family, or fear of being perceived as gay or lesbian for being in a relationship with a transgender individual.

Although resources exist to promote awareness of transgender issues in anti-violence services (Courvant & Cook-Daniels, 1998; Goldberg, 2006; Goldberg & White, 2004; Munson & Cook-Daniels, 2003; White, 2003; White & Goldberg, 2006, in press), no guidelines currently exist for transgender-specific abuse prevention or treatment of victims and perpetrators of violence and abuse. Further work is needed in this area.

While not all transgender individuals experience overt violence or abuse, for many the daily trials of living in a society that does not sufficiently understand, accept, or accommodate their transgender identity constitutes an ongoing source of distress. For some, this distress becomes traumatic. Others experience the physical or emotional distress associated with the conflict between their sex assigned at birth and their gender identity as profoundly traumatic. This may result in symptoms of Post Traumatic Stress Disorder (American Psychiatric Association, 2000). Regardless of the severity of distress, it may be helpful to consider a trauma framework in understanding and treating the related mental health concerns of transgender individuals.

CONCLUDING REMARKS

Transgender persons and their loved ones are an underserved community in need of empathic, comprehensive, and clinically competent care. Health and social service providers engaged in mental health care will likely be approached for assistance by transgender community members at some point in their practice. Mental health professionals can have a significant positive influence in helping transgender people and loved ones address their gender and mental health concerns, build resilience in coping with social stigma, and reach their full potential. We hope this article helps clinicians feel more prepared and confident in clinical practice with the transgender community.

REFERENCES

American Psychiatric Association (2000). *Diagnostic and statistical manual of mental disorders* (4th ed., Text Revision ed.). Washington, DC: Author.

American Psychiatric Association (2003). *Practice guideline for the assessment and treatment of patients with suicidal behaviors.* Arlington, VA: Author.

Anderson, B. F. (1997). Ethical implications for psychotherapy with individuals seeking gender reassignment. In G. E. Israel & D. E. I. Tarver (Eds.), *Transgender care: Recommended guidelines, practical information and personal accounts* (pp. 185-189). Philadelphia, PA: Temple University Press.

Appelbaum, P., & Grisso, T. (1988). Assessing patients' capacities to consent to treatment. *New England Journal of Medicine, 319,* 1635-1638.

Ashbee, O., & Goldberg, J. M. (2006a). *Hormones: A guide for FTMs.* Vancouver, BC: Vancouver Coastal Health Authority. Available online at http://www.vch.ca/transhealth/resources/library/tcpdocs/consumer/hormones-FTM.pdf

Ashbee, O., & Goldberg, J. M. (2006a). *Hormones: A guide for MTFs.* Vancouver, BC: Vancouver Coastal Health Authority. Available online at http://www.vch.ca/transhealth/resources/library/tcpdocs/consumer/hormones-MTF.pdf

Asscheman, H., Gooren, L. J. G., & Eklund, P. L. (1989). Mortality and morbidity in transsexual patients with cross-gender hormone treatment. *Metabolism, 38,* 869-873.

Bakker, A., van Kesteren, P. J., Gooren, L. J. G., & Bezemer, P. D. (1993). The prevalence of transsexualism in the Netherlands. *Acta Psychiatrica Scandinavica, 87,* 237-238.

Barbara, A., & Doctor, F. (2004). *Asking the right questions 2: Talking with clients about sexual orientation and gender identity in mental health, counselling, and addiction settings.* Toronto, ONT: Centre for Addiction and Mental Health.

Blanchard, R. (1994). A structural equation model for age at clinical presentation in nonhomosexual male gender dysphorics. *Archives of Sexual Behavior, 23,* 311-320.

Bockting, W. O. (1997). The assessment and treatment of gender dysphoria. *Directions in Clinical & Counseling Psychology, 7,* 11-3 to 11-22.

Bockting, W. O. (1999). From construction to context: Gender through the eyes of the transgendered. *SIECUS Report, 28,* 3-7.

Bockting, W. O. (2003). *Transgender identity, sexuality, and coming out: Implications for HIV risk and prevention.* Proceedings of the NIDA-sponsored satellite sessions in association with the XIV International AIDS Conference, Barcelona, Spain, July 7-11, 2002 (pp. 163-172). Bethesda, MD: National Institute on Drug Abuse, U. S. Department of Health and Human Services, National Institutes of Health.

Bockting, W., & Coleman, E. (in press). Developmental stages of the transgender coming out process: Toward an integrated identity. In R. Ettner, S. Monstrey, & E. Eyler (Eds.), *Principles of transgender medicine and surgery.* New York: The Haworth Press, Inc.

Bockting, W., Coleman, E., Huang, C.-Y., & Ding, H. (2006). *Stigma, mental health, and resilience in an online sample of the U.S. transgender population.* Manuscript in preparation.

Bockting, W. O., & Ehrbar, R. D. (2006). Commentary: Gender variance, dissonance, or identity disorder. *Journal of Psychology & Human Sexuality, 17,* 125-134.

Bockting, W. O., & Fung, L. C. T. (2005). Genital reconstruction and gender identity disorders. In D. Sarwer, T. Pruzinsky, T. Cash, J. Persing, R. Goldwyn, & L. Whitaker (Eds.). *The psychological aspects of cosmetic and reconstructive plastic surgery* (pp. 207-229). Philadelphia, PA: Lippincott, Williams, and Wilkins.

Bockting, W. O., Huang, C.-Y., Ding, H., Robinson, B., & Rosser, B. R. S. (2005). Are transgender persons at higher risk for HIV than other sexual minorities? A comparison of HIV prevalence and risks. *International Journal of Transgenderism, 8,* 123-132.

Bockting, W. O., Miner, M., Robinson, B. E., Rosser, B. R. S., & Coleman, E. (2005). *Transgender Identity Survey.* Minneapolis, MN: University of Minnesota, Program in Human Sexuality.

Bockting, W. O., Robinson, B. E., Benner, A., & Scheltema, K. (2004). Patient satisfaction with transgender health services. *Journal of Sex and Marital Therapy, 30,* 277-294.

Bockting, W. O., Robinson, B. E., Forberg, J., & Scheltema, K. (2005). Evaluation of a sexual health approach to reducing HIV/STD risk in the transgender community. *AIDS Care, 17,* 289-303.

Bockting, W. O., Robinson, B. E., & Rosser, B. R. S. (1998). Transgender HIV prevention: A qualitative needs assessment. *AIDS Care, 10,* 505-526.

Bodlund, O., Kullgren, G., Sundbom, E., & Höjerback, T. (1993). Personality traits and disorders among transsexuals. *Acta Psychiatrica Scandinavica, 88,* 322-327.

Bolin, A. (1988). *In search of Eve: Transsexual rites of passage.* New York: Bergin & Garvey Publishers, Inc.

Boyce, P., Carter, G., Penrose-Wall, J., Wilhelm, K., & Goldney, R. (2003). Summary: Australian and New Zealand clinical practice guideline for the management of adult deliberate self-harm. *Australasian Psychiatry, 11,* 150-155.

Brown, G. R. (2001). *Sex reassignment surgery in a patient with Gender Identity Disorder and Dissociative Identity Disorders: Report of a successful case.* Paper presented at 17th Biennial Symposium of the Harry Benjamin Gender Dysphoria Association, Galveston, TX.

Brown, M. L., & Rounsley, C. A. (1996). *True selves: Understanding transsexualism–For families, friends, coworkers, and helping professionals.* San Francisco, CA: Jossey-Bass.

Bullough, V. L. & Weinberg, T. S. (1988). Women married to transvestites: Problems and adjustments. *Journal of Psychology & Human Sexuality, 1,* 83-104.

Cameron, L. (1996). *Body alchemy: Transsexual portraits.* San Francisco: Cleis Press.

Campo, J. M., Nijman, H., Evers, C., Merckelbach, H. L., & Decker, I. (2001). Gender identity disorders as a symptom of psychosis, schizophrenia in particular. *Nederlands Tijdschrift Voor Geneeskunde, 145,* 1876-1880.

Clements-Nolle, K., Katz, M. H., & Marx, R. (1999). *Transgender Community Health Project: Descriptive results.* San Francisco: San Francisco Department of Public Health.

Clements-Nolle, K., Marx, R., Guzman, R., & Katz, M. (2001). HIV prevalence, risk behaviors, health care use, and mental health status of transgender persons: Implications for public health intervention. *American Journal of Public Health, 91,* 915-921.

Cole, C. M., O'Boyle, M., Emory, L. E., & Meyer, W. J., III (1997). Comorbidity of gender dysphoria and other major psychiatric diagnoses. *Archives of Sexual Behavior, 26,* 13-26.

Cole, S. S., Denny, D., Eyler, A. E., & Samons, S. L. (2000). Issues of transgender. In L. T. Szuchman & F. Muscarella (Eds.), *Psychological perspectives on human sexuality* (pp. 149-195). New York: John Wiley.

Coleman, E. (1987). Assessment of sexual orientation. *Journal of Homosexuality, 14,* 9-24.

Coleman, E., Bockting, W. O., & Gooren, L. J. G. (1993). Homosexual and bisexual identity in sex-reassigned female-to-male transsexuals. *Archives of Sexual Behavior, 22,* 37-50.

Coleman, E., Miner, M., Ohlerking, F., & Raymond, N. (2001). Compulsive sexual behavior inventory: A preliminary study of reliability and validity. *Journal of Sex & Marital Therapy, 27,* 325-332.

Cook-Daniels, L. (2001). *SOFFA questions and answers.* Glendale, WI: For Ourselves Reworking Gender Expression.

Cook-Daniels, L. (2003). *Trans/SOFFA specific power and control tactics.* Glendale, WI: Transgender Aging Network.

Courvant, D., & Cook-Daniels, L. (1998). *Trans and intersex survivors of domestic violence: Defining terms, barriers, and responsibilities.* Portland, OR: Survivor Project.

Covin, A. (1999). Dee and Anni's story. In M. Boenke (Ed.), *Trans forming families: Real stories about transgendered loved ones* (pp. 92-93). Imperial Beach, CA: Walter Trook.

Currah, P., & Minter, S. (2000). *Transgender equality: A handbook for activists and policymakers.* New York, NY: National Gay and Lesbian Task Force and The National Center for Lesbian Rights.

Dahl, M., Feldman, J., Goldberg, J. M., & Jaberi, A. (2006). Physical aspects of transgender endocrine therapy. *International Journal of Transgenderism, 9*(3/4), 111-134.

Daskalos, C. T. (1998). Changes in the sexual orientation of six heterosexual male-to-female transsexuals. *Archives of Sexual Behavior, 27,* 605-614.

Davis, D. L. (1998). The sexual and gender identity disorders. *Transcultural Psychiatry, 35,* 401-412.

de Jong, P., & Berg, I. K. (2001). Co-constructing cooperation with mandated clients. *Social Work, 46,* 361-374.

de Vries, A. L. C., Cohen-Kettenis, P. T., & Delemarre-van de Waal, H. (2006). Clinical management of gender dysphoria in adolescents. *International Journal of Transgenderism, 9*(3/4), 83-94.

De Sutter, P., Kira, K., Verschoor, A., & Hotimsky, A. (2002). The desire to have children and the preservation of fertility in transsexual women: A survey. *International Journal of Transgenderism, 6.* Retrieved January 1, 2005, from http://www.symposion.com/ijt/ijtvo06no03_02.htm

Derogatis, L. R., & Melisaratos, N. (1979). The DSFI: a multidimensional measure of sexual functioning. *Journal of Sex & Marital Therapy, 5,* 244-281.

Devor, H. (1993). Sexual orientation identities, attractions, and practices of female-to-male transsexuals. *Journal of Sex Research, 30,* 303-315.

Devor, H. (1994). Transsexualism, dissociation, and child abuse: An initial discussion based on nonclinical data. *Journal of Psychology & Human Sexuality, 6,* 49-72.

Docter, R. F., & Fleming, J. S. (2001). Measures of transgender behavior. *Archives of Sexual Behavior, 30,* 255-271.

Dzelme, K., & Jones, R. A. (2001). Male cross-dressers in therapy: A solution-focused perspective for marriage and family therapists. *American Journal of Family Therapy, 29,* 293-305.

Ellis, K. M., & Eriksen, K. (2002). Transsexual and transgenderist experiences and treatment options. *The Family Journal: Counseling and Therapy for Couples and Families, 10,* 289-299.

Emerson, S. & Rosenfeld, C. (1996). Stages of adjustment in family members of transgender individuals. *Journal of Family Psychotherapy, 7,* 1-12.

Esterling, B. A., L'Abate, L., Murray, E., & Pennebaker, J. W. (1999). Empirical foundations for writing in prevention and psychotherapy: Mental and physical health outcome. *Clinical Psychology Review, 19,* 79-96.

Etchells, E., Darzins, P., Silberfeld, M., Singer, P. A., McKenny, J., Naglie, G., Katz, M., Guyatt, G. H., Molloy, D. W., & Strang, D. (1999). Assessment of patient capacity to consent to treatment. *Journal of General Internal Medicine, 14,* 27-34.

Faulk, M. (1990). Psychosis in a transsexual. *British Journal of Psychiatry, 156,* 285-286.

Feldman, J., & Bockting, W. O. (2003). Transgender health. *Minnesota Medicine, 86,* 25-32.

Feldman, J. (2005). *Masculinizing hormone therapy with testosterone 1% topical gel.* Paper presented at the XIX Biennial Symposium of the Harry Benjamin International Gender Dysphoria Association, Bologna, Italy.

Fernández-Aranda, F., Peri, J. M., Navarro, V., Badía-Casanovas, A., Turón-Gil, V., & Vallejo-Ruiloba, J. (2000). Transsexualism and anorexia nervosa: A case report. *Eating Disorders: The Journal of Treatment & Prevention, 8,* 63-66.

Flaherty, C., Franicevich, J., Freeman, M., Klein, P., Kohler, L., Lusardi, C., Martinez, L., Monihan, M., Vormohr, J., & Zevin, B. (2001). *Protocols for hormonal reassignment of gender.* San Francisco: San Francisco Department of Public Health. Retrieved January 1, 2005, from http://www.dph.sf.ca.us/chn/HlthCtrs/HlthCtrDocs/TransGendprotocols.pdf

Fleming, M. Z., & Feinbloom, D. (1984). Similarities in becoming: Transsexuals and adolescents. *Adolescence, 19,* 729-748.

Fraser, L. (2005). Therapy with transgender people across the life-span. *American Psychological Association Division 44 Newsletter, 21,* 14-16.

Gapka, S. & Raj, R. (2003). *Trans Health Project: A position paper and resolution adopted by the Ontario Public Health Association* (Rep. No. 2003-06 (PP)). Toronto, ONT, Canada: Ontario Public Health Association. Available online at http://www.opha.on.ca/ppres/2003-06_pp.pdf

Goffman, E. (1963). *Stigma: Notes on the management of spoiled identity.* Englewood Cliffs, NJ: Prentice-Hall.

Goldberg, J. M. (2006). *Making the transition: Providing services to trans survivors of violence and abuse.* Vancouver, BC: Justice Institute of BC.

Goldberg, J. M., Matte, N., MacMillan, M., & Hudspith, M. (2003). *Community survey: Transition/crossdressing services in BC–Final report.* Vancouver, BC: Vancouver Coastal Health Authority and Transcend Transgender Support & Education Society.

Goldberg, J. M. & White, C. (2004). Expanding our understanding of gendered violence: Violence against trans people and loved ones. *Aware: The Newsletter of the BC Institute Against Family Violence, 11,* 21-25.

Green, R., & Fleming, D. (1990). Transsexual surgery follow-up: Status in the 1990s. *Annual Review of Sex Research, 1,* 163-174.

Grimaldi, J. M., & Jacobs, J. (1996, July). *HIV/AIDS transgender support group: Improving care delivery and creating a community.* Paper presented at XI International Conference on AIDS, Vancouver, BC, Canada.

Hansbury, G. (2005). Mourning the loss of the idealized self: A transsexual passage. *Psychoanalytic Social Work, 12,* 19-35.

Hepp, U., & Milos, G. (2002). Gender identity disorder and eating disorders. *International Journal of Eating Disorders, 32,* 473-478.

Hill, D. B., Rozanski, C., Cargainni, J., & Willoughby, B. (2003, May). Gender Identity Disorder in children and adolescents: A critical review. In D. Karasic & J. Drescher (Co-Chairs), *Sexual and gender identity disorders: Questions for DSM-V.* Symposium conducted at the 156th Annual Meeting of the American Psychiatric Association, San Francisco, CA. Transcript retrieved January 1, 2005, from http://www.tsroadmap.com/info/div-44-roundtable.html

Horton, M. A. (2001). *Checklist for transitioning in the workplace.* Retrieved January 1, 2005, from http://www.tgender.net/taw/tggl/checklist.html

Hughes, T. L., & Eliason, M. (2002). Substance use and abuse in lesbian, gay, bisexual and transgender populations. *Journal of Primary Prevention, 22,* 263-298.

Israel, G. E. & Tarver, D. E. I. (1997). *Transgender care: Recommended guidelines, practical information, and personal accounts.* Philadephia, PA: Temple University Press.

Keatley, J., Nemoto, T., Operario, D., & Soma, T. (2002, July). *The impact of transphobia on HIV risk behaviors among male to female transgenders in San Francisco.* Poster presented at XVI International AIDS Conference, Barcelona, Spain.

Keatley, J., Nemoto, T., Sevelius, J., & Ventura, A. (2004, November). *Expanding mental health services for transgender people.* Poster presented at the 132nd Annual Meeting of the American Public Health Association, Washington, DC. Retrieved January 1, 2005, from http://www.caps.ucsf.edu/pdfs/APHA_Keatley.pdf

Kenagy, G. P. (2002). HIV among transgendered people. *AIDS Care, 14,* 127-134.

Kenagy, G. P. (2005). Transgender health: Findings from two needs assessment studies in Philadelphia. *Health & Social Work, 30,* 19-26.

Kesteren, P.J. van, Gooren, L.J., & Megens, J.A. (1996). An epidemiological and demographic study of transsexuals in the Netherlands. *Archives of Sexual Behavior, 25*(6), 589-600.

Koetting, M. E. (2004). Beginning practice with preoperative male-to-female transgender clients. *Journal of Gay & Lesbian Social Services: Issues in Practice, Policy & Research, 16,* 99-104.

Kopala, L. (2003). *Recommendations for a transgender health program.* Vancouver, BC: Vancouver Coastal Health Authority.

Kotula, D. (2002). *The phallus palace: Female-to-male transsexuals.* Los Angeles: Alyson Publications.

Kübler-Ross, E. (1969). *On death and dying.* New York: Simon & Schuster.

Landen, M., Walinder, J., Hambert, G., & Lundstrom, B. (1998). Factors predictive of regret in sex reassignment. *Acta Psychiatrica Scandinavica, 97,* 284-289.

Langström, N., & Zucker, K. J. (2005). Transvestic fetishism in the general population. *Journal of Sex & Marital Therapy, 31,* 87-95.

Lantz, B. (1999). Is the journey worth the pain? In M. Boenke (Ed.), *Trans forming families: Real stories about transgendered loved ones* (pp. 13-18). Imperial Beach, CA: Walter Trook.

Lawrence, A. A. (2003). Factors associated with satisfaction or regret following male-to-female sex reassignment surgery. *Archives of Sexual Behavior, 32,* 299-315.

Lawrence, A. A. (2005). Sexuality before and after male-to-female sex reassignment surgery. *Archives of Sexual Behavior, 34,* 147-166.

Leslie, D. R., Perina, B. A., & Maqueda, M. C. (2001). Clinical issues with transgender individuals. In U.S. Department of Health and Human Services Center for Substance Abuse Treatments (Ed.), *A provider's introduction to substance abuse treatment for lesbian, gay, bisexual, and transgender individuals* (pp. 91-98). Rockville, MD: U.S. Department of Health and Human Services.

Lev, A. I. (2004). *Transgender emergence: Therapeutic guidelines for working with gender-variant people and their families.* Binghamton, NY: The Haworth Clinical Practice Press.

Linehan, M. M., Armstrong, H. E., Suarez, A., Allmon, D., & Heard, H. L. (1991). Cognitive-behavioral treatment of chronically parasuicidal borderline patients. *Archives of General Psychiatry, 48,* 1060-1064.

Lombardi, E. L., & van Servellen, G. (2000). Building culturally sensitive substance use prevention and treatment programs for transgendered populations. *Journal of Substance Abuse Treatment, 19,* 291-296.

Lombardi, E. L., Wilchins, R. A., Priesing, D., & Malouf, D. (2001). Gender violence: Transgender experiences with violence and discrimination. *Journal of Homosexuality, 42,* 89-101.

Macfarlane, D. (2003). *LGBT communities and substance use–What health has to do with it: A report on consultations with LGBT communities.* Vancouver, BC: LGBT Health Association of BC.

Mallett, P., Marshall, E. J., & Blacker, C. V. (1989). "Puerperal psychosis" following male-to-female sex reassignment? *British Journal of Psychiatry, 155,* 257-259.

Manderson, L., & Kumar, S. (2001). Gender identity disorder as a rare manifestation of schizophrenia. *Australian and New Zealand Journal of Psychiatry, 35,* 546-547.

Martin, T., & Gattaz, W. F. (1991). Psychiatric aspects of male genital self-mutilation. *Psychopathology, 24,* 170-178.

Mason, T. H., Connors, M. M., & Kammerer, C. A. (1995). *Transgenders and HIV risks: Needs assessment.* Boston, MA: Gender Identity Support Services for Transgenders, prepared for the Massachusetts Department of Public Health, HIV/AIDS Bureau.

Mathy, R. M. (2002). Transgender identity and suicidality in a nonclinical sample: Sexual orientation, psychiatric history, and compulsive behaviors. *Journal of Psychology & Human Sexuality, 14,* 47-65.

McGovern, S. J. (1995). Self-castration in a transsexual. *Journal of Accident and Emergency Medicine, 12,* 57-58.

McGowan, C. K. (1999). *Transgender needs assessment.* New York City, NY: Prevention Planning Unit, New York City Department of Health.

Mellon, C. D., Barlow, C., Cook, J., & Clark, L. D. (1989). Autocastration and autopenectomy in a patient with transsexualism and schizophrenia. *Journal of Sex Research, 26,* 125-130.

Meyer, W. J., III, Bockting, W. O., Cohen-Kettenis, P. T., Coleman, E., Di Ceglie, D., Devor, H., Gooren, L., Hage, J. J., Kirk, S., Kuiper, B., Laub, D., Lawrence, A., Menard, Y., Monstrey, S., Patton, J., Schaefer, L., Webb, A., & Wheeler, C. C. (2001). *The standards of care for Gender Identity Disorders* (6th ed.). Minneapolis, MN: Harry Benjamin International Gender Dysphoria Association.

Michel, A., Ansseau, M., Legros, J. J., Pitchot, W., & Mormont, C. (2002). The transsexual: What about the future? *European Psychiatry, 17,* 353-362.

Milrod, C. (2000). Issues of countertransference in therapy with transgender clients. Los Angeles, CA: Southern California Transgender Counseling. Retrieved January 1, 2005, from http://www.transgendercounseling.com/trans1.htm

Moser, C. K., & Kleinplatz, J. (2003, May). DSM-IV-TR and the paraphilias: An argument for removal. In D. Karasic & J. Drescher (Co-Chairs), *Sexual and gender identity disorders: Questions for DSM-V.* Symposium conducted at the 156th Annual Meeting of the American Psychiatric Association, San Francisco, CA. Transcript retrieved January 1, 2005, from http://www.tsroadmap.com/info/div-44-roundtable.html

Munson, M., & Cook-Daniels, L. (2003). *Transgender/SOFFA: Domestic violence/sexual assault resource sheet.* Milwaukee, WI: For Ourselves Reworking Gender Expression.

Murphy, D., Murphy, M., & Grainger, R. (2001). Self-castration. *Irish Journal of Medical Science, 170,* 195.

Nemoto, T., Operario, D., Keatley, J., Nguyen, H., & Sugano, E. (2005). Promoting health for transgender women: Transgender Resources and Neighborhood Space (TRANS) program in San Francisco. *American Journal of Public Health, 95,* 382-384.

Nemoto, T., Operario, D., Keatley, J., & Villegas, D. (2004). Social context of HIV risk behaviors among male-to-female transgenders of colour. *AIDS Care, 16,* 724-735.

Nemoto, T., Operario, D., Sevelius, J., Keatley, J., Han, L., & Nguyen, H. (2004, November). *Transphobia among transgenders of color*. Poster presented at the 132nd Annual Meeting of the American Public Health Association, Washington, DC. Retrieved January 1, 2005, from http://www.caps.ucsf.edu/pdfs/APHA_Nemoto.pdf

Nemoto, T., Sugano, E., Operario, D., & Keatley, J. (2004, July). *Psychosocial factors influencing HIV risk among male-to-female transgenders in San Francisco*. Poster presented at XV International AIDS Conference, Bangkok, Thailand.

Nuttbrock, L., Rosenblum, A., & Blumenstein, R. (2002). Transgender identity affirmation and mental health. *International Journal of Transgenderism, 6*(4). (Retrieved January 1, 2005, from http://www.symposium.com/ijt/ijtvo06no04_03.htm)

O'Brien, M. (2003). *Keeping it real: Transgender inclusion in safe sex education–Notes for risk reduction educators and outreach workers*. Retrieved January 1, 2005, from http://www.deadletters.biz/real.html

Odo, C. F. O. (2002). *The combination of culturally-relevant prevention case management, community building activities and OraSure testing proves effective for Native Hawaiian transgenders*. Poster presented at XIV International AIDS Conference, Barcelona, Spain.

Oggins, J. & Eichenbaum, J. (2002). Engaging transgender substance users in substance use treatment. *International Journal of Transgenderism, 6*. Retrieved January 1, 2005, from http://www.symposion.com/ijt/ijtvo06no02_03.htm

Olsson, S. E., & Möller, A. R. (2003). On the incidence and sex ratio of transsexualism in Sweden, 1972-2002. *Archives of Sexual Behavior, 32*, 381-386.

Osher, F. C. & Drake, R. E. (1996). Reversing a history of unmet needs: Approaches to care for persons with co-occurring addictive and mental disorders. *American Journal of Orthopsychiatry, 66*, 4-11.

Pasillas, A., Anderson, B., & Fraser, L. (2000, May). *Addressing psychosocial issues in the transgender client*. Panel discussion, Transgender Care Conference, San Francisco, CA.

Pfäfflin, F. (1992). Regrets after sex reassignment surgery. In W. O. Bockting & E. Coleman (Eds.), *Gender dysphoria: Interdisciplinary approaches in clinical management* (pp. 69-85). Binghamton, NY: The Haworth Press, Inc.

Pfäfflin, F., & Junge, A. (1998). *Sex reassignment–Thirty years of international follow-up studies; SRS: A comprehensive review, 1961-1991* (R. B. Jacobson & A. B. Meier, Trans.). Düsseldorf, Germany: Symposion Publishing. (Original work published 1992)

Rachlin, K. (2002). Transgender individuals' experiences of psychotherapy. *International Journal of Transgenderism, 6*. Retrieved January 1, 2005, from http://www.symposion.com/ijt/ijtvo06no01_03.htm

Raj, R. (2002). Towards a transpositive therapeutic model: Developing clinical sensitivity and cultural competence in the effective support of transsexual and transgendered clients. *International Journal of Transgenderism, 6*. Retrieved January 1, 2005, from http://www.symposion.com/ijt/ijtvo06no02_04.htm

Ramet, S. P. (1996). *Gender reversals and gender cultures: Anthropological and historical perspectives*. London: Routledge.

Reback, C. J., Simon, P. A., Bemis, C. C., & Gatson, B. (2001). *The Los Angeles Transgender Health Study: Community report*. Los Angeles, CA: University of California at Los Angeles.

Reynolds, A. L., & Caron, S. L. (2000). How intimate relationships are impacted when heterosexual men crossdress. *Journal of Psychology & Human Sexuality, 12*, 63-77.

Risser, J., & Shelton, A. (2002). *Behavioral assessment of the transgender population, Houston, Texas*. Galveston, TX: University of Texas School of Public Health.

Robinow, O., & Knudson, G. (2005, April). *Asperger's Disorder and gender dysphoria*. Paper presented at 19th Biennial Symposium of the Harry Benjamin International Gender Dysphoria Association, Bologna, Italy.

Sachsse, U., Von der Heyde, S., & Huether, G. (2002). Stress regulation and self-mutilation. *American Journal of Psychiatry, 159*, 672.

Samson, A. (1999). Mom, Dad, we need to talk. In M. Boenke (Ed.), *Trans forming families: Real stories about transgendered loved ones* (pp. 56-60). Imperial Beach, CA: Walter Trook.

Schrock, D., Holden, D., & Reid, L. (2004). Creating emotional resonance: Interpersonal emotion work and motivational framing in a transgender community. *Social Problems, 51*, 61-81.

Sheridan, V. (2002). *Crossing over: Liberating the transgendered Christian*. Cleveland, OH: The Pilgrim Press.

Simpson, A. J., & Goldberg, J. M. (2006a). *Surgery: A guide for FTMs*. Vancouver, BC: Vancouver Coastal Health Authority. Available online at http://www.vch.ca/transhealth/resources/library/tcpdocs/consumer/surgery-FTM.pdf

Simpson, A. J., & Goldberg, J. M. (2006b). *Surgery: A guide for MTFs*. Vancouver, BC: Vancouver Coastal Health Authority. Available online at http://www.vch.ca/transhealth/resources/library/tcpdocs/consumer/surgery-MTF.pdf

Steinbeck, A. (1997). Hormonal medication for transsexuals. *Venereology: Interdisciplinary, International Journal of Sexual Health, 10*, 175-177.

Surgenor, L. J., & Fear, J. L. (1998). Eating disorder in a transgendered patient: A case report. *International Journal of Eating Disorders, 24*, 449-452.

Tunzi, M. (2001). Can the patient decide? Evaluating patient capacity in practice. *American Family Physician, 64*, 299-306.

Vitale, A. (2004). Couples therapy when the male partner crossdresses. *T-Note, 11*. Retrieved January 1, 2005, from http://www.avitale.com/cdcouples.htm

Volkmar, F., Cook, E. H. Jr., Pomeroy, J., Realmuto, G., & Tanguay, P. (1999). Practice parameters for the assessment and treatment of children, adolescents, and adults with autism and other pervasive developmental disorders. *Journal of the American Academy of Child & Adolescent Psychiatry, 38,* S32-S54.

Weinberg, T. S., & Bullough, V. L. (1988). Alienation, self-image, and the importance of support groups for the wives of transvestites. *Journal of Sex Research, 24,* 262.

White Holman, C., & Goldberg, J. M. (2006a). Ethical, legal, and psychosocial issues in care of transgender adolescents. *International Journal of Transgenderism, 9*(3/4), 95-110.

White Holman, C., & Goldberg, J. M. (2006b). Social and medical transgender case advocacy. *International Journal of Transgenderism, 9*(3/4), 197-217.

White, C. (2003). *Re/defining gender and sex: Educating for trans, transsexual, and intersex access and inclusion to sexual assault centres and transition houses.* Unpublished master's thesis, University of British Columbia, Vancouver, BC.

White, C., & Goldberg, J. M. (2006, February). Understanding support for trans people and their loved ones. *Communiqué: The Newsletter of the BC/Yukon Society of Transition Houses,* 36-38.

White, C., & Goldberg, J. M. (2007-in press). Safety assessment and planning in abusive trans relationships. In G. Reid (Ed.), *Aid to Safety Assessment and Planning.* Vancouver, BC: BC Institute Against Family Violence.

Williamson, I., & Hartley, P. (1998). British research into the increased vulnerability of young gay men to eating disturbance and body dissatisfaction. *European Eating Disorders Review, 6,* 160-170.

Wilson, K., & Lev, A. I. (2003, May). Disordering gender identity: Issues of diagnostic reform. In D. Karasic & J. Drescher (Co-Chairs), *Sexual and gender identity disorders: Questions for DSM-V.* Symposium conducted at the 156th Annual Meeting of the American Psychiatric Association, San Francisco, CA. Transcript retrieved January 1, 2005, from http://www.tsroadmap.com/info/div-44-roundtable.html

Winston, A. P., Acharya, S., Chaudhuri, S., & Fellowes, L. (2004). Anorexia nervosa and gender identity disorder in biologic males: A report of two cases. *International Journal of Eating Disorders, 36,* 109-113.

Xavier, J. (2000). *The Washington, DC Transgender Needs Assessment Survey: Final report for phase two–Tabulation of the survey questionnaires, presentation of findings and analysis of the survey results, and recommendations.* Washington, DC: Administration for HIV and AIDS, District of Columbia Department of Health.

Yelland, C., & Tiggemann, M. (2003). Muscularity and the gay ideal: Body dissatisfaction and disordered eating in homosexual men. *Eating Behaviors, 4,* 107-116.

doi:10.1300/J485v09n03_03

APPENDIX A. Case Vignettes

The following case vignettes are from the first two authors' clinical practices. Names and identifying details have been changed to protect client anonymity.

The first case is of "Jake," who presented seeking assistance to pursue hormones and surgery as part of sex reassignment. The second case is of "Carlos," who came for treatment to deal with obsessive/compulsive features of his crossdressing and gender dysphoria. Although Carlos has, to date, decided not to change gender roles or undergo sex reassignment, some clients with similar profiles do so after the obsessive/compulsive features have been sufficiently alleviated. The third case, of "Anne," illustrates the quest for affirmation of gender identity. A physical change usually does not suffice to alleviate the impact of gender dysphoria and social stigma on one's mental health; psychotherapy and peer support play a key role in confronting internalized transphobia. The fourth case of "Jamie" illustrates how such mental illness as Schizo-affective Disorder may complicate treatment of gender dysphoria, yet does not necessarily constitute a contraindication for medical intervention. Rather, treatment of both conditions reinforce one another and result in improved stability and psychosocial adjustment. Finally, the fifth case, of "Patricia," illustrates gender dysphoria in a client with Asperger's Disorder. This case illustrates the difficulty in assessing a client with limited ability for psychotherapeutic interaction with the therapist.

The case vignettes reflect the diversity in transgender identities found among the transgender population, but illustrate the more complex cases in which gender identity concerns co-exist with other mental health and psychosocial concerns. Hence, these cases are not equally representative of the overall population of transgender clients. For example, the first case (Jake) is far more typical of FTM clients seeking hormones or surgery than the fourth case (Jamie).

The length of therapy and treatment in these cases varied widely. The first case (Jake) involved a straightforward assessment completed in three sessions. In the other four cases, the types of changes described took a considerable amount of time to emerge.

Jake (Female-to-Male)

Jake presented at age 23 seeking assistance to pursue hormones and surgery as part of sex reassignment. Jake started living as a man when he moved from Regina to Vancouver 18 months earlier. By the time he sought assessment he was already dressing as a man and using the men's restroom at work and in public settings. Jake sought chest surgery as he found it difficult to pass as a man during the summer and found it uncomfortable to bind his chest tightly, especially during warm weather. He also was hoping to start hormone therapy as soon as possible and to undergo a hysterectomy.

At the time of his first appointment, Jake lived alone and had been working as a manager of a fast food restaurant for the past year. Six years ago, he emigrated from Uganda to Regina and lived with his family until he decided to move out on his own to Vancouver.

Jake grew up in a Bahá'í family. Throughout Jake's childhood he was considered to be a tomboy and fought to be able to wear boys' shoes and clothes. Jake described himself as a loner throughout his childhood, not associating much with either boys or girls. He explained always wanting to be a boy and dreaming about getting married to a woman when he grew older. Prior to age 14 he had done well at school and was consistently at the top of his class. When his breasts started growing and he started menstruating, he became very distressed and his academic performance dropped so he was in the bottom third of his class. He subsequently became depressed and described having suicidal thoughts as a regular part of daily life (but not making any attempts). He described being sad about how difficult his life had been as a young woman and feeling that a mistake regarding his gender had been made.

Jake's father died of kidney complications secondary to diabetes when Jake was 15 years old. His mother and brothers moved to Regina two years later. Shortly after the move, Jake discovered information about transsexualism and spoke with his mother about wanting to have surgery. His mother could not accept this, and at age 18 Jake moved out to live with other relatives. It was at this point that he began to request that people call him Jake and that they refer to him as a man. Most members of his family were able to accept this.

After a series of three appointments involving discussion of Jake's gender feelings and personal and family history, it was agreed that the testosterone, chest surgery, and hysterectomy sought by Jake were appropriate treatments. A letter recommending hormone therapy was written to Jake's family physician. Jake described his doctor as supportive, but lacking experience in transgender medicine. Accordingly, a list of endocrinologists with experience in treating transgender individuals was provided for Jake to discuss with his physician for possible referral. Requirements for surgery were discussed with Jake and information regarding surgery was provided to his family physician. Jake returned for a specific assessment for transgender surgery after another year of living in the male gender role, and proceeded with chest surgery shortly thereafter. A hysterectomy was not performed until another year later as Jake was concerned about having sufficient time off work for recovery after the surgery.

Carlos

Carlos (age 41) presented with gender dysphoria and a request for sex reassignment. The mental health history revealed that he had a history of Dysthymia. Psychological testing indicated current symptoms of anxiety and depression. Carlos described a long history of crossdressing. He used to become sexually aroused and masturbate to an article of women's clothing. However, over time, he gradually needed more and more feminine accessories such as wigs, make-up, high heels, and jewelry to satisfy his urges. He described sexual fantasies of himself changing sex. Recently, on several occasions, he stayed up all night when his wife was out of town, impersonating a woman, and calling phone lines advertised in the local newspaper to talk to and meet men for sex. He explained that sex with a man made him feel more feminine, completing the image of himself as a woman. He shared this information with intense shame. He finally mustered the courage to come to therapy to pursue sex reassignment to resolve his situation.

Carlos met criteria for diagnoses of Dysthymia and Transvestic Fetishism with Gender Dysphoria. Individual psychotherapy was recommended to explore his crossdressing and gender dysphoria further. Pharmacotherapy was recommended to alleviate symptoms of anxiety and depression, and to alleviate obsessive/compulsive features of his crossdressing and gender dysphoria. Carlos began taking fluoxetine, and along with the psychotherapy sessions, this eased his feelings of despair. He brought his wife to therapy and shared the concerns with her. She was shocked, yet appreciated her husband's efforts to get help. When she learned that this had been a problem of Carlos dating back to the time before their marriage, she felt betrayed and was angry at Carlos for not telling her sooner.

Carlos began writing his personal and sexual history. It became clear that his crossgender feelings dated back to childhood. He described his family of origin as rather cold. Expressing one's emotions was deemed a sign of weakness. Carlos described much pressure from his family, particularly his father, to be "a man." He kept his crossgender feelings secret, fantasized about waking up one day as a girl, and these fantasies became more sexual in puberty. He secretly put on clothes of his sister, which added to sexual arousal, followed by masturbation. Over the course of his life, his fantasies became more elaborate, and so did his crossdressing. He described fantasies of his body changing from male to female, with breasts and a vagina appearing. He also fantasized about being admired and romanced as a woman by men.

What was particularly problematic for Carlos was that these fantasies at times became so intense that he would stay up most of the night pursuing their fulfillment. The fantasies took on the characteristics of an obsession, interfering with the responsibilities toward his family and job. To address these obsessive/compulsive features, Carlos joined a therapy group for men with compulsive sexual behavior. In this group, he shared his story which helped to alleviate shame. He made a commitment to this group to no longer call phone lines or seek sex with men to affirm his femininity. Carlos discovered that continuing to crossdress made it hard for him to adhere to these boundaries, and crossdressing without these activities became less and less appealing. Eventually, Carlos decided to stop crossdressing altogether. His gender dysphoria persisted, albeit in a more manageable way. He began to read and attend educational events about transgenderism. He eventually became at peace with himself identifying as "a crossdresser who does not crossdress," integrating his transgender feelings into the male gender role. He recommitted himself to the sexual relationship with his wife, and broadened his sexual fantasies to include her as well as other women. Finally, he developed lasting friendships with members of his therapy group.

Anne (Male-to-Female)

Anne (age 24) was referred for treatment of Gender Identity Disorder after completing an inpatient substance abuse treatment program. Her history revealed that she grew up as a gender-role-nonconforming boy. This led to substantial conflict with parents and with peers in school. Her father put pressure on Anne to act more masculine, and forced her to join an all boys hockey team. Peers in school made fun of Anne, calling her a "fag" and a "queer."

At age 15 she dropped out of school and, shortly thereafter, ran away from home. After spending time in a shelter for runaway youth, she returned home and from then on lived in the female gender role. At age 18, she left home permanently. She met other transgender women, who provided her with illicitly procured feminizing hormones and introduced her to sex work. She participated in "pump parties" where peers injected silicone into her body to further feminize her appearance. They affirmed how beautiful she was, and for the first time in her life, Anne felt attractive and wanted. The attention from heterosexual men was initially very exciting; however, soon the hazards of working in the sex industry became overwhelming and she began to use drugs to cope. At age 20, she attempted suicide and was subsequently hospitalized and referred to substance use treatment.

Anne requested medically assisted hormone therapy, along with breast augmentation. Anne clearly met criteria for Gender Identity Disorder. In addition, she met criteria for Major Depression and for Histrionic Personality Disorder. Despite passing extremely well as a woman, she felt very insecure about herself and was hypervigilant about being discovered as transgender. The care plan included individual psychotherapy, group psychotherapy, pharmacotherapy for depression, and hormone therapy. In individual therapy, the depth and sources of Anne's self-hatred were exposed. Group therapy was difficult for Anne. She was unable to be vulnerable or accept help from others. She felt like she did not fit in and discontinued group therapy prematurely. Anne was then encouraged to bring her family into therapy. Both parents had been very concerned about Anne's welfare, and were glad to see that she was getting help. Anne's transgenderism was, at this point, the least of their concerns; they wanted to see Anne stay abstinent from drugs and alcohol, and find happiness.

Anne struggled to let go of her involvement in the sex industry. On the one hand, she recognized the negative impact of sex work on her self esteem and on her ability to establish a primary relationship. On the other hand, sex work provided her with income without having to face her fear and insecurity of finding and functioning in mainstream employment as a transgender woman. After a number of missed therapy appointments, Anne explained that it had been hard for her to come to therapy because "coming here makes me feel so transgendered." She further explained that she consulted with another therapist who recommended vaginoplasty to alleviate this feeling. Moreover, Anne unfolded extensive plans for feminizing surgery of her face, and how she had been working hard to save money for this surgery. Rather than supporting her in pursuing these procedures, the therapist empathized and gently confronted Anne's internalized transphobia. Anne was able to see that no matter how much surgery she would have, she would always be transgender. While she meets the WPATH *Standards of Care* for genital surgery, Anne has so far opted not to undergo this procedure. She did opt for breast augmentation. Anne enrolled in school and eventually found employment outside of the sex industry.

Jamie (Female-to-Male)

Jamie (age 26) presented with questions about his sexual orientation and identity. He was very tense and slow to answer interview questions. It took several sessions to develop adequate trust to obtain sufficient information to conclude that Jamie struggled with gender dysphoria. In one of the extended intake evaluation sessions, Jamie shut down to the extent that the therapist became concerned about his safety; upon probing, Jamie admitted he felt suicidal. During the hospitalization that followed, Jamie was diagnosed with Schizo-affective Disorder. Upon release from the hospital, he was referred to a psychiatrist who had experience working with transgender clients and was able to separate gender identity issues from symptoms of Jamie's Schizo-affective Disorder. Jamie struggled with both. Pharmacotherapy was able to stabilize him.

Jamie lived with his mother, and she was invited to join him in therapy. Jamie's mother explained that Jamie was a loner. He worked in a factory on the assembly line and frequently changed jobs because once colleagues warmed up to him, he would become uncomfortable and quit. His mother also revealed that she divorced Jamie's father because he sexually abused Jamie when he was a child. In individual therapy, this was followed up on and Jamie was able to describe what happened. He felt that since his father had left, he had to be the man in the household and take care of his mother. Working through these issues in therapy did not change Jamie's resolve to live in the male gender role and pursue chest surgery and hormones.

Once Jamie had become more comfortable talking with his therapist, he joined a group with other transgender clients. In this group, he learned a great deal about what it is like to be transgender, what was involved in a gender role transition, and how to deal with people's reactions. He began living full-time in the male gender role and bound his breasts. Although Jamie's mental health had improved, his interpersonal functioning remained impaired. Therefore, once he met the WPATH *Standards of Care*, a competency evaluation was conducted determin-ing that Jamie was competent to make an informed decision about chest surgery.

Jamie did not want to wait the two years required for public health coverage for chest surgery and saved every penny to pay privately. Upon its completion, he was visibly relieved and became more and more comfortable with himself. Subsequently, he requested support for hormone therapy. Because several clients with similar mental health concerns had destabilized after starting testosterone therapy, the possibility of this happening was discussed with Jamie. On the basis of this information, he decided to forego hormone therapy as he did not want to take the risk that his mental health would deteriorate. Jamie subsequently left home and fulfilled his life-long dream of moving to an area with a warmer climate. Since he left, he has kept his therapist informed of his whereabouts and appears to be content and doing well.

Patricia (Male-to-Female)

Patricia (age 19) was referred for assessment by her family physician. Patricia had researched the referral process via the Internet, where she spent most of her time. Since junior high school she had had few friends, socializing primarily on-line where she adopted a female identity. The diagnosis of Asperger's Disorder became obvious after the first two or three sessions; unfortunately, this had not been detected earlier by the school or the family physician.

Patricia's mental health history included two bouts of depression in her mid-teens which were treated with an antidepressant. She was also hospitalized on one occasion after a suicide attempt. There was no history of abuse but the mother left the father because of his alcohol dependence. Patricia denied using alcohol and drugs.

The most difficult task was to assess the degree of gender dysphoria or to diagnose Gender Identity Disorder as Patricia's ability to participate in the interview was limited. This was somewhat remedied by asking her to write about her process. With her permission, we also interviewed family members and a school guidance counselor for collateral information.

Patricia graduated from high school with an opportunity to study computing science at a university. She wanted to go to the university as a woman, and began her real-life experience in the summer prior to starting college on hormone therapy in the fall. She presented to therapy in clothing that was feminine but a few years younger than her peers would have been wearing. However, as time passed, her clothing became more age-appropriate. Although she did not pass well, this did not seem to be of concern to Patricia in terms of her identity or general social acceptance. She was, however, concerned with the potential for violence perpetrated against her.

Throughout the course of treatment Patricia continued to live at home with her mother and doing casual work repairing computers. She did not socialize any more than she used to but felt more content with her life. She continued to spend much time on the computer, and attended college on a part-time basis. There was no recurrence of the depressive episodes or suicide attempts. Therapy sessions continued to be therapist-driven with little input from Patricia; however, she continued to dialogue with the therapist through computer assignments. She went on to complete two years of "real life experience" and subsequently had genital surgery.

APPENDIX B. Sample Gender Assessments

All clinician and client names in the sample assessments are fictional, as are the depicted client characteristics. They are included for illustrative purposes only.

Female-to-Male Sample Assessment

Dear Dr. Smith:
Re: Majida Khattari
DOB: August 10, 1952
Reason for Referral: Client is a 52-year-old natal female who identifies as a man and who hopes to have a bilateral mastectomy/chest reconstruction surgery as part of gender transition.

Thank you for asking me to see your 52-year-old patient in consultation. The following letter represents a summary of my assessment of Majida over three sessions (November 14, December 12, and January 31). Majida was referred to me for gender assessment and to assess eligibility and readiness for chest surgery.

History of Gender Identity

Out of deference to Majida's gender identity, I will use male pronouns throughout this assessment. Majida has been masculine since early childhood. His preferred playmates were boys and his preferred games involved physical activities with boys such as football and hockey. As a child, he wore unisex or boys' clothing. He was often perceived as a boy by strangers and by teachers.

As puberty commenced, Majida remembers his male friends becoming uncomfortable with his masculine appearance, and less interested in spending time with him. To fit in, Majida began growing his hair, wearing make-up and more feminine clothing, and attempting to socialize with teenage girls and date boys. Romantic attempts with males were unsatisfying as he was not interested in boys in a sexual context, although he continued to prefer the social company of men.

In 1975 Majida began working at a mattress factory and became friends with a co-worker who was a butch lesbian. Majida became involved in the local lesbian community, participating in dances and other social events, and dating women. He returned to dressing in a more masculine fashion, and came out to his family as lesbian. He remembers this as an exciting time of self-discovery and clarity relating to his identity.

In recent years, through supporting some of his butch friends through their process of exploring their gender identity and options for gender transition, Majida came to realize that his self-concept is more of himself as a man in a female body rather than a masculine female. In his current life Majida avoids situations such as swimming that would require him to reveal his female body. In his sexual relations he does not remove his top, and imagines himself as having a male body. He binds his breasts using a spandex back brace.

As a very masculine-appearing person, Majida feels little dissonance between his identity and his role. However, to facilitate his comfort he would like to pursue chest reconstruction. He is not interested in testosterone as he has a history of chronic liver disease, and feels the risks of side effects would outweigh the possible benefits. Additionally, he has already gone through menopause so no longer feels any discomfort relating to menstruation.

Majida has a strong supportive circle around him. He has told many of his friends of his transgendered feelings and has received positive feedback.

Medical History

1. cigarette smoking–25 years, currently one pack a day
2. obesity
3. Hepatitis C

Medications

1. has taken interferon for Hepatitis C–not currently taking any medication
2. no known drug allergies

Mental Health History

Majida sought counseling in 1992 to deal with issues relating to being molested by a neighbor at age 10. He reports being depressed and suicidal at that time, but having stable mental health in the years since.

Substance Use

Majida started drinking alcohol at parties in high school and continued to drink recreationally through the 1980s and early 1990s. In the mid-1980s he experimented with amphetamines to assist in working night shifts. His use gradually increased and he reports being addicted for several years. He went through an amphetamine addiction program in 1991 and has not been using recreational drugs since that time. In 1993 he was diagnosed with Hepatitis C and has not been drinking alcohol since that time. He typically smokes one pack of cigarettes and drinks several cups of coffee per day.

Personal History

Majida was born and raised in Nanaimo. He has two younger twin brothers age 42, and an older sister age 53. His parents and grandparents are deceased. As a child Majida spent much time with his family fishing, camping, and playing sports. As both his parents worked during Majida's childhood, his grandparents and aunt were primary caregivers. He remains close with his aunt.

Majida began his career doing heavy physical labor in factories in the 1980s. In the late 1980s he lost his job as the result of difficulties relating to amphetamine addiction, and made his living through selling drugs. In the early 1990s after going through an addiction program he started driving taxis. Fatigue related to Hepatitis C has become increasingly debilitating and Majida is no longer able to work. He is currently receiving disability benefits through the Ministry of Human Resources.

Majida has had sexual relationships in the past but is not dating at this time. He is sexually attracted to women.

Summary and Treatment Plan

Majida does not experience clinically significant distress relating to his gender role or gender identity, as his physical masculinity has enabled him to live in a way that is congruent with his strong masculine identity. However, Majida does report distress relating to his female body. Specifically, he feels he would be more comfortable with a more masculine appearing chest and that it would enable him to be more comfortable in sexual relations and other activities that may involve disrobing. Majida is a mature individual who has carefully considered the pros and cons of surgical intervention, and he has been cross-living for many years. In my opinion, Majida meets both the eligibility and readiness criteria of the World Professional Association for Transgender Health *Standards of Care*. I do not find any mental health considerations that would negatively impact his ability to make an informed decision regarding chest surgery.

Please do not hesitate to contact me with any questions you may have.

Male-to-Female Sample Assessment

Dear Dr. Smith:
Re: Sandeep Singh
DOB: January 15, 1970
Reason for Referral: Client is a 34-year-old natal male who identifies as a woman and is seeking assistance to resolve gender confusion.

Thank you for asking me to see your patient in consultation. I saw Sandeep on three occasions (January 12, February 2, and February 20, 2005) and the following letter represents a summary of these sessions.

Sandeep is a 34-year-old anatomical male who identifies as a woman (out of deference for her gender preference I will refer to her as "she" throughout this letter). Sandeep is a 34-year-old agricultural worker who has been married for 15 years and has two daughters age 8 and 11. Her wife Parmit works as a school teacher. Sandeep presents today wanting to explore options for resolution of her gender confusion.

History of Gender Identity

Sandeep was the youngest child in a family of four, with three older sisters. As a young child, she lived in a rural area of the Fraser Valley and played most of the time with her sisters. All of the children in the family were expected to participate in helping the mother work at a berry farm on the weekends, while the father worked in a local lumber mill.

At age 8, Sandeep began wearing female undergarments under her clothes to school. She was afraid of being caught with these articles on, and tried to either avoid physical education class or change in the cubicle. As she went through puberty, she was very distressed by the erections and nocturnal emissions she experienced, and started to tape down her penis.

At age 19, Sandeep married Parmit, and did not discuss any of the crossdressing activity or gender identity concerns with her. Sandeep put all of her energies into her work and family in hope that her feelings about being a woman would disappear. Four years into the marriage, Sandeep and Parmit had a daughter and Sandeep wished that she would have been the one to bear the child. Both were happy in the parenting role, and they had another child three years later. Throughout this time Sandeep continued to crossdress in private, and continued to struggle with feeling a conflict between her public life as a man and her private identity as a woman.

Shortly after the birth of their second child, Sandeep's mother was diagnosed with breast cancer and died within a year of the diagnosis. The time with her mother prior to her death made Sandeep re-evaluate her life, and she disclosed both the crossdressing and her conflict over her identity to her wife. Parmit was very angry and upset but did not want to lose Sandeep as her partner and wanted the family to remain together. They sought counseling and Parmit decided that she would not be able to stay with Sandeep if she were to live her public life as a woman. Sandeep at this time also did not want to lose the family and so she continued to crossdress in private for the next six years. As time progressed, she realized that she did not want to continue living as she was, and so she is presenting today with hopes of discussing her marital situation as well as getting information about options for transition.

Medical History

1. Tonsillectomy at age 9

Medications

1. No medications
2. No known drug allergies

Substance Use

Sandeep reports not smoking, drinking alcohol or caffeinated drinks, or using recreational drugs.

Mental Health History

Sandeep suffered from depression after the death of her mother and was treated with sertraline for one year, after which time the depression had been alleviated sufficiently to stop this medication.

Personal History

Sandeep started school when she was 6 years old. She remembers disliking school as the few Sikhs in the class were frequently teased by the White boys. She left school at age 15 to work full-time.

Sandeep has been close to her three sisters throughout her life, and maintains a close connection to them and to their families. None of them are aware of Sandeep's gender identity concerns. Sandeep is not currently close with her father. She has always found it difficult to connect emotionally with him, and in recent years the father has become more reclusive following the death of his wife.

Sandeep has little connection with the transgender community as she lives in a rural area where there are no peer support groups. She has seen a documentary on transsexuals and would like to explore the possibility of hormones and surgery. She does not have any detailed information at this time relating to either option, nor is she certain what she wants to pursue.

Summary and Treatment Plan

Sandeep is a 34-year-old anatomical male who identifies as a woman. She presents with a history of strong and persistent cross-gender identification, persistent discomfort in the male gender role, and clinically significant distress relating to her gender concerns. She has limited support from the people around her, who are either unaware of her gender identity or are opposed to her transition. She presents today to obtain information about hormones and transitioning but is reluctant to move forward at this time, particularly until an agreement is made with her wife relating to their marriage. She agrees that it is premature at this time to consider hormone therapy and will enter a course of relationship counseling that will hopefully include her wife Parmit.

Please do not hesitate to contact me with any questions you may have.

APPENDIX C. Sample Letter to Client Prior to Assessment for Hormone Therapy

Dear client:

This letter is intended to explain what to expect from the hormone eligibility and readiness assessment process and help you prepare for the first appointment.

Purpose of the Assessment

The clinician providing the assessment will:

1. Determine whether you meet the eligibility and readiness criteria for hormone therapy outlined in the current version of the World Professional Association for Transgender Health (WPATH)'s *Standards of Care*.

2. Make a recommendation to the prescribing physician about whether or not they feel hormone therapy is appropriate in your treatment.

Eligibility Criteria

1. Able to provide fully informed consent to medical treatment.
2. Demonstrable knowledge of what hormones medically can and cannot do and their social benefits and risks.
3. Either a documented "real life experience" of at least three months prior to the administration of hormones, OR a period of psychotherapy of a duration specified by the mental health professional after the initial evaluation. This may be waived in some special situations.

Readiness Criteria

1. Further consolidation of gender identity during the real-life experience or psychotherapy.
2. Progress in mastering other identified problems, leading to improving or continuing stable mental health.
3. Likelihood of taking hormones in a responsible manner.

Assessment Sessions

Appointments are 50 minutes long. Assessment may take one or more appointments to complete. Discussion topics may include:

- general personal history: who you are, home life, what you do during the day, education, work, friends, family, hobbies, interests
- history of gender identity concerns, from start to present day
- medical and mental health history, including medications taken in past/present
- substance use history
- gender transition process thus far, and future plans
- any questions or concerns you have

Documentation to Bring to First Session

You will need to bring your health insurance card and picture identification (e.g., passport, driver's license). The picture identification is necessary to confirm that you are the person being assessed. It is not required that you have had a legal name change, but if you have, please bring documentation of this name change.

If you want assistance with documentation or support relating to the assessment process, peer support and advocacy groups are listed below.

APPENDIX D. Sample Letter to Client Seeking Sex Reassignment Surgery

Dear client:

This letter is intended to explain what to expect from the surgery eligibility and readiness assessment process and help you prepare for the first appointment.

Purpose of the Assessment

The clinician providing the assessment will:

1. Determine whether you meet the eligibility and readiness criteria for sex reassignment surgery outlined in the current version of The World Professional Association for Transgender Health (WPATH)'s *Standards of Care*.
2. Make a recommendation to the surgeon about whether or not they feel surgery is appropriate in your treatment.

Eligibility Criteria

For all types of sex reassignment surgery:

1. Able to provide fully informed consent to medical treatment.
2. Demonstrable knowledge of what sex reassignment surgery medically can and cannot do; potential benefits, risks, and complications; approximate cost; expected time in hospital; aftercare requirements; and surgeon options.

For female-to-male (FTM) chest surgery, assessment by one mental health professional who meets the competency requirements outlined in the WPATH *Standards of Care* is sufficient. In addition to the general criteria, FTM transgender persons seeking chest surgery must:

3. Have completed either a documented real-life experience of at least 3 months prior to chest surgery, OR a period of psychotherapy of a duration specified by the mental health professional after the initial evaluation.

For male-to-female (MTF) breast surgery, assessment by one mental health professional who meets the competency requirements outlined in the

WPATH *Standards of Care* is sufficient. In addition to the general criteria, MTF transgender persons seeking breast augmentation must:

3. Have completed either a documented "real-life experience" of at least 3 months prior to breast surgery, OR a period of psychotherapy of a duration specified by the mental health professional after the initial evaluation.
4. Have taken feminizing hormones for at least 18 months before surgery to allow for maximal hormonal breast growth, unless there are medical contraindications to hormone therapy.

For genital surgery (FTM or MTF) or removal of the ovaries and uterus (FTM), assessment by two mental health professionals who meet the competency requirements outlined in the WPATH *Standards of Care* is required. In addition to the general criteria, individuals seeking "lower surgery" must have:

3. Completed at least 1 year "real life experience" (RLE).
4. Taken hormones continuously for at least 12 months, unless there are medical contraindications to hormone therapy.
5. Completed any psychotherapy required by the mental health assessor.

Readiness Criteria

1. Further consolidation of gender identity during the real-life experience or psychotherapy.
2. Progress in mastering other identified problems, leading to improving or continuing stable mental health.

Number of Sessions

Appointments usually are 50 minutes long. Assessment may take one or more appointments to complete. Discussion topics may include:

- general personal history: who you are, who you live with, what you do during the day, education, work, friends, hobbies, interests
- history of gender identity concerns, from start to present day
- medical and mental health history, including medications taken in past/present
- substance use history
- gender transition process thus far, and future plans
- any questions or concerns you have

Documentation to Bring to First Session

You will need to bring your health insurance card and picture identification (e.g., passport, driver's license). The picture identification is necessary to confirm that you are the person being assessed. It is not required that you have had a legal name change, but if you have, bring your documentation of this name change.

If you have completed "real life experience" (i.e., living as the gender you identify as), it is helpful to bring documents to confirm the length of time that you have done this. For example:

- Pay stubs or a letter from your supervisor indicating the length of time you have been employed
- A letter from your academic advisor or teacher indicating the length of time you have been in school, and/or a school transcript
- A letter from your supervisor in a volunteer position indicating the length of time you have been involved in volunteering
- If you are unable to work, attend school, or volunteer, bring a letter from your doctor explaining your circumstances and confirming that to the best of their knowledge you are living full-time in the gender you identify as

It is not necessary to disclose your gender history to your employer, teacher, or supervisor: you can tell them you need a general reference letter without saying what it is for. The letter can be a short statement that includes your name, the gender pronoun you are called, and the length of time you have been working, volunteering, in school. For example:

- "I have known John Doe for two years. He began work for me on (date) and has worked full-time since then."
- "Jane Doe has volunteered ten hours a week for (name of organization) for over two years. She began as a volunteer here on (date)."
- "Jan Doe has been taking a full academic courseload since (date)."

If you wish, you can include letters from friends, relatives, neighbors, or others who you interact with socially as additional evidence of completion of the real life experience.

Letters must be *signed originals*, and transcripts or pay stubs must be original copies. We encourage you to make a photocopy of all documents for your records prior to the appointment, as the originals will be kept in your file.

If you want assistance with documentation or support relating to the assessment process, peer support and advocacy groups are listed below.

APPENDIX E. Sample Letter to Prescribing Clinician, Recommending Hormone Therapy

All clinician and client names are fictional, as are the depicted client characteristics. They are included for illustrative purposes only.

Dear Dr. Smith:
Re: Saul Cohen (a.k.a. Sarah Cohen)
DOB: April 23, 1980
Reason for Referral: Client is a 23-year-old natal female who identifies as a man and seeks medically monitored testosterone therapy as part of gender transition.

I am writing to support my client's request for testosterone therapy. Saul (whose legal name is Sarah) is a 23-year-old anatomical female who identifies as a man. He has been my client since January 12, 2003 when he sought my services to assess for suitability for hormone prescription as part of gender transition. I am a registered clinical counselor in private practice, working with other professionals who have an interest in transgender health but not as part of a formal gender team.

I have seen Mr. Cohen in two 50-minute counseling sessions. In those sessions we have discussed Saul's gender identity, as well as his overall psychosocial history and current status. I note that Saul does not see his identity as a type of mental illness and thus does not want to be labeled as having Gender Identity Disorder, despite having a strong cross-gender identity.

In the last year Saul has come to strongly identify as a gay man. For the past 2 months has been taking testosterone he purchased from the Internet, to alleviate discomfort he feels when he is perceived as a woman and also to change his voice and appearance to be more congruent with his sense of self. Thus far Saul reports a deepened voice, enlarged and sensitized clitoris, heightened libido, and acne as a result of the testosterone he has taken. Saul is pleased by these changes and is eager for other changes, particularly cessation of menses and growth of facial hair. He cannot currently afford to legally change his name from Sarah to Saul, but does prefer that Saul be used.

Saul is aware of the risks of taking testosterone without medical assistance, and wishes to have regular medical monitoring from this point onward. According to Saul, he started taking testosterone without medical assistance because there was a lengthy wait to see a family physician with expertise in transgender medicine.

Saul is well-informed about the female-to-male (FTM) community, having read several articles on hormonal and surgical options (including the World Professional Association for Transgender Health's *Standards of Care*) and also participating in a FTM Internet mailing list. I believe that Saul understands his options for peer and professional support should he need assistance to adjust to any of the changes that occur as a result of taking testosterone.

In closing, while Saul has not yet been cross-living or attending psychotherapy for the full 3 months recommended in the World Professional Association for Transgender Health's *Standards of Care*, I am confident that he does meet the other eligibility and readiness criteria defined in the *Standards of Care*, and I believe it would be beneficial for him to move from medically unsupervised use to medically supported use of testosterone. I feel confident that Saul understands the permanence of continuing to take testosterone, and that he will take hormones in a responsible manner.

If you have any questions or concerns, please do not hesitate to contact me.

APPENDIX F. Sample Letter to Surgeon, Recommending Sex Reassignment Surgery

All clinician and client names are fictional, as are the depicted client characteristics. They are included for illustrative purposes only.

Dear Dr. Smith:
Re: Shirley Alexander
DOB: September 9, 1959
Reason for Referral: Client is a 45-year-old natal male who identifies as a woman and who hopes to have vaginoplasty as part of gender transition.

This letter will introduce Ms. Shirley Alexander, a 45-year-old anatomical male who identifies as a woman, whom I would like to refer for vaginoplasty as part of sex reassignment. Ms. Alexander has been my client since January 2, 2003 when she was referred to me by her family physician. I am a psychiatrist in private practice, working with other professionals who have an interest in transgender health but not as part of a formal gender team.

After an initial assessment of three sessions, I diagnosed Ms. Alexander with Gender Identity Disorder. Since then I have been seeing her every three weeks and she has been engaged in therapy focusing on family of origin issues.

Ms. Alexander began facial electrolysis in May 2002, and with the support of her family physician (Dr. John Bigelow) was started on feminizing hormone therapy by endocrinologist Dr. Doris Reinbolt on April 1, 2003. She began her "real life experience" May 15, 2003, and her legal name change was granted June 15, 2003. Psychologist Dr. Robert Jones completed a second assessment on April 3, 2005 and concurred with my initial diagnosis. Contact information for all professionals involved in Ms. Alexander's care relating to Gender Identity Disorder is included at the end of this letter; if you have not already received reports from them, you should be receiving them soon.

Past medical history includes Type II diabetes (controlled by diet and exercise), exercise-induced asthma, ankle fracture at age 11, and an appendectomy at age 10. Ms. Alexander is physically fit and is a non-smoker. Current medications include transdermal estradiol patch (0.2 mg/24 hours, applied twice per week), spironolactone 300 mg po daily, and ventolin inhaler PRN. She has no known drug allergies.

In closing, Ms. Alexander meets the criteria for Gender Identity Disorder. She has been living as a woman full-time for over two years and has adjusted well to this role. I have discussed the risks and benefits of vaginoplasty with Shirley and feel confident that she understands the seriousness and permanence of the surgery. I also feel confident that she will undertake the appropriate self-care that is necessary after vaginoplasty.

If you have any questions or concerns, please do not hesitate to contact me.

Clinical Management of Gender Dysphoria in Adolescents

Annelou L. C. de Vries, MD, PhD
Peggy T. Cohen-Kettenis, PhD
Henriette Delemarre-van de Waal, MD, PhD

SUMMARY. This paper aims to provide professionals working with adolescents with gender-dysphoric feelings practical clinical guidelines for diagnosis and treatment. The different phases of the assessment procedure and treatment process are described. Differential diagnostic considerations and possible psychotherapeutic treatment options are given. Physical interventions, including GnRH analogues to inhibit puberty and cross-sex hormones, are described with consideration of eligibility and readiness issues. We end with discussion of post-treatment evaluation. doi:10.1300/J485v09n03_04 *[Article copies available for a fee from The Haworth Document Delivery Service: 1-800-HAWORTH. E-mail address: <docdelivery@haworthpress.com> Website: <http://www. HaworthPress.com> © 2006 by The Haworth Press, Inc. All rights reserved.]*

KEYWORDS. Gender identity disorder, gender dysphoria, adolescents, clinical guidelines, treatment

This chapter aims to provide professionals working with adolescents with gender-dysphoric feelings practical clinical guidelines for diagnosis and treatment. *Gender dysphoria* refers to distress caused by discrepancy between sense of self (gender identity) and the aspects of the body associated with sex/gender, other people's misidentification of one's gender, and the social roles associated with gender (Fisk, 1973). Apart from psychotherapy or other psychological interventions, treatment may include hormonal intervention, surgery, or other *sex reassignment* procedures to feminize/masculinize primary or secondary sexual characteristics to facilitate ease with self and presentation congruent with identity.

Ideally, work with gender dysphoric adolescents is done by a team of professionals from various disciplines, such as adolescent psychiatry and clinical psychology, psychotherapy, family therapy, and pediatric endocrinology. Clinicians who diagnose and treat gender

Annelou L. C. de Vries, MD, PhD, Peggy T. Cohen-Kettenis, PhD, and Henriette Delemarre-van de Waal, MD, PhD, are affiliated with the Vrije Universiteit Medical Center.

Address correspondence to: Dr. Annelou L. C. de Vries, Department of Medical Psychology, PO Box 7057, 1007 MB Amsterdam, The Netherlands (E-mail: alc.devries@vumc.nl).

This manuscript was created for the Trans Care Project, a joint initiative of Transcend Transgender Support & Education Society and Vancouver Coastal Health's Transgender Health Program, with funding from the Canadian Rainbow Health Coalition. The authors would like to thank Sheila Kelton, Roey Malleson, Gerald P. Mallon, Edgardo J. Menvielle, Daniel L. Metzger, Jorge L. Pinzon, and Wallace Wong for comments on an earlier draft.

[Haworth co-indexing entry note]: "Clinical Management of Gender Dysphoria in Adolescents." de Vries, Annelou L. C., Peggy T. Cohen-Kettenis, and Henriette Delemarre-van de Waal. Co-published simultaneously in *International Journal of Transgenderism* (The Haworth Medical Press, an imprint of The Haworth Press, Inc.) Vol. 9, No. 3/4, 2006, pp. 83-94; and: *Guidelines for Transgender Care* (ed: Walter O. Bockting, and Joshua M. Goldberg) The Haworth Medical Press, an imprint of The Haworth Press, Inc., 2006, pp. 83-94. Single or multiple copies of this article are available for a fee from The Haworth Document Delivery Service [1-800-HAWORTH, 9:00 a.m. - 5:00 p.m. (EST). E-mail address: docdelivery@haworthpress.com].

dysphoric adolescents should have training in adolescent psychiatry or clinical psychology and experience diagnosing and treating the ordinary problems of adolescents (Meyer et al., 2001). The clinician must also be knowledgeable about transgender identity development, and the specialized counseling needs of family members and other significant others, as discussed in general terms elsewhere (Bockting, Knudson, & Goldberg, 2006). This document focuses on the specific issues involved in care of adolescents.

First, we will describe the different phases of the assessment procedure and treatment process. Differential diagnostic considerations and possible psychotherapeutic treatment options are given. Physical interventions, including GnRH analogues to inhibit puberty and cross-sex hormones, are described with consideration of eligibility and readiness issues. We end with discussion of post-treatment evaluation.

The recommendations in this document are based on published literature and the authors' clinical experience. These guidelines are consistent with but not entirely similar to the *Standards of Care* of the World Professional Association for Transgender Health (Meyer et al., 2001) and the Royal College of Psychiatrists' guidelines for management of gender identity disorders in adolescents (Di Ceglie, Sturge, & Sutton, 1998). This document expands on both of these previously published works, including discussion of early diagnosis and intervention. Results of a May 2005 consensus meeting of pediatric endocrinologists, child psychologists, child psychiatrists, and ethicists (from Australia, North America, and Europe) on the hormonal treatment of gender dysphoric adolescents are incorporated (Gender Identity Research and Education Society, 2005). Ongoing interdisciplinary research and collegial meetings are important in further developing practice protocols.

CLINICAL PICTURE

Prevalence data are lacking for prepubertal children. Most epidemiological studies include older adolescents, but no separate data exist for this age group.

The clinician should be aware of the different sex ratios according to age. The majority of the prepubertal children attending gender clinics are biological males; this is believed to be primarily due to lower social acceptability of cross-gender behaviour in boys than in girls (Bradley & Zucker, 1997). The sex ratio of adolescents, however, approaches a 1:1 relationship.

Not all prepubertal children with gender concerns will seek sex reassignment after puberty. Unlike adolescent Gender Identity Disorder (American Psychiatric Association, 2000), Gender Identity Disorder (GID) in childhood is believed to be more strongly predictive of homosexuality than transsexualism (Bradley & Zucker, 1997). So a clinician meeting a child with GID is more likely seeing a future gay/lesbian than a future transsexual. Additionally, while adolescents with GID have usually had gender concerns since childhood, not all children with GID continue to have gender concerns in adolescence or adulthood (Zucker & Bradley, 1995). For this reason, it is important to understand the clinical picture for adolescents who may be in need of intervention, and to make a distinction between prepubertal children and adolescents.

Adolescents who seek treatment for gender dysphoria have often shown signs of gender dysphoria from very early in age. They may have repeatedly stated that they were members of the other sex, have had cross-gender preferences, and have been unhappy if not allowed to act on these preferences. When older, but still prepubertal, they might have stopped talking about their cross-gender feelings out of shame, and might also have shown less cross-gender behaviours in an attempt to conform to societal norms. Biological males who look or behave feminine are frequently teased or bullied, which increases the risk of developing social or other problems. Biological females who look or behave masculine tend to be less ostracized and teased in childhood, as cross-gender behaviour is far more accepted in girls than in boys (Cohen-Kettenis & Pfäfflin, 2003).

Adolescents with gender dysphoria may suffer deeply from fears relating to the physical changes of puberty or, for older adolescents, distress relating to the changes already experienced in puberty. Some already cross-live by the time they seek sex reassignment and take age-appropriate developmental steps (e.g. dating). Other adolescents try to conform to gender typical norms, behaving as inconspicuously as possible.

Although many gender dysphoric adolescents who seek treatment already have a strong and persistent wish for sex reassignment, it is important to note that these adolescents are a *heterogeneous* group who may:

- request sex reassignment but have ambivalence about it
- express a strong wish for sex reassignment during the intake phase, but change their minds later
- have no real sex reassignment request, but are merely confused about their gender feelings
- have gender concerns secondary to a co-existing condition (e.g., pervasive developmental disorder)

THE DESIRABILITY OF SEX REASSIGNMENT FOR ADOLESCENTS: THREE VIEWS

The desirability of sex reassignment as a resolution for the psychological suffering of people with gender dysphoria, has, irrespective of the person's age, been controversial since the first surgeries were performed. Because gender identity seems to be fixed in most individuals after puberty, and psychological treatments are not particularly successful in changing gender identity once it is consolidated, changing the body to match the identity is often the treatment of choice for very gender dysphoric adults.

As discussed earlier, the outcome for children with gender concerns is far more variable than for adults (i.e., some have gender dysphoria that resolves spontaneously as the child ages). Additionally, it is extremely important to take into account that children and adolescents are in a rapidly changing developmental process. For this reason, there is clinical consensus that pre-pubertal children with GID should not be offered any physical treatment–although psychotherapy may be indicated (Cohen-Kettenis & Pfäfflin, 2003)–and that surgery should not be performed before the age of 18. Although ex-

perts agree that mental or emotional maturity would probably be a more appropriate criterion for determining surgery eligibility than setting an arbitrary age, at this time there are no clear and objective criteria for how to define and assess readiness for sex reassignment surgery in adolescents. Because of the current stage of knowledge regarding the effects of irreversible interventions, most professionals consider it premature to perform surgery before the age of 18, irrespective of legislation in some regions relating to adolescent competence to make decisions relating to medical care.

At the aforementioned expert-meeting in London (Gender Identity Research and Education Society, 2005) it became clear that three different views exist on the hormonal treatment for adolescents between the ages of 12 and 18 who are seeking sex reassignment:

1. *No physical treatment, including hormones, should be given before legal adulthood* (defined by most countries as 18 years of age). Clinicians holding this view argue that adolescents should experience all physical puberty stages and fully experience their adult physical characteristics. Only then are they believed to be able to fully appreciate their gender identity and capable of deciding on any physical treatment (Meyenburg, 1994).

2. *Adolescents should experience puberty at least to Tanner Stage 4 or 5* (typically 15-16 years of age). They are eligible for GnRH analogues if they fulfill the DSM-IV criteria for GID, have had a strong cross-gender identity from an early age, are psychologically relatively stable, and live in a supportive environment (Cohen-Kettenis & Pfäfflin, 2003; Cohen-Kettenis & Van Goozen, 1998). At this time GnRH analogues may be given to prevent further pubertal physical development, and cross-sex hormones might or might not be added soon after (Viner, Brain, Carmichael, & Di Ceglie, 2005). Studies on the effects of this treatment policy show good results with disappearance of the gender dysphoric feelings, no regret relating to the reassignment, and psychological well-being in the normal range (Smith, Van Goozen, & Cohen-Kettenis, 2001).

3. *Adolescents may be eligible for hormonal suppression of puberty after Tanner Stage 2 or 3* (typically 12-13 years of age) if they fulfill the DSM-IV criteria for GID, have had a strong cross-gender identity from an early age, are psychologically relatively stable, and live in a supportive environment (Cohen-Kettenis & Pfäfflin, 2003; Cohen-Kettenis & Van Goozen, 1998). Because thus far little is known about the psychological effects of pubertal sex hormones in adolescents with GID, the current policy is to start pubertal suppression only after Tanner Stage 2 or 3 has been reached.

There are several advantages for adolescents with GID receiving puberty-inhibiting hormones (Cohen-Kettenis & Van Goozen, 1998). First, it is a fully reversible process: if there is a change of mind during the process, the pubertal delay can be brought to end and the patient can continue to live in the gender role associated with phenotypic sex. Second, psychotherapy to more deeply explore gender concerns is easier if puberty is delayed, because the adolescent is free of fear of further physical development and has more psychological room to explore the inner world. Third, the delay provides more time to decide upon further treatment without having to commit to cross-gender living (although some already choose to do so and are able to function quite well). It has been our experience that whether the young adolescent is already cross-living or not, in both cases the chance of developmental problems and reactive depressive symptoms seems to diminish with this early intervention. Fourth, the suppression of puberty is considered as a useful aid in the diagnostic procedure: i.e., if the distress is eased by suppression of pubertal changes, this suggests that gender dysphoria is a primary cause of the distress. Fifth, for those who do go on to a full transition, the prevention of the development of unwanted and irreversible (after Tanner Stage 2 or 3) changes in secondary sex characteristics typically means less medical intervention is needed to remove these features

(as is the case when interventions start later in life).

These different views on hormonal treatment are rooted in large part in varying perceptions of adolescence and puberty. A decision about which to adhere to depends on the individual adolescent, the guiding principles of the institution or system in which a clinician works, and the personal view of the clinician. In every case a thoughtful decision should be made about what is best to offer the adolescent. In our clinical experience it is clear that waiting until the age of 18 for any physical treatment is not an option for adolescents with severe gender dysphoria, although it can be a reasonable course of action in other cases and may be the only option if the clinical picture is so complicated by co-existing conditions that a clear diagnosis cannot be made. The decision to postpone medical treatment until an adolescent with GID has experienced either puberty Tanner Stage 2 or 3 or puberty Tanner Stage 4 or 5 has to be made in the absence of objective criteria and consensus among professionals.

THE PROCEDURE: DIAGNOSTIC ASSESSMENT AND TREATMENT

Although most cross-gendered adolescents come to clinics with a straightforward wish for sex reassignment, some have more open questions regarding their identity. In every adolescent the gender problem and potential underlying or related problems have to be examined comprehensively in the diagnostic phase.

The First (Diagnostic) Phase

Procedure

In this phase, information is obtained from both the adolescent and the parents/guardians on various aspects of the general and psychosexual development of the adolescent. Current cross-gender feelings and behaviour, current school functioning, peer relations, and family functioning have to be assessed (Goldenring & Rosen, 2004). With regards to sexuality, the subjective meaning of crossdressing, the type of crossdressing, sexual experiences, sexual behaviour and fantasies, sexual attractions, and body image should be explored.

In this diagnostic phase, the adolescent also has to be thoroughly informed about the possibilities and limitations of sex reassignment and other kinds of treatment to prevent unrealistically high expectations. This information is best given soon after the first sessions if the youth presents with a strong wish for sex reassignment. If the youth presents with confusion/ambivalence, or has gender problems but is not interested in sex reassignment, information on sex reassignment is postponed until this seems to become a realistic option. The way a patient responds to their understanding of the reality of sex reassignment can be informative diagnostically.

It is important to realize that even extremely cross-gender identified adolescents may lack the support or psychological resilience to handle the drastic life changes that accompany sex reassignment. Thus one should take potential psychological and social risk factors into account when making decisions relating to appropriateness of early interventions.

Instruments

Most instruments that measure aspects of GID have been developed for adults. Specific instruments that can also be used for adolescents are scarce. Some experience exists with the *Utrecht Gender Dysphoria Scale* (Cohen-Kettenis & Van Goozen, 1997), which is a short questionnaire dealing with the distress persons feel when confronted in daily life with the fact that they belong to their biological sex (see Appendix A). *The Body Image Scale* (Lindgren & Pauly, 1975), on which an individual can mark satisfaction with many different body parts as well as a wish to change these body parts, can be used. A *Gender Identity Questionnaire* for adolescents has been developed by Zucker et al. (2005), consisting of questions concerning cross-sex behaviour and gender identity in the last 12 months and over the entire lifetime. On the *Draw-a-Person* test (Rekers, Rosen, & Morey, 1990), both children and adolescents with GID usually draw a person of their wished (other) sex first when asked to draw a person. This last instrument is primarily interesting because of its qualitative information, but it is not a diagnostic instrument with good psychometric properties. (For a recent review of mea-

surements of gender identity and gender role at various ages, see Zucker, 2005.) Besides these specific instruments, regular instruments (personality scales, structured psychiatric interviews, intelligence tests) are also needed for the assessment of the adolescent's intellectual, emotional, and social strengths and weaknesses.

Differential Diagnosis

As noted before, not all adolescents with gender concerns have a clear and explicit wish for sex reassignment. Some may simply be confused regarding aspects of their gender. For example, some young gays/lesbians/bisexuals have a history of cross-gender interests and behaviours (Green, 1987; Rottnek, 1999) and may have difficulty distinguishing sexual orientation issues from gender concerns. Individuals with transient stress-related crossdressing (crossdressing used in a ritualized fashion to alleviate stress) or compulsive crossdressing (for sexual or other reasons) may mistake their interest in crossdressing for a need for sex reassignment. This may also happen in patients suffering from severe psychiatric conditions (e.g., schizophrenia), accompanied by delusions of belonging to the other sex.

In cases involving confusion about gender feelings, psychotherapy and peer support can be helpful in resolving the confusion and coming to self-acceptance. If the wish for sex reassignment exists in an adolescent who has been extremely cross-gendered from early on and still exists after the other problems are adequately treated, it is likely the GID and other psychological problems co-occur. However, in cases of severe psychopathology one should be even more careful with sex reassignment than in other cases. Typically sex reassignment is postponed until a clear clinical picture emerges. In practice, this may imply that interventions do not take place before adulthood, to allow the evolution of the course of the psychiatric disorder and the level of psychosocial functioning to be evaluated over time.

Some individuals with gender dysphoria do not seek complete sex reassignment. Instead they try to integrate masculine and feminine aspects of the self, adopting an androgynous or bi-gendered form of expression. In such cases hormones or some form of surgery may be sought to minimize existing masculine or feminine physiologic characteristics (rather than to promote cross-sex development). In the experience of most clinicians, however, such a treatment wish is rare in adolescents. This might be because people who experience onset at earlier ages typically have more severe and extreme forms of gender dysphoria. Because the normal developmental process of adolescence often involves experimentation relating to identity and self-expression, caution is indicated if an adolescent presents seeking partial change.

The Second Phase: "Real Life Experience" and Treatment

As explained earlier, different views exist about the appropriate age for initiation of sex reassignment. In each individual case, it is key to decide whether early physical treatment will be beneficial or that the risk of regret or adverse outcome will be too high. Adolescents who are merely gender-confused or whose wish for sex reassignment seems to originate from factors other than a genuine and complete cross-gender identity are served best by psychological interventions. Even in adolescents with clear GID, if psychological resiliency or adequate social supports are lacking sometimes it is better to postpone medical intervention and use psychosocial interventions to try to create the conditions that will be conducive to a positive outcome for eventual sex reassignment. In other cases the gender dysphoria must be treated concurrent with other interventions.

Psychological Interventions

Psychotherapeutic treatment can be helpful both for adolescents who are unsure of the direction they want to take and also for those who have a clear wish to pursue sex reassignment. As there are numerous possible underlying concerns, the range of treatment goals is equally large.

Individual therapy is usually the treatment of choice, but for individuals who want to explore their options for coping with gender dysphoria, group therapy has also been advocated. The observation of other adolescents dealing with their gender concerns, the sharing of information, and the peer support seem to be particularly beneficial to group members. In the Netherlands a volunteer organization organizes meetings for 12-18 year old adolescents with gender dysphoria. These meetings do not have a therapeutic goal. Instead, the meetings give the opportunity to meet gender dysphoric peers in a safe and informal social setting.

For applicants who pursue sex reassignment, the process of sex reassignment is lengthy and intensive and even the diagnostic phase contains therapeutic elements. Adolescents with gender dysphoria need time to reflect on any unresolved personal issues or doubts regarding sex reassignment before embarking on somatic treatment. Any form of psychotherapy offered to adolescents who are considering sex reassignment should be supportive. This means that the clinician makes clear to the adolescent that any outcome of therapy (ranging from acceptance of living in the social role congruent with the phenotypic sex to sex reassignment) is acceptable as long as it ultimately contributes to the well being of the adolescent. After all, for the adolescent, a false negative decision (no medical treatment for someone who needs it) is as disastrous as a false positive decision (sex reassignment for someone who should not have it). Only in a supportive environment will an adolescent be likely to explore any doubts and ambivalence that may exist.

Therapists need to be knowledgeable about the different treatment options to be able to explain all the consequences of sex reassignment. They also should be accustomed to working with this age group and be able to discuss sensitive topics. During the diagnostic phase but also later, when some form of hormone treatment has been initiated, various issues have to be brought up repeatedly–including relationships, sexuality, and infertility. Views and experiences of the adolescent often change over time. A 13-year-old interested in dating but not genital sexual touching or penetration will likely experience less discomfort relating to genital incongruence (or will find it easier to suppress the discomfort) than an 18-year-old who is more interested in pursuing sexual relationships.

It has been our experience that quite a few adolescents with GID entirely refrain from dating and sexual activity. The adolescent may feel uncertain because they are afraid to tell the partner about their gender identity problem (if they still live in the original gender role) or about their biological sex (if they have already made the role change). If reluctance to disclose transgender identity to a partner only seems to be a matter of communication skill, it may be helpful to discuss pros and cons of various options, and to role-play or rehearse explanations to imaginary partners. There is no single 'right moment' or 'right way' for disclosure, but the better prepared and the more confident an adolescent is, the easier it will be to overcome the barriers. If other underlying factors–personality characteristics such as shyness, self-consciousness, or extreme perfectionism ("I can only have a relationship if my treatment is completed"); psychopathology (e.g., depression or personality disorders); or external factors (e.g., religious/cultural prohibitions)–are an issue, they should be addressed first.

Like other adolescents, adolescents with gender problems need adequate information about sexuality in general, including prevention of HIV and other sexually transmitted infections. If they are not very capable in judging other persons and situations, it may be necessary to point out the chances of aggressive reactions when they engage in sexual encounters, especially if the sexual partners are not aware of the adolescent's sex of birth.

A very difficult matter that has an impact not only on relationships but also on many aspects of the self is body image. If secondary sex characteristics have hardly developed and an early social role change has been made, unhappiness about unwanted characteristics such as beard growth and a low voice (male-to-female, abbreviated as MTF) or breasts (female-to-male, abbreviated as FTM), typical concerns in older adolescents/adults, are virtually non-existent. Yet many adolescents who have had pubertal delay treatment feel frustrated even in the absence of unwanted secondary sex characteristics because, in their opinion, they have to wait too long for their estrogen or androgen treatment to feminize/masculinize in the same ways as their age peers. There are usually more internal conflicts and more intense negative emotions if secondary sex characteristics have already developed prior to treatment starting; this may result in breast binding (FTM) and wrapping the penis or testicles (MTF). In these cases

there might be shame, frustration, and regret that treatment had not started earlier. Some adolescents undergoing sex reassignment find it increasingly confusing that they still have genitals of their original sex over time.

Another subject that has to be discussed repeatedly and over time is the life-long impact of sex reassignment. Adolescents who have been fortunate to have supporting parents, a protective school, and have been treated so early that they have no unwanted secondary sex characteristics do not always realize that life may be less easy in adulthood. Colleagues or acquaintances may discover the situation and be less accepting than their parents and current friends. When involved in serious relationships, they will always have to inform the partners about their infertility and, most probably, their sex reassignment. Conversely, adolescents who have been exposed to teasing and bullying, or who have a non-accepting family, may feel shameful about their cross-genderedness and overestimate the negative impact of sex reassignment on their lives. Adolescents will benefit most from having a balanced view of the short- and long-term costs and benefits of sex reassignment. Therapists may be helpful in establishing the youth with such a view.

Both adolescents who are eligible for sex reassignment as well as those who are not may need psychotherapy to address the impact of teasing, bullying, violence, and social isolation (Burgess, 1999). As with other youth who have had similar experiences, such life histories may seriously hamper the development of a healthy self-esteem or trust in other people. It may even cause an internalized transphobia. In severe cases, clinicians may have to reduce the negative impact of these experiences before they can continue with the diagnostic work.

Family therapy may, in some instances, help to resolve conflicts between family members. For example, some adolescents want to be open about transgender feelings or express their gender in ways that other family members are not comfortable with; conversely, if an adolescent is already cross-living, parents may fear aggressive reactions if friends who are not informed discover the adolescent's history of transition. Another common cause of conflicts is that the family members find it hard to make a distinction between what is related to gender dysphoria and what is not; some families (the adolescents included) tend to attribute every mishap to gender issues, whereas other families tend to underestimate the impact of gender dysphoria on the adolescent's development. It may be helpful to emphasize that all adolescents, including those with gender problems, have certain responsibilities–having gender dysphoria is no excuse for not washing the dishes or failing to complete homework. However, this does not mean that parents should not try to be sensitive to the special needs of their children. Family therapists or family counselors should try to help parents determine realistic demands and to work on the development of healthy boundaries and limits. Conflicts may also arise between parents when they have different views about how to handle their child. Fathers often find it harder to accept cross-gender behavior of their children, especially the boys, than mothers do; if the mother tries to protect her child against the criticism or aggression of the father, marital conflicts may occur. The adolescent may feel guilty about causing the marital discord. A family therapist or counselor may help in finding solutions for such disagreements.

In the Netherlands, there is an organization of parents of gender dysphoric children and/or adolescents. At their regular meetings they exchange experiences, try to support each other and sometimes invite professionals to give relevant presentations. Although not all parents attend the meetings and some do so only a few times, most parents find it very useful to know of other parents who are familiar with the problems a family with a gender dysphoric child may encounter.

Real Life Experience (RLE)

During the "real-life experience" (RLE) phase, adolescents live full-time in the role they are transitioning to, if they were not already doing so. The World Professional Association for Transgender Health (WPATH)'s *Standards of Care* define the RLE as "the act of fully adopting a new or evolving gender role or gender presentation in everyday life," with the intention of experiencing *in vivo* the familial, interpersonal, socioeconomic, and legal consequences of transition (Meyer et al., 2001). The *Standards*

of Care explicitly state that RLE is not a diagnostic test to evaluate whether gender concerns are present, but that the process tests "the person's resolve, the capacity to function in the preferred gender, and the adequacy of social, economic, and psychological supports." A fundamental premise of the RLE is that the person should experience life in the desired role before making irreversible physical changes.

For adolescents seeking sex reassignment, RLE includes informing family, friends, school and other social contacts about the wish for sex reassignment and the intention to undergo gender transition. Usually, a new name congruent with the adolescent's gender identity is chosen, and there is a concurrent switch in gender pronouns. There may also be a change in clothing, hairstyle, and gender-specific behaviours (including the use of the boys' washroom for FTMs, and the girls' washroom for MTFs). Essentially it is expected that the adolescent live as if physical transformation had already taken place.

During the RLE, the adolescent's feelings about the social transformation, including coping with the responses of others, is a major focus of the discussions and counseling. This is obviously less the case when an adolescent already lived in the desired role before applying for sex reassignment. It is difficult to give a general rule for the start of the RLE, as the personalities and life circumstances of adolescents are so different. Some wait until they have graduated from school, or after the feminization/masculinization of cross-sex hormones begins (after age 16). Others begin living in the desired role even before they have started with puberty-delaying hormones.

Physical Interventions

Physical intervention (hormonal and/or surgical feminization/masculinization, discussed below) is a long-term process. It is a very strong recommendation that the adolescent undergoing physical treatment have adequate familial support and stability, both to ensure attendance at medical appointments and also to help cope with psychosocial stresses. The psychological and social burden placed on adolescents during the sex reassignment procedure deserves adult care and support.

Mental health professional involvement is a requirement for physical intervention in adolescence. The objective of this involvement is that treatment is thoughtfully and recurrently considered over time. Each developmental phase might bring up new issues and the consequences of sex reassignment as well as the wish for sex reassignment should be reconsidered and discussed again.

Informed consent is essential (as it is for any type of physical intervention). The different steps in physical interventions and the long duration of the process require that treatment information is repeatedly given and discussed. Each phase of this process results in a letter of recommendation from the mental health professional to the prescribing physician or surgeon.

The guidelines of the Royal College of Psychiatrists (Di Ceglie et al., 1998) and the WPATH *Standards of Care* (Meyer et al., 2001) distinguish between fully reversible, partially reversible, and irreversible stages of physical interventions for adolescents.

Fully reversible interventions: Pubertal delay. As discussed previously, different views exist on at what age and at what pubertal stage to start with puberty-delaying hormones. To let adolescents experience their physical puberty at least to some extent, some clinicians choose to wait until Tanner stage 2 or 3, whereas others believe it is better to wait until Tanner stage 4 or 5. In addition to standard readiness criteria relating to psychological stability sufficient to withstand the stresses of sex reassignment, three additional criteria must be met for pubertal delay: (a) throughout childhood the adolescent has demonstrated an intense pattern of cross-gender behaviours and cross-gender identity, (b) the adolescent has gender dysphoria that is significantly increased with the onset of puberty, and (c) parents or guardians must consent to and participate in the therapy.

Puberty-delaying hormone treatment should not be viewed as a first step that inevitably leads to gender transition, but as a diagnostic aid. Therefore, "real life experience" is not required prior to or during hormonal treatment at this stage.

Typically, gonadotropin releasing hormone (GnRH) analogues such as leuprolide or triptorelin are used to delay/suppress puberty

(Gooren & Delemarre-van de Waal, 1996). These compounds bind so strongly to the pituitary GnRH receptors that the secretion of luteinizing hormone and follicle-stimulating hormone is blocked. Eventually the gonadal production of sex steroids discontinues and a prepubertal state is (again) achieved. Height and bone density growth will be tapered off during GnRH analogue treatment, but there is some preliminary evidence that, once cross-sex hormone treatment is started and puberty of the opposite sex is induced, bone density recovers (Delemarre-van de Waal, Van Weissenbruch, & Cohen-Kettenis, 2004). GnRH analogues should be prescribed by a pediatrician specialized in endocrinology who can carefully decide which dose to give, following important body measures like height, weight, Tanner stages, bone age, skin folds, laboratory endocrine as well as metabolic blood parameters and bone density. More detailed guidelines on the treatment with GnRH analogues for GID are not available yet in print, but a publication on the procedure and the physical effects is in preparation and will be submitted for publication soon.

Alternatives may be preferred to delay specific elements of pubertal development. For example, low-dose progestins (e.g., 0.5 mg lynestrenol po qd) have been used to suppress menstruation in FTMs (Gooren & Delemarre-van de Waal, 1996). Cyproterone acetate has been suggested as a reversible intervention for MTFs seeking to avoid the development of spontaneous erections and nocturnal emissions (Gooren & Delemarre-van de Waal, 1996), but as androgen antagonists can also promote irreversible breast development we do not consider this to be a fully reversible form of treatment. Additionally, there is some concern that neutralization of all androgen effects may not be healthy for developing adolescents.

Partially reversible interventions: Cross-sex hormone therapy. Feminizing/masculinizing hormone therapy (estrogens/anti-androgens/progestins for MTFs, androgens for FTMs) is considered partially reversible, as some of the changes persist even if hormone therapy is discontinued. Some changes (breast growth in MTFs, pitch drop and facial hair growth in FTMs) require surgery or other treatment to "reverse." It is not known whether hormonally-induced sterility is reversible. The expected effects and possible risks of cross-sex hormone therapy are discussed in detail by Dahl and colleagues (2006).

Because of the risks involved in feminizing/masculinizing hormone therapy, it typically does not begin until the adolescent is 16 years or older. From a pediatric endocrinologist's point of view, it is argued that, irrespective of Tanner stage at presentation for treatment, adolescents undergoing sex reassignment should be treated with GnRH analogues first to keep their own sex-hormone production low. Cross-sex hormones are then gradually added to induce puberty of the desired sex.

As per the WPATH *Standards of Care*, the mental health professional coordinating care should be involved with the adolescent (and family, for younger adolescents) for a minimum of six months prior to making a recommendation to begin hormonal feminization/masculinization (Meyer et al., 2001). The number of sessions during this six-month period depends upon the clinician's judgment.

Irreversible interventions: Surgery. The details of surgical feminization/masculinization are explained elsewhere (Bowman & Goldberg, 2006). As discussed earlier, sex reassignment surgery is not carried out prior to adulthood. There is international clinical consensus that the risks of early surgical intervention far outweigh the potential benefits in virtually all cases.

The WPATH *Standards of Care* emphasize that the "threshold of 18 should be seen as an eligibility criterion and not an indication in itself for active intervention" (Meyer et al., 2001). At age 18, the eligibility for sex reassignment surgery should be reconsidered and discussed. If the adolescent is not functioning well, is ambivalent about the social role change or has experienced no relief relating to the changes brought about by hormones, there should be no referral for surgery.

As per the WPATH *Standards of Care*, a minimum of two years "real life experience" is necessary prior to surgery in an older adolescent. An 18-year-old who is felt to be a suitable candidate for surgery must have been cross-living since age 16 (or earlier). When an adolescent turns 19 the guidelines for adults will be followed (Bockting et al., 2006).

If a MTF adolescent has taken GnRH analogues from an early age it is possible that not enough penile skin will be available to allow for a deep vagina using the penile inversion method. In that case, additional skin may need to be used from other parts of the body, such as the groin or abdominal wall. This will be evaluated by the surgeon as part of treatment planning.

Other Treatment

MTFs who have gone into puberty at a very young age or have started with GnRH analogues at a relatively late age might already have developed unwanted facial hair or gone through pubertal changes to voice by the time they present for treatment. There are currently no adolescent-specific guidelines for the provision of hair removal or speech therapy treatment as part of gender transition.

Hormonal treatment does not completely stop facial hair growth in adult MTFs. If facial hair persists, electrolysis, laser treatment, or other depilation treatments may be necessary.

As part of puberty, biological males experience numerous physiologic changes to the vocal tract that result in lowered pitch and changes to resonance and vocal quality. Additionally, there are gender-based differences in articulation, intonation, pragmatics, and other aspects of speech/voice. Speech therapy and pitch-elevating surgery as part of gender transition are discussed in detail elsewhere (Davies & Goldberg, 2006).

POST-TREATMENT EVALUATION

Psychotherapy for adolescents may be necessary during the whole sex reassignment period, including after surgery. Even after treatment psychosocial challenges may arise. For clinicians who work only with children and adolescents, care planning includes identification of resources the patient can call on as they transition from adolescence to adulthood. Clinicians who work with all age groups may be consulted by a patient long after gender transition has taken place, as there is already therapeutic rapport, trust, and an understanding of the history of a patient's transition process. For this reason, it is recommended that those who work with adolescents with gender dysphoria also have an understanding of issues that can emerge for transgender adults (Bockting et al., 2006).

REFERENCES

American Psychiatric Association (2000). *Diagnostic and statistical manual of mental disorders (DSM-IV-TR)* (4th Ed., Text Revision ed.). Washington, DC: American Psychiatric Association.

Bockting, W. O., Knudson, G., & Goldberg, J. M. (2006). Counseling and mental health care for transgender adults and loved ones. *International Journal of Transgenderism, 9*(3/4), 35-82.

Bowman, C. & Goldberg, J. M. (2006). Care of the patient undergoing sex reassignment surgery. *International Journal of Transgenderism, 9*(3/4), 135-165.

Bradley, S. J. & Zucker, K. J. (1997). Gender identity disorder: a review of the past 10 years. *Journal of the American Academy of Child and Adolescent Psychiatry, 36*, 872-880.

Burgess, C. (1999). Internal and external stress factors associated with the identity development of transgendered youth. In G. P. Mallon (Ed.), *Social services with transgendered youth* (pp. 35-47). Binghamton, NY: Harrington Park Press.

Cohen-Kettenis, P. T. & Pfäfflin, F. (2003). *Transgenderism and intersexuality in childhood and adolescence: Making choices.* Thousand Oaks, CA: Sage Publications.

Cohen-Kettenis, P. T. & Van Goozen, S. H. M. (1997). Sex reassignment of adolescent transsexuals: a follow-up study. *Journal of the American Academy of Child and Adolescent Psychiatry, 36*, 263-271.

Cohen-Kettenis, P. T. & Van Goozen, S. H. M. (1998). Pubertal delay as an aid in diagnosis and treatment of a transsexual adolescent. *European Child and Adolescent Psychiatry, 7*, 246-248.

Dahl, M., Feldman, J., Goldberg, J. M., & Jaberi, A. (2006). Physical aspects of transgender endocrine therapy. *International Journal of Transgenderism, 9*(3/4), 111-134.

Davies, S. & Goldberg, J. M. (2006). Clinical aspects of transgender speech feminization and masculinization. *International Journal of Transgenderism, 9*(3/4), 167-196.

Delemarre-van de Waal, H., Van Weissenbruch, M. M., & Cohen-Kettenis, P. T. (2004). Management of puberty in transsexual boys and girls. Poster presentation at 43rd Annual Meeting of the European Society for Paediatric Endocrinology (ESPE), Basel, Switzerland. Abstract published in *Hormone Research, 62*(Suppl. 2), 75.

Di Ceglie, D., Sturge, C., & Sutton, A. (1998). *Gender identity disorders in children and adolescents: Guid-*

ance for management (Rep. No. Council Report CR63). London, England: Royal College of Psychiatrists.

Fisk, N. (1973). Gender dysphoria syndrome (the how, what and why of the disease). In D. Laub & P. Gandy (Eds.), *Second Interdisciplinary Symposium on Gender Dysphoria Syndrome* (pp. 7-14). Palo Alto, CA: Stanford University Press.

Gender Identity Research and Education Society (2005). Hormonal medication for adolescents: Developing guidelines for endocrinological intervention in the gender identity development treatment of adolescents. Retrieved October 31, 2005, from http://www.gires.org.uk/Web_Page_Assets/Hormonal_Medication.htm

Goldenring, J. M. & Rosen, D. S. (2004). Getting into adolescent heads: An essential update. *Contemporary Pediatrics, 21*, 64-90.

Gooren, L. J. G. & Delemarre-van de Waal, H. (1996). The feasibility of endocrine interventions in juvenile transsexuals. *Journal of Psychology & Human Sexuality, 8*, 69-74.

Green, R. (1987). *The "sissy boy syndrome" and the development of homosexuality.* New Haven, CT: Yale University Press.

Lindgren, T. W. & Pauly, I. B. (1975). A body image scale for evaluating transsexuals. *Archives of Sexual Behavior, 4*, 639-656.

Meyenburg, B. (1994). Kritik der hormonellen behandlung jugendlichen mit geslächtsidentitätsstörungen. *Zeitschrift für Sexualforschung, 7*, 343-349.

Meyer, W. J., III, Bockting, W. O., Cohen-Kettenis, P. T., Coleman, E., Di Ceglie, D., Devor, H., Gooren, L., Hage, J. J., Kirk, S., Kuiper, B., Laub, D., Lawrence, A., Menard, Y., Monstrey, S., Patton, J., Schaefer, L., Webb, A., & Wheeler, C. C. (2001). *The standards of care for Gender Identity Disorders* (6th ed.). Minneapolis, MN: Harry Benjamin International Gender Dysphoria Association.

Rekers, G. A., Rosen, A. C., & Morey, S. M. (1990). Projective test findings for boys with gender disturbance: Draw-A-Person Test, IT scale, and Make-A-Picture Story Test. *Perceptual and Motor Skills, 71*, 771-779.

Rottnek, M. (1999). *Sissies & tomboys: Gender nonconformity & homosexual childhood.* New York, NY: New York University Press.

Smith, Y. L. S., Van Goozen, S. H. M., & Cohen-Kettenis, P. T. (2001). Adolescents with gender identity disorder who were accepted or rejected for sex reassignment surgery: A prospective follow-up study. *Journal of the American Academy of Child and Adolescent Psychiatry, 40*, 472-481.

Viner, R. M., Brain, C., Carmichael, P., & Di Ceglie, D. (2005). Sex on the brain: Dilemmas in the endocrine management of children and adolescents with gender identity disorder. *Archives of Disease in Childhood, 90*, A77-A81.

Zucker, K. J., & Bradley, S. J. (1995). *Gender Identity Disorder and psychosexual problems in children and adolescents*. New York: Guilford Press.

Zucker, K. J., Deogracias, J. J., Johnson, L. L., Meyer-Bahlburg, H. F., Kessler, S. J., & Schober, J. M.

(2005). *The Gender Identity Questionnaire for Adults and the Recalled Childhood Gender Questionnaire-Revised: Final analyses.* Poster presentation, Meeting of the International Academy of Sex Research, Ottawa, ONT.

doi:10.1300/J485v09n03_04

APPENDIX A. Utrecht Gender Dysphoria Scale, Adolescent Version

Female-to-Male Version

Response categories are: agree completely, agree somewhat, neutral, disagree somewhat, disagree completely. Items 1, 2, 4-6 and 10-12 are scored from 5-1; items 3 and 7-9 are scored from 1-5.

1. I prefer to behave like a boy.
2. Every time someone treats me like a girl I feel hurt.
3. I love to live as a girl.
4. I continuously want to be treated like a boy.
5. A boy's life is more attractive for me than a girl's life.
6. I feel unhappy because I have to behave like a girl.
7. Living as a girl is something positive for me.
8. I enjoy seeing my naked body in the mirror.
9. I like to behave sexually as a girl.
10. I hate menstruating because it makes me feel like a girl.
11. I hate having breasts.
12. I wish I had been born as a boy.

Male-to-Female Version

Response categories are: agree completely, agree somewhat, neutral, disagree somewhat, disagree completely. Items are all scored from 5-1.

1. My life would be meaningless if I would have to live as a boy.
2. Every time someone treats me like a boy I feel hurt.
3. I feel unhappy if someone calls me a boy.
4. I feel unhappy because I have a male body.
5. The idea that I will always be a boy gives me a sinking feeling.
6. I hate myself because I'm a boy.
7. I feel uncomfortable behaving like a boy, always and everywhere.
8. Only as a girl my life would be worth living.
9. I dislike urinating in a standing position.
10. I am dissatisfied with my beard growth because it makes me look like a boy.
11. I dislike having erections.
12. It would be better not to live than to live as a boy.

Scoring and Evaluation

As can be expected most non-transsexuals score close to the minimum score, which is 12. Most transsexuals score close to the maximum score, which is 60. Problematic applicants in terms of eligibility for sex reassignment and in terms of treatment course tend to score in the middle range of the scale.

Ethical, Legal, and Psychosocial Issues in Care of Transgender Adolescents

Catherine White Holman

Joshua M. Goldberg

SUMMARY. Complete care for transgender adolescents must be considered in the context of a holistic approach that includes comprehensive primary care as well as cultural, economic, psychosocial, sexual, and spiritual influences on health. Not all transgender adolescents have gender dysphoria or wish to undergo sex reassignment. In this article we focus on general care of transgender adolescents by the non-specialist working in primary care, family services, schools, child welfare, mental health, and other community settings. doi:10.1300/J485v09n03_05 *[Article copies available for a fee from The Haworth Document Delivery Service: 1-800-HAWORTH. E-mail address: <docdelivery@haworthpress.com> Website: <http://www.HaworthPress.com> © 2007 by The Haworth Press, Inc. All rights reserved.]*

KEYWORDS. Transgender, transsexual, crossdressing, gender variance, adolescent, adolescence

This article is a companion piece to *Clinical Management of Gender Dysphoria in Adolescents* (de Vries, Cohen-Kettenis, & Delemarre-van de Waal, 2006). That article, written by advanced practitioners, offers important advice for gender specialists working with adolescents who need specialty care relating to gender dysphoria. However, not all transgender adolescents have gender dysphoria or wish to undergo sex reassignment. In this article we focus on general care of transgender adolescents by the non-specialist working in primary care, family services, schools, child welfare, mental health, and other community settings.

Complete care for transgender adolescents must be considered in the context of a holistic approach that includes comprehensive primary care as well as cultural, economic, psychosocial, sexual, and spiritual influences on health. The non-specialist can facilitate peer and family interactions that help the transgender adolescent learn emotional and rela-

Catherine White Holman is Community Counselor at Three Bridges Community Health Centre and Joshua Goldberg is Education Consultant at the Transgender Health Program, Vancouver, BC, Canada.

Address correspondence to: Catherine White Holman, Three Bridges Community Health Centre, 1292 Hornby Street, Vancouver, BC, Canada V6Z 1W2 (E-mail: Catherine.WhiteHoman@vch.ca).

This manuscript was created for the Trans Care Project, a joint initiative of Transcend Transgender Support & Education Society and Vancouver Coastal Health's Transgender Health Program, with funding from the Canadian Rainbow Health Coalition. The authors thank Sheila Kelton, Roey Malleson, Gerald P. Mallon, Edgardo J. Menvielle, Daniel L. Metzger, Jorge L. Pinzon, and Wallace Wong for comments on an earlier draft, and Donna Lindenberg, Olivia Ashbee, A. J. Simpson, and Rodney Hunt for research assistance.

[Haworth co-indexing entry note]: "Ethical, Legal, and Psychosocial Issues in Care of Transgender Adolescents." Holman, Catherine White, and Joshua M. Goldberg. Co-published simultaneously in *International Journal of Transgenderism* (The Haworth Medical Press, an imprint of The Haworth Press, Inc.) Vol. 9, No. 3/4, 2006, pp. 95-110; and: *Guidelines for Transgender Care* (ed: Walter O. Bockting, and Joshua M. Goldberg) The Haworth Medical Press, an imprint of The Haworth Press, Inc., 2006, pp. 95-110. Single or multiple copies of this article are available for a fee from The Haworth Document Delivery Service [1-800-HAWORTH, 9:00 a.m. - 5:00 p.m. (EST). E-mail address: docdelivery@haworthpress.com].

tional skills, including tools to recognize, express, and manage emotion; resolve conflicts constructively; and work cooperatively with others (American Psychological Association, 2002). A positive youth development approach that focuses on building the adolescent's competence, confidence, and social connectedness can help promote resilience and healthy development (Lerner, 2002; Tonkin, 2002).

Adolescent health is an interdisciplinary field, and our recommendations are accordingly broad. Many of the discipline-specific protocols and recommendations discussed in other articles (e.g., Bockting, Knudson, & Goldberg, 2006; Feldman & Goldberg, 2006) are also applicable to clinicians who work with older adolescents. We encourage adaptation of our recommendations to fit the specifics of clinical practice.

THE CLINICAL PICTURE

To date, most demographic information about transgender adolescents is derived from research performed by specialized clinics for gender dysphoric children and adolescents in Canada, England, and The Netherlands (Bradley & Zucker, 1990; Cohen, de Ruiter, Ringelberg, & Cohen-Kettenis, 1997; Di Ceglie, Freedman, McPherson, & Richardson, 2002; Zucker, 2004). There is no systematic documentation of transgender adolescents who are not gender dysphoric, or who pursue sex reassignment outside the gender clinic system (e.g., obtaining hormones through Internet purchase, friends, or street trade). In the absence of information about the broader spectrum of transgender adolescents, we can only comment on trends within the population we have worked with, noting in particular differences between our client base and the clinical picture described by de Vries and colleagues (2006). Further work is needed to document trends among the diverse range of transgender adolescents, both locally and in other regions.

Fluidity of Gender Identity

The Amsterdam team (de Vries et al., 2006) works primarily with adolescents who are strongly cross-identified transsexuals (i.e., na-

tal males who identify as young women and natal females who identify as young men). Many of our transgender adolescent clients–including those who have sought sex reassignment–have identified outside a gender binary of male/female, using terms such as *gender-fluid, gender-bending, genderqueer*, and *pangender* to describe their sense of self. A similar trend was noted by clinicians at the Dimensions youth clinic in San Francisco (Dimensions, 2000a; Dimensions, 2000b), as well as by clinicians at other North American health centres who were interviewed as part of the Trans Care Project. It may be that this is a population trend specific to North America; it is also possible that transgender youth who are not transsexual tend to engage with the health and social service system in ways that are different than transsexual youth.

Initial Presentation

In a gender clinic or other trans-specialty service, clients are obviously transgender and have been referred for help to deal with gender concerns. This is not necessarily the case in a general community service setting, where the client base and the reasons for seeking service are far more diverse. As professionals providing advocacy, crisis intervention, and counseling for people of all ages in urban community-based service settings, it is not surprising that the types of services sought by out transgender clients are different than the patients entering the Amsterdam team's specialized hospital clinic for gender dysphoric children and adolescents.

Few of our transgender adolescent clients have sought our help specifically to deal with gender identity concerns. Most have presented seeking assistance for the same range of concerns as non-transgender adolescents–abuse, anxiety, depression, difficulty at school, disordered eating, drug and alcohol use, family stress, financial worries, homelessness, loneliness, peer or relationship violence, questions about sexual orientation, relationship difficulties, and suicidal ideation. In some situations transgender identity has had no bearing on our client's concern, while in others there have been trans-specific components requiring evaluation and incorporation into the care plan.

Regardless of the presenting concern, we have found it important to evaluate the impact of trans-specific issues on the adolescent's overall health and well-being. This can be challenging in the community setting when gender concerns are suspected but the adolescent has not disclosed transgender identity.

FACILITATING DISCUSSION OF TRANSGENDER ISSUES

While some transgender adolescents are open about being transgender and may talk about this on the first visit, others are more wary initially, or unsure how to discuss it. We have found the following strategies useful in creating an environment conducive to discussion of transgender issues with adolescents.

Promoting Adolescent Awareness of Transgender Issues

Although public awareness of transgenderism has greatly increased in the last decade, many individuals with transgender feelings do not know how to articulate their concerns. Trans-specific posters, magazines that include articles about transgender youth, and consumer information that describes terms relating to the diversity of transgender identity and experience can help adolescents name and express their feelings. Inclusion of transgender brochures and posters in public education materials also demonstrates a trans-positive and trans-inclusive approach. It is important that materials be reflective of the diversity within the transgender community (e.g., ethnicity, disability).

Active Demonstration of Transgender Awareness and Sensitivity

Adolescents may fear a negative reaction upon disclosure of transgender identity, or may assume that the clinician will not be able to relate to their concerns. Emphasis on non-judgmental attitude, reassurance about confidentiality, and active demonstration of transgender awareness and sensitivity helps convey safety and approachability. Inclusion of a statement such as "Transgender people are welcome" in crisis line or resource guide service listings lets adolescents know that you have an active interest in transgender issues.

Asking a question about transgender identity on an intake form is a simple way to encourage disclosure of transgender identity. Some clinicians use "Choose as many as apply: M/F/MTF (male-to-female)/FTM (female-to-male)/other (please specify)," or give the options "M/F/Transgender." This not only demonstrates understanding of transgender issues, but also raises adolescents' consciousness that there are options beyond a binary gender system.

Routinely Screening for Gender Concerns

Internal conflict related to gender identity is not always immediately apparent. To date, no screening tools have been developed to facilitate detection of gender identity concerns in the general community setting. Gender dysphoria measurement instruments (Cohen-Kettenis & Van Goozen, 1997; Lindgren & Pauly, 1975; Zucker et al., 2005) are designed for use by the gender specialist where there is already suspicion of distress about gender identity. In the absence of formal screening tools, we recommend incorporating a brief question about gender into the intake process with all clients, not just those who look gender-variant. We recommend making a short normalizing statement followed by a simple question that can be answered without directly declaring transgender identity. For example: "Many people struggle with gender. Is this an issue for you?" Asking in this indirect way creates an opening for adolescents who are unsure of their identity or are embarrassed or ashamed of transgender feelings, and would be intimidated by a direct question. It also avoids a negative response by non-transgender adolescents who would be confused or angry if asked a direct question about transgender identity. A positive answer should be followed by a more detailed evaluation, as outlined in Table 1.

For the adolescent who is confused, questioning, or unsure about gender issues, counseling by the non-specialist and referral to age-appropriate community resources are often sufficient. As with lesbian, gay, bisexual or questioning adolescents, this level of support typically focuses on normalization of feelings, discussion of options for identification and ex-

TABLE 1. Evaluating Gender Concerns in Adolescents

Topic	Areas to Explore
Nature of gender concerns	• What is the adolescent concerned about (e.g., discrepancy between body and identity, social perceptions, social roles, sexual arousal from crossdressing)? • When did these feelings start? • Are the feelings constant, or do they come and go? Does anything make them better or worse? • How intense are the feelings?
Impact on the adolescent's life	• How are the gender concerns impacting on the adolescent's overall well-being (including mental health and developmental progress)? • What is the impact on peer and family relationships? • What is the impact on school and work? • What are the adolescent's coping strategies? Are there any concerns about escalating substance use, self-harm, binge eating, compulsive exercise, or other potentially harmful coping mechanisms? • How aware is the adolescent of community resources and options for support?
Feelings about transgenderism	• What is the adolescent's belief structure about transgenderism? • How does the adolescent feel about the possibility that they may be transgender? • What is the adolescent's information about transgenderism based on (e.g., talk shows, peer opinion, cultural or religious beliefs, Internet, movies)?
Related or co-existing factors	• Are there any other physical or psychosocial concerns that are contributing to the adolescent's distress? • Do these seem related to the gender concerns? If so, how?

pression, exploration of fears and anxiety, and discussion of non-destructive ways to cope with societal stigma (Fontaine & Hammond, 1996). To alleviate the isolation commonly experienced by gender conflicted adolescents, community peer support groups, internet resources, and other options for social connection should be identified. Evaluation by a mental health clinician specializing in gender identity concerns is recommended if the adolescent (a) is so distressed about gender issues that health and well-being, relationships, school, or work are negatively affected; (b) expresses feelings of gender dysphoria, an aversion to aspects of their body associated with sex or gender, discomfort with gender identity, or a wish to live as the opposite sex; (c) is compulsively crossdressing or pursuing validation of gender identity–for example, through compulsive sexual or online encounters; or (d) has a co-existing or pre-existing condition that complicates evaluation of gender concerns–for example, schizophrenia, personality disorder, or cognitive disability.

Dilemmas in diagnosis of gender concerns in adolescence. The *DSM-IV-TR* (American Psychiatric Association, 2000) defines two conditions relating to gender concerns: Gender Identity Disorder (GID) and Transvestic Fetishism (TF). GID is divided into two age groupings–GID of Childhood (302.6) and GID of Adolescence and Adulthood (302.85)–with both referring to a discrepancy between felt sense of gender and the gender assigned at birth. GID Not Otherwise Specified is used when the client is felt to have GID but does not meet criteria for GID of Adolescence. Transvestic Fetishism (302.3) refers to erotically motivated crossdressing that has become so obsessive or compulsive as to cause problems in other aspects of life.

There is controversy about these diagnoses (Bartlett, Vasey, & Bukowski, 2000; Bockting & Ehrbar, 2005; Burgess, 1999; Hill, Rozanski, Carfagnini, & Willoughby, 2005; Langer & Martin, 2004; Menvielle, 1998; Minter, 1999; Moore, 2002; Newman, 2002; Wilson, Griffin, & Wren, 2002). Some clinicians feel that a diagnosis of GID or TF is fundamentally important in guiding clinical consideration of options for treatment in adolescents, and that a formal diagnosis enables understanding and acceptance that the distress is clinically serious and that treatment may be required. Others have expressed concern that these diagnoses pathologize transgender identity and erotic cross-dressing, fail to differentiate between distress caused by gender dysphoria and distress caused by societal pressures (internalized stigma, societal marginalization, etc.), and are not scientifically valid or reliable as psychiatric diagnoses. The characterization of gender dysphoria as a disorder of identity may lead parents of young gender-variant adolescents to seek "normalizing," "conversion," or "reparative" therapies that reinforce stigma and shame by attempting to change the adolescent's identity or behaviour (Raj, 2002; Rosenberg, 2002).

Regardless of clinical or political position on GID and TF diagnoses, it is important to thoroughly assess the gender-conflicted client's history and current concerns as the basis for an informed opinion relating to care, and to record this in a way that facilitates understanding by other clinicians (to promote continuity of care). This includes formal charting of the nature, severity, and persistence of gender concerns over the duration of a client's care.

By definition, the clinical threshold for GID requires not only cross-gender behaviour but also "clinically significant distress or impairment in social, occupational, or other important areas of functioning." This is a subjective judgment that has been applied to include youth who are unhappy when forced to conform to prevailing gender norms. We do not believe it is helpful to apply the distress criterion to parents' distress that their child is atypical, or to an adolescent's distress about other people's transphobic reactions. These are societally-caused situations that can be addressed by supportive intervention with the parents focused on building acceptance for gender diversity (Menvielle & Tuerk, 2002), along with intervention for the youth to build resilience and address stigma issues.

While untreated gender dysphoria can result in anxiety, depression, and other mental health problems, not all mental health concerns stem from gender dysphoria. Overall, adolescents with gender dysphoria do not show more psychopathology than other adolescents (Cohen et al., 1997; Cohen-Kettenis & Van Goozen, 1997), but there is variation individually (Smith

et al., 2001) and co-existing mental illness should be screened for and appropriately treated as part of the care plan. Behaviours that may have been adopted as mechanisms to cope with gender dysphoria (e.g., cutting, burning, binge eating, substance use) should be addressed and monitored as the dysphoria is treated.

Conducting a Detailed Trans-Inclusive Psychosocial Evaluation

There are various tools that can be used to evaluate psychosocial concerns in adolescents. HEEADSSS is a way of organizing the evaluation of the adolescent to assess psychosocial concerns in eight areas: Home, Education/employment, Eating, Activities, Drugs, Sexuality, Suicide/depression, and Safety (Goldenring & Rosen, 2004). While none of the HEEADSSS questions include trans-specific content, many of the questions are conducive to disclosure of transgender concerns for the closeted adolescent.

For the adolescent who has already disclosed transgender identity, the HEEADSSS interview can be modified to include trans-specific content, as in Table 2. As in the original HEEADSSS protocol, the wording, pacing, and number of questions used should be adapted in consideration of the needs of each client.

COMMON PSYCHOSOCIAL CONCERNS

Many non-dysphoric transgender adolescents struggle with the same psychosocial issues as those described by de Vries and colleagues (2006), such as concerns about body image, relationships, or sexuality. Both dysphoric and non-dysphoric transgender adolescents share psychosocial struggles related to societal marginalization, including identity confusion, internalized stigma, shame, guilt, isolation, discrimination, harassment, and violence. In the following section we briefly identify psychosocial concerns commonly expressed by the transgender adolescents we have worked with.

Safety

Visibly gender-variant people and those who have disclosed their transgender identity

TABLE 2. Sample Trans-Specific Modification of HEEADSSS Psychosocial Interview (adapted from Goldenring & Rosen, 2004)

Topic	Sample questions
Home	• Do the people who live with you know that you are transgender? (Who?) How did they find out, and how did they react? • How much do you feel you can be yourself at home?
Education/ employment	• Do people at school or work know that you are transgender? (Who?) How did they find out, and how did they react? • Are there people at school or work you feel you could talk to if you needed to talk about transgender issues? (Who?) • Do you skip or miss classes? How often? What do you do instead? • Have you ever been harassed or attacked at school or work? • Do you ever worry about your academic or work future as a transgender person? • Has anyone ever offered you money, clothes, alcohol, or drugs in exchange for sex? Has anyone ever tried to get you involved in the sex trade?
Eating	• What do you like and not like about the way you look? Do you wish you looked different? (How?) • Do you ever daydream about your body being different than it is now? What is your ideal image? • Do you eat more (less) when you are under stress?
Activities	• Do any of your friends know that you are transgender? How did they find out, and how did they react? • Do you know any other transgender people? How did you meet them? • How much time do you spend on the Internet in a week?
Drugs	• Do you ever use drugs or alcohol to cope with stress? • What do you think is a safe limit for drug and alcohol use? Have you ever crossed that limit? (How often?) • Have you ever done things when you were drunk or high that you regretted afterwards?
Sexuality	• Have any of the people you've dated known that you are transgender? How did they find out, and how did they react? • Is being transgender part of your sex life? (How?) • Are you attracted to boys, girls, other transgender people? • Are there parts of your body that are off-limits sexually?
Suicide/ depression	• Do you worry about people finding out you are transgender? • Do you ever wish you weren't transgender? • Does thinking about transgender issues ever make you feel stressed, sad, or lonely? • Do you ever feel that your situation is hopeless?
Safety	• Has anyone ever threatened to "out" you as transgender? Do you worry about this happening? • Have you ever been threatened or attacked because you are transgender, or for other reasons? Do you worry about this happening? • How safe do you feel in your neighbourhood or the places where you hang out?

to others are vulnerable to hate-motivated harassment and violence by dates, acquaintances, family members, school-age peers, co-workers, and strangers (Kenagy, 2005; Kosciw & Cullen, 2001; Lombardi, Wilchins, Priesing, & Malouf, 2001; Odo & Hawelu, 2001; Wyss, 2004). Violence against transgender people is not formally tracked in most jurisdictions in North America, but newspaper and anecdotal reports collected by community organizations suggest that transgender people of colour in the male-to-female (MTF) spectrum are particularly vulnerable to violence as a result of the triple burden of transphobia, sexism, and racism

(Currah & Minter, 2000; Goldberg & White, 2004). We have also observed heightened risk of interpersonal violence among transgender people who are financially dependent on another person, cognitively impaired, physically disabled, homeless, or involved in the sex trade. Adolescents are particularly vulnerable to violence due to their limited options for economic independence, the prevalence of age-peer violence in schools, and power differentials between adults and youth.

De Vries and colleagues (2006) note the need to discuss safety relating to disclosure of transgender identity in sexual relationships. We also routinely assess transgender adolescents' potential risks for violence and their perception of safety at school, home, the workplace, and general public settings (e.g., public transit) and, where necessary, create safety plans (e.g., a safe place to go, trans-positive emergency services, and group safety).

Poverty and Homelessness

Within the published literature there is recognition that gender-variant adolescents are vulnerable to abuse, neglect, and parental rejection, with resulting poverty and homelessness (de Castell & Jenson, 2002; Estes & Weiner, 2001; Klein, 1999; Leichtentritt & Arad, 2004). Cross-gender behaviour may be met with scorn, ridicule, abuse, or violence, and the adolescent may have to choose between living in a way that is not congruent with identity or leaving home. The adolescent may attempt to suppress transgender feelings as a way of coping, or may leave home or be forced to leave. Gender dysphoric adolescents without family support face numerous psychological and socioeconomic challenges and it may be impractical to begin sex reassignment until stability has been regained. In other instances the clinician and client may feel that sex reassignment should proceed along with interventions focused on psychosocial stability.

Transgender adolescents who have left home voluntarily or involuntarily may struggle to find safe and affordable housing. While some homeless transgender adolescents may wish to reunite with their families of origin, for others reunification is not appropriate (e.g., high risk of familial abuse) or feasible (e.g., no willing-

ness to accept the adolescent back into the home). Adolescents whose family members were unaware of transgender identity prior to leaving home and who wish to reconnect with family members may need support around management of disclosure. Trans-specific advocacy relating to foster care and emergency shelter is discussed elsewhere (White Holman & Goldberg, 2006).

Sex Work

For both MTF and FTM adolescents without financial support from family, the sex trade may offer a means of financial survival (Klein, 1999; Pazos, 1999). A study of North American adolescents in the sex trade concluded that the financial costs of sex reassignment and the low earning power of adolescents left transsexual youth without family economic support few choices other than the sex trade (Estes & Weiner, 2001). In addition, the sex trade can appeal to young transgender women as a way to find community, validate identity as a woman, and feel desirable (Worth, 2000). In British Columbia, the combined impacts of colonization, poverty, racism, and violence as well as a lack of accessible and relevant supports have led to high numbers of Aboriginal youth among adolescents involved in the sex trade (Social Services and Community Safety Division–Justice Institute of British Columbia, 2002).

In Canada, provincial governments typically define exchange of sex for drugs, money, food, shelter, or other goods as commercial sexual exploitation (CSE) if a youth 18 years or younger is involved (Assistant Deputy Ministers' Committee on Prostitution and the Sexual Exploitation of Youth, 2000). While in British Columbia the term "sexual exploitation" is used by some former sex workers who are now advocates (Tubman & Bramly, 1998), transgender adolescents involved in the sex trade typically do not use the term "sexual exploitation" to describe their situation (Klein, 1999), and many of the adolescents we have worked with reject the term as patronizing. Like Klein, we have found adolescents are most receptive to discussing involvement in the sex trade when they are confident that the clinician is non-judgmental about their involvement in sex work. For this reason we use the term "sex trade" here rather than CSE.

In our experience there is great diversity of gender identity among adolescents who work in the sex trade. We have worked with three different populations of transgender adolescents in the sex trade:

1. *Adolescent MTFs who strongly identify as women*: Some work as women, while others feel it is too dangerous to do so prior to genital surgery and work in the sex trade as men (but present in other settings as women). A small number have been able to work openly as transgender women in escort agencies or on the street "tranny track." In our experience the trans-specific concerns of this group primarily relate to validation of female identity and obtaining sex reassignment.
2. *Adolescent males who do not identify as women, but work crossdressed*: This group crossdresses only for work purposes, and outside of work identifies as male. Many of our clients in this circumstance did not identify as transgender but wanted support relating to transphobic violence or harassment they experienced while working. Some also sought counseling relating to confusion about gender identity or sexual orientation.
3. *Adolescent FTMs working as women*: We have worked with a few FTMs who, while personally identifying strongly as masculine or male and living as male in their personal and social life, worked in the sex trade as women. FTMs in the sex trade have been a more hidden population and it may well be that some FTM adolescents are able to work as men, despite not having access to genital surgery. The number of FTM sex workers in our client base is too small to identify service themes.

Clinicians working with transgender adolescents have the opportunity to engage in positive interventions that make it possible for youth to get sufficient social and economic supports to have alternatives to the sex trade, and also provide support for transgender adolescents already involved in the sex trade (Social Services and Community Safety Division–Justice Institute of British Columbia, 2002). A detailed discussion of prevention and support strategies is outside the realm of this document, but clinicians working with transgender adolescents should be aware of the possibility of sex trade involvement, and ensure that services for transgender adolescents are both relevant and accessible to youth who are involved in the sex trade. Klein (1999) suggests services for transgender youth in the sex trade should include assistance with education, employment, and life skill development; psychotherapeutic interventions aimed at exploring transgender identity and building resilience to deal with conflict, relationships, shame, stigma, depression, safer sex, and peer pressure; and facilitation of connections with peer support. It is also important that involvement in the sex trade not be considered an exclusionary criterion for youth who are seeking sex reassignment, as this leaves adolescents who are economically dependent on the sex trade unable to access care (Raj, 2002).

Sexual Health

De Vries and colleagues (2006) identified the need to discuss sexuality with adolescents undergoing sex reassignment. In our experience this is also a key issue for transgender adolescents who are not undergoing reassignment.

Sexual health education with transgender adolescents should involve frank, explicit, and sex-positive discussion about the actual practices an adolescent is engaged in, with no assumptions about the gender of partner(s) or sexual activities. While some transgender adolescents are strongly dysphoric about their genitals, others are not. Both MTFs and FTMs may engage in receptive or insertive oral, vaginal, and anal intercourse, as well as sexual activities that do not involve penetration. The same sexual health topics that are routinely discussed with non-transgender adolescents (e.g., sexually transmitted infections, contraception) should also be discussed with transgender adolescents, using language that corresponds to the adolescent's identity (i.e., ask the adolescent what words they use for their genitals). While cross-sex hormones decrease fertility and may cause permanent sterility, hormones taken as part of sex reassignment are not failsafe contraceptives (Feldman & Goldberg, 2006). MTF adolescents who are taking feminizing hormones and engage in penile penetration should be aware that the hormones typically reduce erectile firmness, and condoms may therefore be more likely to slip or leak.

Body image. As noted by de Vries and colleagues (2006), body image problems are common in adolescents with gender dysphoria. It has been our experience that non-dysphoric transgender adolescents who have had few positive transgender role models also tend to have a distorted self-image, compounded by media stereotypes of MTFs and the invisibility of FTMs in popular culture. General societal norms and standards for non-transgender women and men also affect transgender people. In particular we have noticed a struggle with North American values of thinness and standards of attractiveness among adolescent MTFs, with high value placed on ability to "pass" as a non-transgender woman and conformity to beauty norms for non-transgender women. Exploration of transgender identity may be important as part of intervention. Transgender community involvement and peer support may also be useful in exploring myths and stereotypes about transgender "attractiveness" and worth.

For adolescents with intense frustration or distress about body image, in addition to a general screening tool for eating disorders such as the SCOFF questionnaire or the Eating Disorder Screen for Primary Care (Kagan & Melrose, 2003) it may be appropriate to inquire about excessively tight breast binding (FTM) or tucking of the penis and testicles (MTF). If binding or tucking is causing pain or skin rash, peer support or information resources may be helpful in discussing less physically harmful techniques that can be used.

SUPPORTING TRANSGENDER EMERGENCE IN ADOLESCENCE

Even in the absence of gender dysphoria, transgender youth may struggle with identity development. Lev (2004) characterizes *transgender emergence* as a developmental process of realizing, discovering, identifying, or naming one's gender identity. This does not necessarily mean a transition from male-to-female or female-to-male; for some adolescents (and adults) transition involves emergence as a bi-gender, pan-gender, or androgynous person—a challenging task in a society that has a binary and polarized gender schema.

The distinction of transgender emergence from typical gender identity development is a culturally-derived phenomenon, stemming from the societal assumption that there are two genders (corresponding to two sexes) and that there are norms of appearance and behaviour for each. While in our experience transgender adolescents have not typically struggled with denial, avoidance, or repression for the same length of time or to the same degree as transgender adults (Lev, 2004), youth who do not fit the dominant gender norms must still find a way to consciously articulate their difference and find language to express their identity.

Transgender emergence is often considered analogous to the process of "coming out" as lesbian, gay, or bisexual. While both processes involve disclosure of a personal secret that may evoke a negative response by others, transgender emergence is not just a matter of declaring membership in a stigmatized group. The existence of homosexuality and bisexuality is generally recognized; in contrast, transgenderism is not widely recognized or understood, and challenges societal beliefs about sex, gender, and sexuality in a way that can be disorienting to the transgender individual and the people around them (Brown & Rounsley, 1996). For most transgender individuals, a search for language is a key element in the emergence process.

The following discussion of interventions to support transgender emergence in adolescence is adapted from Lev (2004)'s model of six stages of transgender emergence in adults undergoing gender transition. The levels of intervention described below are not intended as a model for transgender adolescent development, but rather to help the non-specialist consider appropriate strategies for clinical assistance. A "stages of change" approach (Prochaska, DiClemente, & Norcross, 1992) may also be useful in guiding clinical interventions.

Awareness of Diversity of Gender Identity and Expression

Some adolescents have only been exposed to information about transsexuality and are not aware of other options for transgender identity or of ways other than physical change to express or affirm a transgender identity. With adolescents who have already made a decision to pursue sex reassignment, we do not try to dissuade them but do try to focus on keeping options open and promoting awareness of diverse possibilities for gender identity and expression. Books and movies that include transsexual and non-transsexual transgender individuals can be useful in demonstrating a breadth of identity and expression. Contact with a diverse range of transgender individuals (appropriately screened age peers as well as older role models) can also help demonstrate options for gender identity and expression that include but are not limited to sex reassignment. This includes discussion of challenges, risks, and societal limits if the adolescent expresses increasing interest in moving beyond private exploration to integrate transgender identity or expression into life at home, school, or work.

With adolescents who are in early stages of questioning or exploring their gender, we encourage ways of exploring identity and experimenting that do not involve disclosing transgender identity to others or making decisions about transition or sex reassignment (Lev, 2004). If asked we provide information about transition options, but the focus is exploration rather than decision-making. This may include journaling, collage or other creative expressions; trying out a new name or pronoun in the clinical setting to see how it feels; reading or watching movies that portray various kinds of gender expression; or attending trans-themed community events (e.g., drag performances). It has been our experience that many youth who are early in exploration or questioning find peer contact overwhelming and need time to explore on their own; others are more social and want peer contact earlier in the process.

With transgender adolescents who have a generally stable core sense of self (i.e., no evidence of dissociation, thought disorder, or personality disorder) we actively encourage experimentation with fluidity of gender identification and expression as part of the exploration process. This may include experimentation with gender pronouns, name, and aspects of appearance. Some adolescents who are considering gender transition bring cross-gender

clothing, wigs, shoes, or makeup to our appointments to try interacting with another person as their imagined self. We do not suggest that adolescents try a form of gender expression they are uncomfortable with, but rather encourage them to try experimenting as a way of deciding who they are and what feels right. We find that adolescents usually relate easily to the concept of experimentation and are excited by the possibility of trying out ways of expressing themselves that are in keeping with their (possibly shifting) sense of self.

For both questioning adolescents and those who already have a strong sense of self, the emphasis is on self-understanding rather than reaching towards a preset goal. If there are concerns about fragmentation of identity or if the process of experimentation seems to be increasing distress, we suggest involvement of an advanced mental health clinician with experience in treatment of co-existing gender concerns and mental illness.

Increasing Congruence Between Gender Identity and Daily Life

For the adolescent who has a clear and consistent sense of self, the next step is the identification of strategies to reconcile discrepancies between identity and daily life. The hormonal and surgical interventions discussed by de Vries and colleagues (2006) are, for many gender dysphoric adolescents, a necessary treatment to alleviate the dysphoria. However, not all transgender adolescents are dysphoric, and sex reassignment is not the only course of action a transgender adolescent may take to bring daily life into closer congruence with felt sense of self.s

The World Professional Association for Transgender Health's (WPATH) *Standards of Care* (Meyer et al., 2001) identify a range of non-medical possibilities transgender individuals may explore, spontaneously or with professional support: (a) learning about transgenderism from the Internet, lay and professional literature, or peers; (b) participating in peer support or self-help groups, or in the transgender community; (c) counseling to explore gender identity and to deal with psychosocial pressures; (d) disclosing transgender identity to family, friends, and other loved ones ("coming out"); (e) integrating of transgender awareness into daily living; (f) changing gender pronoun or name; (g) episodic crossdressing or cross-living; and (h) undertaking temporary and potentially reversible changes to gender expression, such as changing hairstyle, makeup, or clothing; removing facial and body hair, or applying facial hair; wearing prosthetic breasts or penile prosthesis; binding the chest or tucking the genitals; and changing speech and voice. This list is not meant to be exhaustive, but simply to illustrate that there are multiple options that may be considered by transgender adolescents. Some options require a high level of cognitive and social sophistication and will likely not be spontaneously pursued by young adolescents. Whatever options are considered, there should be thought as to how changes will realistically be integrated into daily life, and what reactions there might be by others.

Disclosing transgender identity to others. For some transgender adolescents, increased congruence between identity and daily life involves disclosing transgender identity to others. "Coming out" as transgender may be prompted by a desire to make feelings or identity known to others, or by planned changes in social role or appearance. Disclosure is not only an issue early in transgender emergence: throughout life, transgender adolescents need to consider how much to disclose. Clarity about what the adolescent wants to convey is an important part of decision-making regarding disclosure.

In "coming out" literature there is often an emphasis on disclosure as a necessary stage in self-acceptance, and adolescents may feel they have to come out to be a "real" transgender person. In our experience it is viable for some transgender individuals to live comfortably and in a congruent way without disclosing their identity to others. The decision not to disclose is not necessarily evidence of shame or embarrassment; it may be based on concern about the likely response of others, or may be a reflection of the adolescent's feeling that this aspect of their identity is private. We encourage adolescents to consider disclosure as only one of many possible paths in transgender emergence, and to focus on self-acceptance as the primary goal.

The adolescent who is considering disclosure should be supported to think about the likely reactions of the people they are telling, and potential resources to help facilitate understanding and adjustment. Loved ones often go through stages of adjustment involving feelings of shock, disbelief, denial, fear, anger, and betrayal, followed by sadness and possibly eventual acceptance (Ellis & Eriksen, 2002; Emerson & Rosenfeld, 1996). This is important for transgender people of all ages to be aware of but is particularly important to discuss with adolescents, as there is often dependence on others for financial and emotional support.

In our experience adolescents are often aware of potential risks of disclosure and are willing to engage in discussion about possible negative reactions. When there are concerns about possible violence or eviction from the home we include a crisis and safety plan as part of the preparation for disclosure. In some circumstances a safety plan includes discussion of the possible consequences of involuntary discovery of transgender status. For example, we have worked with several adolescents who transitioned early in life and whose teachers and age peers were not aware of transsexual history; as genital surgery is not recommended prior to age 18, there is a risk for any cross-living adolescent that their transgender status will be discovered. In these types of situations the benefits of controlled disclosure are important to discuss.

With the adolescent's consent, the clinician may be involved in the disclosure process. For example, the clinician may offer to meet with family members or other professionals in the adolescent's life to provide information about transgender issues or referral to peer or professional resources. Family therapy can be useful in helping both the transgender adolescent and their family members reach a deeper understanding of each other's perspectives and concerns.

Ethical and legal issues relating to parental consent to treatment. Transgender adolescents who are questioning or exploring their gender identity are often fearful that the clinician will disclose information to family members, teachers, social workers, or others involved in care. As with any other sensitive area of care (e.g., substance use, sexual health) the adolescent should be reassured that clinical professions have strict rules governing confidentiality and privacy. We have found it helpful to candidly review the legal limits of confidentiality (e.g., duty to report child abuse), and the process that we use when there is information that must be disclosed to a third party.

Legislation relating to consent by parents or guardians in medical treatment of adolescents varies greatly across jurisdictions. In British Columbia, as with any other type of non-emergency medical treatment, sex reassignment of adolescents is governed by the *Infants Act*. Medical treatment for mature minors (defined in provincial legislation as a person under the age of 19) can be provided in the absence of parental consent if (a) the health provider has explained the treatment options to the adolescent and is satisfied that the adolescent "understands the nature and consequences and the reasonably foreseeable benefits and risks"; (b) the health provider has made "reasonable efforts to determine and has concluded that the health care is in the infant's best interests," and (c) the patient has provided consent.

With sex reassignment, decisions about the risk and benefits of proceeding without parental consent must be carefully considered, as there is the potential for negative psychological, social, and economic consequences in addition to the normal health risks of any medical procedure. De Vries and colleagues (2006) "strongly recommend" that adolescents undergoing sex reassignment have adequate familial support and stability. For adolescents who are already living independently when treatment starts, it may be appropriate to assess social supports independent of family, particularly if the adolescent is estranged from the family-of-origin.

Managing the "real life experience" (RLE) at school and work. Adolescents who are not already cross-living prior to sex reassignment will undergo "real life experience" (RLE)–living as the desired gender in every aspect of life–as part of the reassignment process (de Vries et al., 2006; Meyer et al., 2001). For adolescents this often involves transition at school and work settings.

Some transgender youth undergo role transition prior to puberty and enter high school already cross-living full-time. For adolescents whose puberty has been suppressed, while there may be teasing or gossip about the lack of development of secondary sex characteristics, a noticeable transition will not be an issue. For adolescents who were not cross-living prior to starting high school, the transition from male-to-female or female-to-male is more complex. Advocacy with teachers and school administrators is often necessary during this stage of the transition process, particularly if the adolescent wants to remain at the same school throughout transition or has no alternative (e.g., in rural areas). Discussion topics with school staff may include decisions relating to disclosure (to staff and students); the need for accommodation relating to washrooms, change rooms, and gender-specific activities; change of name on school records and in verbal interactions; use of preferred pronoun; and, if there are concerns about peer violence, anti-harassment and safety planning measures (White Holman & Goldberg, 2006).

We have worked with several adolescents whose schools were sufficiently supportive to make it possible to stay during the process of change. In other situations, the harassment experienced at early stages of transition was so intense that our clients have decided to drop out of school and start fresh at a new school where peers are not aware they are transgender. Some clients have waited until hormonal changes had reduced their visibility as a gender-variant person before starting at a new school.

In some circumstances adolescents have already left school by the time they seek treatment, and may be living independently outside the parental home. While human rights legislation in some jurisdictions offers protection against termination of employment on the basis of sex, gender, and disability, even when these grounds are held to extend to transgender individuals (or there is explicit protection against discrimination on the basis of gender identity or expression) it is not uncommon for transgender people (of all ages) to experience employment discrimination, including termination of employment and difficulty finding work (findlay, Laframboise, Brady, Burnham, & Skolney-Elverson, 1996; Lombardi et al., 2001; Nemoto, Operario, Keatley, & Villegas, 2004; Odo & Hawelu, 2001). This possibility should be discussed with the adolescent and thought given to possible strategies that could be used to prepare an employer, disclose identity to co-workers, and otherwise manage the workplace transition. With adolescents who are new to the workforce we may provide information relating to employees' rights and responsibilities, and discuss trans-specific issues (such as asking an employer for time off for sex reassignment procedures).

Some of our older adolescent clients have been strongly dysphoric, committed to transition, and yet unable to cross-live in their current employment or school. In difficult situations such as these the clinician must consider whether the inability to live full-time in the desired role is simply a mature and reasonable accommodation of difficult circumstances, or ambivalence about full-time cross-living. Planning around RLE must include consideration of the adolescent's safety and the relative risks and benefits of undergoing RLE.

Feminizing or masculinizing hormones. There are documented reports of transgender individuals obtaining hormones without medical approval (Dean et al., 2000; Hope-Mason, Conners, & Kammerer, 1995), and the WPATH *Standards of Care* (Meyer et al., 2001) also recognize this risk. Estrogen and testosterone can be purchased illicitly or through the internet, or shared among friends. The risks associated with cross-sex hormones are exponentially increased when there is no screening for health conditions that may be made worse by hormone use, or regular medical monitoring of adverse effects after hormones are started (Dahl, Feldman, Goldberg, & Jaberi, 2006). Non-prescription-grade hormones may be poor quality and may be diluted with toxic substances. For those taking hormones by injection, improper injection technique or needle sharing poses additional health hazards such as abscess and transmission of HIV and Hepatitis C.

It has been our experience that transgender individuals who take hormones without medical assistance often do so because they don't know who to approach for help, cannot access hormones in any other way, or believe that the process for hormone assessment is so lengthy that their transition will be greatly delayed. Adolescents who are considering hormone therapy should be informed of local service options. Appropriately screened peer mentors may be helpful in explaining what to expect from the hormone assessment process, and in providing

perspective about the temporary wait that is typically involved while the hormone assessment is completed. Expedited referrals to clinicians who can provide medical monitoring should be considered for the adolescent who has disclosed use of hormones without medical assistance.

Feminizing or masculinizing surgery. While sex reassignment surgery is typically not indicated prior to age 18 (de Vries et al., 2006), it is important to begin discussion about surgery early on if the adolescent has expressed a clear intention to transition. Treatment options, impacts, and limitations should be clearly explained, as some adolescents believe that surgery is a simple process that will magically resolve all of their problems. Consumer education materials appropriate for older adolescents have recently been developed as part of the Trans Care Project (Simpson & Goldberg, 2006a; Simpson & Goldberg, 2006b).

Discussion about surgery should include information about costs and options for payment. In jurisdictions where private or public health insurance is an option, the eligibility criteria and process for application should be discussed. In many jurisdictions insurance explicitly excludes coverage for sex reassignment surgery, and adolescents should be made aware of this so they understand that they may not be able to obtain surgery at age 18. For adolescents in this situation, appropriately screened experienced peer mentors may be helpful in sharing information about ways to cope with not having access to needed surgery.

Integration of Transgender Identity into Core Identity

Integration relates to awareness of the self as a whole person, of which transgender identity is a part rather than the consuming focus (Lev, 2004). Transgender issues are not necessarily completely resolved or static, but the adolescent feels relatively settled and content in terms of gender issues. Some clients describe this as being "able to imagine a future."

Integration does not necessarily mean development of a fixed gender identity. Some individuals retain a fluid identity throughout life, or have periods of ambivalence about identity. For some adolescents integration includes acceptance of ambiguity and the shifting nature of their feelings. When these shifts occur without distress, integration has been achieved.

For the adolescent undergoing sex reassignment, integration does not always depend on completion of surgical changes. As Lev (2004) states,

> In the beginning of this journey some transsexuals focused exclusively on "getting the surgery," as if surgery validated their gender transition . . . In the integration stage, most transsexuals, including those who are postsurgical, accept that "the surgery" is neither the end all or be all of their identity. Although they may choose surgery, their gender identity does not depend on their genitalia, but on who they know themselves to be. (p. 268)

The clinician's role in this stage depends on the adolescent's overall development. In some circumstances regular appointments stop because the adolescent no longer needs clinical assistance. For other adolescents, resolution of gender issues reveals areas of development that have been hampered by concerns about gender identity (e.g., development of social skills) or the existence of psychosocial concerns unrelated to transgender concerns. As discussed in the preceding chapter, psychotherapy may continue after surgery.

In our experience integration is a long-term process that is rarely achieved during adolescence. We are encouraged by outcome data from the Amsterdam clinic (Cohen-Kettenis & Van Goozen, 1997; Smith, Cohen, & Cohen-Kettenis, 2002), where supportive treatment of gender-variant adolescents is more easily accessed at an earlier age. These studies suggest that with appropriate treatment and supports, even highly dysphoric transgender adolescents can reach an integrated state.

CONCLUDING REMARKS

Synchronized care for transgender adolescents is a challenge for clinicians working in community settings. Careful communication is needed to ensure that transgender and gender-questioning adolescents have adequate access to clinical and peer resources, particularly in rural regions. While specialists should coordinate care of youth who are gender dysphoric or highly distressed about gender identity issues, the non-specialist should expect to be involved in care of transgender adolescents at some point in their practice. Both the specialist and the non-specialist can have a significant positive influence in promoting healthy development of transgender adolescents. We hope this article helps non-specialists to feel more confident in working with this underserved population.

REFERENCES

American Psychiatric Association (2000). *Diagnostic and statistical manual of mental disorders (DSM-IV-TR)* (4th Ed., Text Revision ed.). Washington, DC: Author.

American Psychological Association (2002). *Developing adolescents: A reference for professionals*. Washington, DC: Author.

Assistant Deputy Ministers' Committee on Prostitution and the Sexual Exploitation of Youth (2000). *Sexual exploitation of youth in British Columbia* (Rep. No. C00-960303-4). Victoria, BC, Canada: BC Ministry of Health.

Bartlett, N. H., Vasey, P. L., & Bukowski, W. M. (2000). Is Gender Identity Disorder in children a mental disorder? *Sex Roles, 43*, 753-785.

Bockting, W.O., & Ehrbar, R. (2005). Commentary: Gender variance, dissonance, or identity disorder. *Journal of Psychology and Human Sexuality, 17*(3/4), 125-134.

Bockting, W. O., Knudson, G., & Goldberg, J. M. (2006). Counseling and mental health care for transgender adults and loved ones. *International Journal of Transgenderism, 9*(3/4), 35-82.

Bradley, S. J., & Zucker, K. J. (1990). Gender identity disorder and psychosexual problems in children and adolescents. *Canadian Journal of Psychiatry, 35*, 477-486.

Brown, M. L., & Rounsley, C. A. (1996). *True selves: Understanding transsexualism–For families, friends, coworkers, and helping professionals*. San Francisco, CA: Jossey-Bass.

Burgess, C. (1999). Internal and external stress factors associated with the identity development of transgendered youth. In G. P. Mallon (Ed.), *Social services with transgendered youth* (pp. 35-47). Binghamton, NY: Harrington Park Press.

Cohen, L., de Ruiter, C., Ringelberg, H., & Cohen-Kettenis, P. T. (1997). Psychological functioning of

Catherine White Holman and Joshua M. Goldberg 109

adolescent transsexuals: Personality and psychopathology. *Journal of Clinical Psychology, 53,* 187-196.

Cohen-Kettenis, P. T., & Van Goozen, S. H. M. (1997). Sex reassignment of adolescent transsexuals: a follow-up study. *Journal of the American Academy of Child and Adolescent Psychiatry, 36,* 263-271.

Currah, P., & Minter, S. (2000). *Transgender equality: A handbook for activists and policymakers.* New York, NY: National Gay and Lesbian Task Force and The National Center for Lesbian Rights.

Dahl, M., Feldman, J., Goldberg, J. M., & Jaberi, A. (2006). Physical aspects of transgender endocrine therapy. *International Journal of Transgenderism, 9*(3/4), 111-134.

de Castell, S. & Jenson, J. (2002). *No place like home: Final research report on the Pridehouse Project.* Burnaby, BC, Canada: Simon Fraser University.

de Vries, A. L. C., Cohen-Kettenis, P. T., & Delemarre-van de Waal, H. (2006). Clinical management of gender dysphoria in adolescents. *International Journal of Transgenderism, 9*(3/4), 83-94.

Dean, L., Meyer, I. H., Robinson, K., Sell, R. L., Sember, R., Silenzio, V. M. B., Bowen, D. J., Bradford, J., Rothblum, E., White, J., Dunn, P., Lawrence, A., Wolfe, D., & Xavier, J. (2000). Lesbian, gay, bisexual, and transgender health: Findings and concerns. *Journal of the Gay and Lesbian Medical Association, 4,* 102-151.

Di Ceglie, D., Freedman, D., McPherson, S., & Richardson, P. (2002). Children and adolescents referred to a specialist gender identity development service: Clinical features and demographic characteristics. *International Journal of Transgenderism, 6.* Retrieved January 1, 2005, from http://www.symposion.com/ijt/ijtvo06no01_01.htm

Dimensions (2000a). *Dimensions treatment guidelines for FTM Transition.* Retrieved January 1, 2005, from http://tghealth-critiques.tripod.com/protoc2.htm

Dimensions (2000b). *Dimensions treatment guidelines for MTF transition.* Retrieved January 1, 2005, from http://tghealth-critiques.tripod.com/protoc1.htm

Ellis, K. M., & Eriksen, K. (2002). Transsexual and transgenderist experiences and treatment options. *The Family Journal: Counseling and Therapy for Couples & Families, 10,* 289-299.

Emerson, S., & Rosenfeld, C. (1996). Stages of adjustment in family members of transgender individuals. *Journal of Family Psychotherapy, 7,* 1-12.

Estes, R. J., & Weiner, N. A. (2001). *The commercial sexual exploitation of children in the U.S., Canada, and Mexico.* Philadelphia, PA: University of Pennsylvania.

Feldman, J., & Goldberg, J. M. (2006). Transgender primary medical care. *International Journal of Transgenderism, 9*(3/4), 3-34.

findlay, b., Laframboise, S., Brady, D., Burnham, C. W. G., & Skolney-Elverson, S. R. (1996). *Finding our place: The transgendered law reform project.* Vancouver, BC, Canada: High Risk Project Society.

Fontaine, J. H., & Hammond, N. L. (1996). Counseling issues with gay and lesbian adolescents. *Adolescence, 31,* 817-830.

Goldberg, J. M., & White, C. (2004). Expanding our understanding of gendered violence: Violence against trans people and loved ones. *Aware: The Newsletter of the BC Institute Against Family Violence, 11,* 21-25.

Goldenring, J. M., & Rosen, D. S. (2004). Getting into adolescent heads: An essential update. *Contemporary Pediatrics, 21,* 64-90.

Hill, D. B., Rozanski, C., Carfagnini, J., & Willoughby, B. (2005). Gender identity disorders in childhood and adolescence: A critical inquiry. *Journal of Psychology & Human Sexuality, 17*(3/4), 7-34.

Hope-Mason, T., Conners, M. M., & Kammerer, C. A. (1995). *Transgender and HIV risks: Needs assessment.* Boston, MA: Department of Public Health, HIV/AIDS Bureau.

Kagan, S., & Melrose, C. (2003). The SCOFF questionnaire was less sensitive but more specific than the ESP for detecting eating disorders. *Evidence-Based Nursing, 6,* 118.

Kenagy, G. P. (2005). Transgender health: Findings from two needs assessment studies in Philadelphia. *Health & Social Work, 30,* 19-26.

Klein, R. (1999). Group work practice with transgendered male to female sex workers. In G. P. Mallon (Ed.), *Social services with transgendered youth* (pp. 95-109). Binghamton, NY: The Haworth Press, Inc.

Kosciw, J. G., & Cullen, M. K. (2001). *The GLSEN 2001 National School Climate Survey: The school-related experiences of our nation's lesbian, gay, bisexual and transgender youth.* New York, NY: Gay, Lesbian and Straight Education Network.

Langer, S. J., & Martin, J. I. (2004). How dresses can make you mentally ill: Examining Gender Identity Disorder in children. *Child and Adolescent Social Work Journal, 21,* 5-23.

Leichtentritt, R. D., & Arad, B. D. (2004). Adolescent and young adult male-to-female transsexuals: Pathways to prostitution. *British Journal of Social Work, 34,* 349-374.

Lerner, R. M. (2002). *Adolescence: Development, diversity, context, and application.* Upper Saddle River, NJ: Prentice-Hall.

Lev, A. I. (2004). *Transgender emergence: Therapeutic guidelines for working with gender-variant people and their families.* Binghamton, NY: The Haworth Clinical Practice Press.

Lindgren, T. W., & Pauly, I. B. (1975). A body image scale for evaluating transsexuals. *Archives of Sexual Behavior, 4,* 639-656.

Lombardi, E. L., Wilchins, R. A., Priesing, D., & Malouf, D. (2001). Gender violence: Transgender experiences with violence and discrimination. *Journal of Homosexuality, 42,* 89-101.

Menvielle, E. J. (1998). Gender identity disorder. *Journal of the American Academy of Child & Adolescent Psychiatry, 37*, 243-244.

Menvielle, E. J. & Tuerk, C. (2002). A support group for parents of gender-nonconforming boys. *Journal of the American Academy of Child & Adolescent Psychiatry, 41*, 1010-1013.

Meyer, W. J., III, Bockting, W. O., Cohen-Kettenis, P. T., Coleman, E., Di Ceglie, D., Devor, H., Gooren, L., Hage, J. J., Kirk, S., Kuiper, B., Laub, D., Lawrence, A., Menard, Y., Monstrey, S., Patton, J., Schaefer, L., Webb, A., & Wheeler, C. C. (2001). *The standards of care for Gender Identity Disorders* (6th ed.). Minneapolis, MN: Harry Benjamin International Gender Dysphoria Association.

Minter, S. (1999). Diagnosis and treatment of gender identity disorder in children. In M. Rottnek (Ed.), *Sissies and tomboys: Gender nonconformity and homosexual childhood* (pp. 9-33). New York: New York University Press.

Moore, S. M. (2002). Diagnosis for a straight planet: A critique of gender identity disorder for children and adolescents in the *DSM-IV*. *Dissertation Abstracts International, 63*(4B), 2066. (University Microfilms No. AAI3051898)

Nemoto, T., Operario, D., Keatley, J., & Villegas, D. (2004). Social context of HIV risk behaviours among male-to-female transgenders of colour. *AIDS Care, 16*, 724-735.

Newman, L. K. (2002). Sex, gender and culture: Issues in the definition, assessment and treatment of gender identity disorder. *Clinical Child Psychology & Psychiatry, 7*, 352-359.

Odo, C., & Hawelu, A. (2001). Eo na Mahu o Hawai'i: the extraordinary health needs of Hawai'i's Mahu. *Pacific Health Dialog, 8*, 327-334.

Pazos, S. (1999). Practice with female-to-male transgendered youth. In G. P. Mallon (Ed.), *Social services with transgendered youth* (pp. 65-82). Binghamton, NY: The Haworth Press, Inc.

Prochaska, J. O., DiClemente, C. C., & Norcross, J. C. (1992). In search of how people change: Applications to addictive behaviors. *American Psychologist, 47*, 1102-1114.

Raj, R. (2002). Towards a transpositive therapeutic model: Developing clinical sensitivity and cultural competence in the effective support of transsexual and transgendered clients. *International Journal of Transgenderism, 6*. Retrieved January 1, 2005, from http://www.symposion.com/ijt/ijtvo06no02_04.htm

Rosenberg, M. (2002). Children with gender identity issues and their parents in individual and group treatment. *Journal of the American Academy of Child and Adolescent Psychiatry, 41*, 619-621.

Simpson, A. J., & Goldberg, J. M. (2006). *Surgery: A guide for FTMs*. Vancouver, BC, Canada: Vancouver Coastal Health Authority.

Simpson, A. J., & Goldberg, J. M. (2006). *Surgery: A guide for MTFs*. Vancouver, BC, Canada: Vancouver Coastal Health Authority.

Smith, Y. L. S., Cohen, L., & Cohen-Kettenis, P. T. (2002). Postoperative psychological functioning of adolescent transsexuals: A Rorschach study. *Archives of Sexual Behavior, 31*, 255-261.

Smith, Y. L. S., Van Goozen, S. H. M., & Cohen-Kettenis, P. T. (2001). Adolescents with gender identity disorder who were accepted or rejected for sex reassignment surgery: a prospective follow-up study. *Journal of the American Academy of Child and Adolescent Psychiatry, 40*, 472-481.

Social Services and Community Safety Division - Justice Institute of British Columbia (2002). *Commercial sexual exploitation: Innovative ideas for working with children and youth*. New Westminster, BC, Canada: Justice Institute of British Columbia.

Tonkin, R. S. (2002). *Accenting the positive: A developmental framework for reducing risk and promoting positive outcomes among BC youth*. Vancouver, BC, Canada: McCreary Centre Society.

Tubman, M., & Bramly, L. (1998). *Out from the Shadows: International Summit of Sexually Exploited Youth–Final summit report*. Ottawa, ONT, Canada: Save the Children.

White Holman, C., & Goldberg, J. (2006). Social and medical transgender case advocacy. *International Journal of Transgenderism, 9*(3/4), 197-217.

Wilson, I., Griffin, C., & Wren, B. (2002). The validity of the diagnosis of gender identity disorder (child and adolescent criteria). *Clinical Child Psychology & Psychiatry, 7*, 335-351.

Worth, H. (2000). Up on K Road on Saturday night: Sex, gender and sex work in Auckland. *Venereology: Interdisciplinary, International Journal of Sexual Health, 13*, 15-24.

Wyss, S. E. (2004). 'This was my hell': The violence experienced by gender non-conforming youth in US high schools. *International Journal of Qualitative Studies in Education, 17*, 709-730.

Zucker, K. J. (2004). Gender identity development and issues. *Child and Adolescent Psychiatric Clinics of North America, 13*, 551-568.

Zucker, K. J., Deogracias, J. J., Johnson, L. L., Meyer-Bahlburg, H. F., Kessler, S. J., & Schober, J. M. (2005). *The Gender Identity Questionnaire for Adults and the Recalled Childhood Gender Questionnaire-Revised: Final analyses*. Poster presentation, Meeting of the International Academy of Sex Research, Ottawa, ONT, Canada.

doi:10.1300/J485v09n03_05

Physical Aspects of Transgender Endocrine Therapy

Marshall Dahl, MD, PhD, FRCPC
Jamie L. Feldman, MD, PhD
Joshua M. Goldberg
Afshin Jaberi, BSc (Pharm), RPh

SUMMARY. The goal of transgender endocrine therapy is to change secondary sex characteristics to reduce gender dysphoria and/or facilitate gender presentation that is consistent with the felt sense of self. To maximize desired effects and minimize adverse effects, endocrine therapy must be individualized based on the patient's goals, the risk/benefit ratio of medications, the presence of other medical conditions, and consideration of social and economic issues. In this article we suggest protocols for the prescribing clinician relating to physical assessment, prescription planning, initiation of endocrine therapy, and ongoing maintenance in transgender adults. doi:10.1300/J485v09n03_06 *[Article copies available for a fee from The Haworth Document Delivery Service: 1-800-HAWORTH. E-mail address: <docdelivery@haworthpress.com> Website: <http://www.HaworthPress.com> © 2006 by The Haworth Press, Inc. All rights reserved.]*

KEYWORDS. Transgender, gender dysphoria, sex reassignment, hormones, sex steroids, endocrine therapy

Endocrine therapy is a strongly desired medical intervention for many transgender individuals. The goal of transgender endocrine therapy is to change secondary sex characteristics to reduce gender dysphoria and/or facilitate gender presentation that is consistent with the felt sense of self. While there are risks associated with taking feminizing/masculinizing medications, when appropriately prescribed they can greatly improve mental health and quality of life for transgender people (Kuiper & Cohen-Kettenis, 1988; Leavitt, Berger, Hoeppner, &

Marshall Dahl, MD, PhD, FRCPC, is affiliated with the Division of Endocrinology, Department of Medicine, University of British Columbia, Vancouver, BC, Canada. Jamie L. Feldman, MD, PhD, is Assistant Professor, Department of Family Medicine and Community Health, University of Minnesota Medical School, Minneapolis, MN, USA. Joshua M. Goldberg is Education Consultant of the Transgender Health Program, Vancouver, BC, Canada. Afshin Jaberi, BSc (Pharm), RPh, is affiliated with Reach Community Health Centre, Vancouver, BC, Canada.

Address correspondence to: Dr. Marshall Dahl, 236-575 West 8th Avenue, Vancouver, BC, Canada, V5Z 1C6 (E-mail: marshall.dahl@vch.ca).

This manuscript was created for the Trans Care Project, a joint initiative of Transcend Transgender Support & Education Society and Vancouver Coastal Health's Transgender Health Program, with funding from the Canadian Rainbow Health Coalition. The authors thank Rosemary Basson, Fionna Bayley, Trevor Corneil, Stacy Elliott, Lucretia van den Berg, and Michael van Trotsenburg for their comments on an earlier draft, and Donna Lindenberg, Olivia Ashbee, A. J. Simpson, and Rodney Hunt for research assistance.

[Haworth co-indexing entry note]: "Physical Aspects of Transgender Endocrine Therapy." Dahl, Marshall et al. Co-published simultaneously in *International Journal of Transgenderism* (The Haworth Medical Press, an imprint of The Haworth Press, Inc.) Vol. 9, No. 3/4, 2006, pp. 111-134; and: *Guidelines for Transgender Care* (ed: Walter O. Bockting, and Joshua M. Goldberg) The Haworth Medical Press, an imprint of The Haworth Press, Inc., 2006, pp. 111-134. Single or multiple copies of this article are available for a fee from The Haworth Document Delivery Service [1-800-HAWORTH, 9:00 a.m. - 5:00 p.m. (EST). E-mail address: docdelivery@haworthpress.com].

Northrop, 1980). In addition to inducing physical changes, the act of using cross-sex hormones is itself an affirmation of gender identity–a powerful incentive for this population (Gay and Lesbian Medical Association, 2001; Kammerer, Mason, Connors, & Durkee, 1999).

There is great variation in the extent to which hormonal changes are undertaken or desired. Some individuals seek maximum feminization/masculinization, while others experience relief with an androgynous presentation resulting from minimization of existing secondary sex characteristics. Endocrine therapy must be individualized based on the patient's goals, the risk/benefit ratio of medications, the presence of other medical conditions, and consideration of social and economic issues. As economic factors may be a barrier for patients seeking medications, comparative cost (based on prices in British Columbia, Canada as of 2005) is included as Appendix A.

This article suggests protocols for the prescribing clinician relating to physical assessment, prescription planning, initiation of endocrine therapy, and ongoing maintenance in transgender adults. Assessment of psychological eligibility and readiness prior to initiation of endocrine therapy is discussed elsewhere (Bockting, Knudson, & Goldberg, 2006), as is endocrine treatment of transgender adolescents (de Vries, Cohen-Kettenis, & Delemarre-van de Waal, 2006).

As discussed in The World Professional Association for Transgender Health (WPATH)'s *Standards of Care* (Meyer et al., 2001), transgender endocrine therapy is best undertaken in the context of a complete approach to health that includes comprehensive primary care and a coordinated approach to psychosocial issues. While the WPATH *Standards* do not require psychotherapy prior to initiation of endocrine therapy, ideally a trans-experienced therapist will be available as needed to assist the patient in adjusting to the profound physical and psychosocial changes involved in endocrine therapy. Advocacy may also be required to assist with changes to legal name or identification. Issues in counseling and clinical advocacy are discussed elsewhere (Bockting et al., 2006; White Holman & Goldberg, 2006).

Just as the WPATH *Standards* (Meyer et al., 2001) are intended as a flexible framework to guide the treatment of transgender people, the recommendations made in this article should not be perceived as a rigid set of guidelines. In any clinical practice it is important that protocols be tailored to the specific needs of each patient, and clinicians are encouraged to adapt and modify our suggested protocols to address changing conditions and emerging issues. Research in transgender health is still in its infancy, and there are widely diverging clinical and consumer opinions about "best" practice. Our recommendations are based on a review of transgender health research, a review of protocols used in 16 clinics, interviews with expert clinicians, and the authors' clinical experience. Ongoing research and collegial meetings are needed to further develop practice protocols.

RESPONSIBILITIES OF THE PRESCRIBING CLINICIAN

Feminizing/masculinizing medication is typically prescribed by a family physician, endocrinologist, or nurse practitioner.[1] With appropriate transgender health training, endocrinologic manipulation of secondary sex characteristics can usually be managed by the primary care provider. Medical visits relating to hormone maintenance provide an opportunity for broader care to a population that is often medically underserved, and many of the screening tasks involved in long-term hormone maintenance fall within the scope of primary care rather than specialist care. For this reason we suggest that if hormones are prescribed by an endocrinologist rather than the primary care provider, there be close communication between the two clinicians to ensure adequate care. An expert endocrinologist should be involved if the primary care provider has no experience with transgender health, or if the patient has a pre-existing metabolic or endocrine disorder that may be affected by endocrine therapy.

The WPATH *Standards* (Meyer et al., 2001) state that the prescribing clinician should:

1. perform an initial evaluation that includes health history, physical examination, and relevant laboratory tests

2. explain what feminizing/masculinizing medications do and the possible side effects/health risks

3. confirm that the patient has the capacity to understand the risks and benefits of treatment and to make an informed decision about medical care

4. inform the patient of the HBIGDA *Standards* and eligibility/readiness requirements

5. provide ongoing medical monitoring, including regular physical and laboratory examination to monitor hormone effects and side effects

MALE-TO-FEMALE (MTF) ENDOCRINE THERAPY

Mechanisms of Action

Endocrinologic feminization is achieved by direct or indirect suppression of the effects of androgens, and induction of female physical characteristics (Asscheman & Gooren, 1992; Basson, 2001). Androgen suppression can be achieved by: (a) using agents that suppress the production of gonadotrophic releasing hormone (GnRH) or are GnRH antagonists (e.g., progestational agents), (b) suppressing the production of luteinizing hormone (e.g., progestational agents, cyproterone acetate), (c) interfering with the production of testosterone or metabolism of testosterone to dihydrotestosterone (e.g., spironolactone, finasteride, cyproterone acetate), or (d) interfering with the binding of androgens to receptors in target tissues (e.g., spironolactone, cyproterone acetate, flutamide).

Estrogen is the principal agent used to induce female characteristics, and works primarily by direct stimulation of receptors in target tissues (Moore, Wisniewski, & Dobs, 2003). Although estrogen also suppresses luteinizing hormone (LH), the estrogen dose required for effective LH suppression is dangerously high (Basson, 2001).

Expected Feminizing Effects

Rapidity and degree of change from feminizing endocrine therapy depends on the agents used, dosage, and the patient's responsiveness to endocrine therapy. Typically, within the first 1-6 months there is gradual redistribution of body fat to more closely approximate a female body habitus, decreased muscle mass and decreased upper body strength, softening of skin, decreased libido and possible difficulty reaching orgasm, reduction of ejaculate, and decreased spontaneous/morning erections (Asscheman & Gooren, 1992; Dimensions, 2003a; Futterweit, 1998; Israel & Tarver, 1997; Kirk & Rothblatt, 1995; Meyer et al., 1981; Meyer et al., 2001; Schlatterer, von Werder, & Stalla, 1996; Steinbeck, 1997). Testicular volume is reduced by up to 25% within the first year (Asscheman & Gooren, 1992; Meyer et al., 1986), with gradual reduction up to 50% of the original volume over a long period of time (Jin, Turner, Walters, & Handelsman, 1996). The shrinkage of testes may make them feel softer on palpation (Futterweit, 1998). Testicular atrophy impacts sperm maturation and motility, and this may be permanent (Lubbert, Leo-Rossberg, & Hammerstein, 1992).

Tender breast buds may start to form within 3-6 months, with gradual breast growth (highly variable) and nipple development taking two or more years (Asscheman & Gooren, 1992; Israel & Tarver, 1997; Meyer et al., 1986; Tangpricha, Ducharme, Barber, & Chipkin, 2003). Typically breast growth is not as pronounced in MTFs as in non-transgender women, and it is rare for MTF breasts to reach Tanner Stage 5 appearance (Reutrakul et al., 1998; Sosa et al., 2004). If after 18-24 months of feminizing endocrine therapy breast growth is not sufficient for patient comfort, surgical augmentation may be considered (Bowman & Goldberg, 2006). Weight increase may help promote breast development in thin MTF patients.

Over a period of several years body and facial hair becomes finer and growth is slowed (Asscheman & Gooren, 1992; Basson, 2001; Bromham & Pearson, 1996; Flaherty et al., 2001; Futterweit, 1998; Levy, Crown, & Reid, 2003; Schlatterer et al., 1996; Steinbeck, 1997). However, body and facial hair typically cannot be eliminated by hormones alone, and electrolysis, laser treatments, or other forms of hair removal may be desired (Hage, Bouman, & Bloem, 1992; Paquet, Fumal, Piérard-Franchimont, & Piérard, 2002; Schroeter, Groenewegen, Reineke, & Neumann, 2003; Shenenberger & Utecht,

2002). While feminizing endocrine therapy may gradually slow or stop the progression of male pattern baldness, scalp hair does not completely regrow in bald areas (Asscheman & Gooren, 1992; Bromham & Pearson, 1996; Flaherty et al., 2001; Futterweit, 1998; Meyer et al., 2001).

Most of these changes are reversible if treatment is discontinued. Breast growth and development of the nipple-areolar complex are permanent. As discussed by Feldman and Goldberg (2006), it is not known if changes to fertility are completely reversible, and options for sperm banking should be discussed prior to initiation of endocrine therapy (De Sutter, 2001; Meyer et al., 2001).

Recommended Feminizing Regimen

Table 1 summarizes our recommendations for a basic regimen for the MTF patient who desires maximum feminization. A combination of estrogen and spironolactone (an androgen antagonist) is recommended. Spironolactone has a direct effect of reducing male pattern hair growth and also minimizes the dosage of estrogen needed to suppress testosterone, thereby reducing risks associated with high dose exogenous estrogen (Oriel, 2000; Prior, Vigna, & Watson, 1989; Prior, Vigna, Watson, Diewold, & Robinow, 1986). Finasteride may be added to slow male pattern balding.

Androgen antagonists (a.k.a. "anti-androgens") may be prescribed alone for patients who wish to reduce masculine characteristics for a more androgynous appearance. As spironolactone can induce irreversible gynecomastia, 5α-reductase inhibitors are preferred for those who do not want visible breast development.

With both estrogen and androgen antagonists, the starting dose for patients who are at low risk for adverse effects can be gradually increased to the recommended maximum if needed to achieve the desired changes and to bring free testosterone to the lower half of the female range (Table B1, Appendix B). Following orchiectomy, the dosage should be adjusted as endogenous androgen production is significantly reduced. To preserve bone density following orchiectomy estrogen supplementation should be maintained throughout life (or consider bisphosphonates), and calcium/Vitamin D supplementation is recommended.

Estrogen. There is evidence that MTFs taking estrogen are at increased risk for venous thrombosis, pulmonary embolism, and cholelithiasis (Asscheman, Gooren, & Eklund, 1989; Schlatterer et al., 1998; Toorians, Gooren, & Asscheman, 2001; van Kesteren, Asscheman, Megens & Gooren, 1997). These risks may be mitigated by the type of endocrine agent chosen, the route of administration (transdermal vs. oral), dosage, and by other factors such as

TABLE 1. Basic Feminizing Regimen

| Agent | Estrogen 17β-estradiol | | | Androgen antagonist | |
| | | | | Spironolactone *and/or* | Finasteride |
	Transdermal[a]	*or*	Oral	Oral	Oral
Pre-orchiectomy	Start at 0.1 mg/24 hrs, applied twice per week; gradually increase up to maximum of 0.2 mg/24 hrs, applied twice per week.		Start with 1-2 mg qd; gradually increase up to maximum 4 mg qd.	Start with 50-100 mg qd; increase by 50-100 mg each month up to average 200-300 mg qd (maximum 500 mg qd). Modify if there are risks of adverse effects.[b]	Use 2.5-5.0 mg qd for systemic anti-androgen effect; use 2.5 mg every other day if solely for alopecia androgenetica.
Post-orchiectomy	0.375-0.1 mg/24 hrs, applied twice per week.		1-2 mg qd	25-50 mg qd	2.5 mg qd

[a]Use transdermal estradiol if the patient is > age 40 or is at risk for DVT. Oral estradiol is an option if the patient is < age 40 and is low risk for DVT. [b]If taking ACE-inhibitors or other potassium-sparing medication, spironolactone should not go above 25 mg qd, and serum potassium should be closely monitored. If the patient has low blood pressure or renal insufficiency start at 50 mg and increase by up to 50 mg per week to a maximum of 300 mg qd, with a renal function test 1-2 weeks after each increase.

smoking cessation. Some centres taper or temporarily discontinue estrogen 2-4 weeks before any major surgery to minimize thrombosis risk, restarting after the patient has recovered sufficiently to be significantly mobile (Bromham & Pearson, 1996; Flaherty et al., 2001; Futterweit, 1998; Israel & Tarver, 1997; Tangpricha et al., 2003).

In the absence of empirical evidence that one type of estrogen (esterified vs. conjugated vs. estradiol) is a more effective feminizing agent than another, our recommendation to use 17β-estradiol is based on concerns about thromboembolic risk. Evidence suggests the lowest thromboembolic risk with transdermal estradiol (Scarabin, Oger, & Plu-Bureau, 2003; Toorians et al., 2001; van Kesteren et al., 1997). This is particularly important for those with vascular or thrombotic risks, including smokers and people over age 40, and people with co-morbid conditions. If an oral agent is desired, oral 17β-estradiol is recommended rather than oral ethinyl estradiol or conjugated estrogens due to studies suggesting higher risks of blood clots with the latter forms (Toorians et al., 2003).

The Drug and Poison Information Centre of BC's *Drug Information Reference* (Cadario & Leathem, 2003) lists three clinically significant interactions between estrogen and other medications: anticonvulsants (decreased estrogen effect), rifampin (decreased estrogen effect), and corticosteroids (increased corticosteroid effect). A more detailed list of interactions is available as an online supplement at http://www.vch.ca/transhealth/resources/library/tcpdocs/estrogen-interactions.pdf.

Spironolactone. In the mid-1980s, clinicians at the Vancouver Gender Dysphoria Program began using spironolactone as part of the feminizing regimen for MTFs, based on its anti-androgenic properties and its use for treatment of hirsutism in non-transgender women (Basson, 2001; Prior et al., 1986; Prior et al., 1989). It has since been adopted for use by many other clinicians (Flaherty et al., 2001; Israel & Tarver, 1997; Kirk & Rothblatt, 1995; Levy et al., 2003; Oriel, 2000; Tangpricha et al., 2003). Possible adverse effects of spironolactone include hyperkalemia, renal insufficiency, hypotension, and rash (Futterweit, 1998; Prior et al., 1989). Hyperkalema is a particular

concern if the patient is also taking ACE-inhibitors or Angiotensin Receptor Blockers, or has Type IV renal tubular acidosis.

Alternative Regimens and Agents

Progestins. The inclusion of progestins in MTF feminizing therapy is controversial (Oriel, 2000). Some clinicians believe progestins are necessary for full nipple development (Basson & Prior, 1998). However, a clinical comparison of feminization regimens with and without progestins found that the addition of progestins neither enhanced breast growth nor lowered serum levels of free testosterone (Meyer et al., 1986). There are concerns regarding potential adverse effects of progestins, including weak androgen receptor stimulation, depression, weight gain, and lipid changes (Meyer et al., 1986; Tangpricha et al., 2003); the Women's Health Initiative findings of increased risk of coronary heart disease, stroke, pulmonary embolism, and invasive breast cancer in postmenopausal women taking combined estrogen and progestin HRT (Rossouw et al., 2002) are also noteworthy. Many of the clinical protocols reviewed did not include progestins, and some clinicians explicitly recommended against their use (Bromham & Pearson, 1996; Buffat, 2003; Dimensions, 2000b; Kirk & Rothblatt, 1995; Moore et al., 2003; Schlatterer et al., 1998; Tangpricha et al., 2003). Others included medroxyprogesterone acetate as part of their basic feminizing regimen (Basson, 2001; Futterweit, 1998; Levy et al., 2003).

We do not recommend progestin unless further androgen suppression effects are required after maximum estrogen doses, or the patient cannot tolerate an estrogen-based regimen (Flaherty et al., 2001). Table 2 represents our recommended doses for progestin use in these circumstances.

Alternative forms of estrogen. There is no empirical evidence that one form of estrogen brings about greater feminization than other forms of estrogen. However, it has been observed that intramuscular (IM) estrogen tends to give slightly faster results compared to oral/transdermal estrogen, and patients may therefore request it. IM estrogen is typically not a first choice as IM administration results in larger fluctuations in blood levels than transdermal/

TABLE 2. Progestin Options in a MTF Feminizing Regimen

	Progestin options
Oral	Micronized progesterone: 100-400 mg qd Medroxyprogesterone acetate: 5-30 mg po qd (in divided doses at higher range)
Transdermal single patch	140 ug or 250 ug norethindrone acetate (progestin) with 50 ug 17ß-estradiol[a] twice per week

[a]If also taking estradiol alone, adjust the dosage of estradiol accordingly.

oral administration (with according greater risks of adverse effects and mood lability). We recommend that IM injection only be used if the clinician has high confidence in patient compliance and if the patient is low risk for deep vein thrombosis (DVT). If in the first two years of treatment there is minimal breast development or an early plateau in growth (no change in three months despite being on the maximum dose) some clinicians switch to IM estradiol valerate (20-40 mg IM q 2 weeks) for 3-6 months to see if it is possible to boost breast development. Clinician-administered IM estrogen may also be the preferred agent in conditions where the patient may be pressured to share or sell oral or transdermal medication (e.g., incarceration).

Transdermal estradiol gel is a possible alternative to the transdermal patch for those who experience a skin reaction from the patch. The amount of skin needed for absorption of the required amount of gel is quite large (both legs) so estradiol gel is not a first choice for most patients.

Alternative androgen antagonists. Cyproterone acetate is not available in the USA, but is used by some clinicians in other locations as an alternative to spironolactone (Bromham & Pearson, 1996; Levy et al., 2003; Schlatterer et al., 1998; T'Sjoen, Rubens, De Sutter, & Gooren, 2004). Cyproterone acetate inhibits the production of luteinizing hormone, is a 5α-reductase inhibitor, and interferes with the binding of testosterone at receptor sites. Possible adverse effects include liver enzyme elevation and depression (Basson, 2001), and for this reason we do not recommend it unless spironolactone cannot be tolerated.

Flutamide use (750 mg po qd) has been reported by some clinicians (Israel & Tarver, 1997; Levy et al., 2003). Hepatotoxicity has been reported in men receiving comparable doses of flutamide for treatment of prostate cancer (Wysowski, Freiman, Tourtelot, & Horton, 1993), and for this reason we do not recommend flutamide as part of MTF feminization. A clinical trial of flutamide, finasteride, and spironolactone in the treatment of hirsute non-transgender women found all agents equally effective in reducing facial hair (Moghetti et al., 2000).

Assessment Prior to Initiating MTF Endocrine Therapy

Comprehensive primary care evaluation. A full primary care evaluation (Feldman & Goldberg, 2006) should be completed, with particular attention to risks/history of venous thrombosis, atherosclerotic vascular disease, cholelithiasis, glucose intolerance, dyslipidemia, estrogen-dependent cancer, migraine, and hepatic disease. If there are additional primary care concerns these should be appropriately investigated. When possible, efforts should be made to stabilize and control co-morbid conditions with medication, lifestyle changes, or other suitable interventions prior to initiating hormones.

Cigarette smoking is associated with increased risk for venous thrombosis. We recommend a harm reduction approach that strongly encourages patients to reduce or stop smoking along with a clear recommendation that their estrogen dosage must be kept low as long as they are smoking.

Baseline evaluation. To assist in monitoring of adverse effects, baseline values should be recorded for lipid profile, fasting blood glucose (and glycosylated hemoglobin if diabetes or suspected glucose intolerance), liver enzymes, prolactin, electrolytes, urea, and creatinine. If there are clinical concerns there may be indications for additional tests, including complete blood count, creatinine/eGFR, and coagulation profile.

To assess feminizing effects, laboratory investigation should include baseline free testosterone and baseline measurements of the breasts and hips should be recorded. Breasts should be measured in a standing position (a) vertically from the midclavicular line to the inframammary fold, across the largest portion of the breast, and (b) from the anterior axillary line to the midsternum, across the largest portion of the breast.

Written informed consent document. The WPATH *Standards* (Meyer et al., 2001) state that a written informed consent document reflecting a detailed discussion of the anticipated effects and possible risks of hormone therapy must be included as part of the medical record. Sample informed consent forms for MTF endocrine therapy are included as Appendix C.

Monitoring Recommendations Following Initiation of MTF Endocrine Therapy

At minimum patients should be seen every month after initiating treatment or while adjusting medication dosages, then every 3-4 months for the first year, then every 6 months thereafter. The primary focus of monitoring cross-sex hormone use is to assess the degree of feminization and the possible presence of adverse effects of medication. However, as with monitoring of any long-term medication, monitoring should take place in the context of comprehensive care of all health concerns.

Evaluation of feminization. Feminization takes place gradually over a period of years. Observed changes to male pattern hair growth, breast/nipple development, and testicular volume should be noted; breast and hip measurements recorded; and the patient asked about changes to male pattern hair quality and growth (e.g., mechanical hair-removal frequency), mood, libido, and sexual function. Other changes should also be noted. Breast budding should be discussed in advance to reassure the patient that it is not a malignant process.

Free testosterone level should be checked every 3 months until stable in target range (typically < 7.2 pg/mL or 75 pmol/L; if not achieving desired feminization, try to decrease to low end of female range).

Monitoring of adverse effects. All exams should include careful assessment of cardiovascular and thrombosis risk, including measurement of blood pressure and weight, lung exam, and examination of the extremities for peripheral edema, localized swelling, or pain.

At minimum, laboratory tests should include the following tests, summarized in Table B1 of Appendix B:

1. Liver enzymes: 1 month after starting estrogen or changing dose, 3 months thereafter, and every 6 months once estrogen dose is stable. Investigate rise with abdominal ultrasound and hepatitis serology; discuss alcohol use.

2. Lipid profile: 1 month after starting estrogen or changing dose, 3 months thereafter, and every 12 months once estrogen dose is stable.

3. Fasting glucose: 1 month after starting estrogen or changing dose, 3 months thereafter, and every 6 months once estrogen dose is stable. Monitor more frequently and include evaluation of glycosylated hemoglobin if significant weight gain, increase in fasting glucose levels, or family history of diabetes mellitus.

4. Prolactin: 3 months, 6 months, then annually to 3 years; stop if stable at that point. Hyperprolactinemia is common with estrogen therapy, and is typically mild and reversible if estrogen is reduced or temporarily discontinued. Hyperprolactinemia may also result from antidepressants or other medication, thyroid hypofunction, supplementation with additional estrogen, or prolactin-secreting pituitary adenoma. Further investigation may be warranted if prolactin levels are unusually high or do not reverse with reduction of estrogen dosage.

5. If taking spironolactone: serum potassium, urea, and creatinine 1 week after commencement or dosage change; with other bloodwork if levels and dose have been stable.

Ongoing comprehensive primary care. Feldman and Goldberg (2006) provide detailed protocols for primary care of MTFs undergoing endocrinologic feminization both prior to and following orchiectomy. Cardiovascular risk factors should be aggressively screened for and treated, osteoporosis assessment should be considered for MTFs who are at risk (e.g., thin and age 50+, particularly those who have taken hormones intermittently or have had orchiectomy), and breast cancer screening should be implemented as breast tissue develops. Primary care of the MTF patient includes screening for all other types of cancer (e.g., lung, colorectal, anal) and regular prostate evaluation as for natal males, as well as periodic screening for concerns relating to sexual health, mental health, and substance use.

FEMALE-TO-MALE (FTM) THERAPY

Mechanisms of Action

Endocrinologic masculinization is achieved by the use of testosterone to induce male physical characteristics. Testosterone works primarily by direct stimulation of receptors in target tissues; clinical effects correlate to elevation of serum testosterone level to a male reference range, rather than a decrease in serum estradiol (Moore et al., 2003). Testosterone also has antigonadotropic action in high doses (Asscheman & Gooren, 1992).

Expected Masculinizing Effects

Rapidity and degree of change from masculinizing endocrine therapy depends on the agents used, dosage, and the patient's responsiveness to endocrine therapy. Typically, within the first 1-3 months patients experience redistribution of fat to a more masculine pattern (shifting from the hips and buttocks to the abdomen), increased muscle mass and upper body strength, and oilier skin/acne (Bromham & Pearson, 1996; Elbers, Asscheman, Seidell, & Gooren, 1999; Flaherty et al., 2001; Kirk & Rothblatt, 1995; Schlatterer et al., 1996; Slabbekoorn, Van Goozen, Gooren, & Cohen-Kettenis, 2001; Steinbeck, 1997; Tangpricha et al., 2003). There are case reports of tendon rupture in both FTM patients on testosterone and natal men taking anabolic steroids (Morgenthaler & Weber, 2005; Strauss & Yesalis, 1991), and FTMs who are involved in strength training should be cautioned to increase weight load gradually, with an emphasis on repetitions rather than weight.

The voice often starts to crack and deepen within the first 3-6 months, but it can take a year or more for the voice pitch to fully drop (Kirk & Rothblatt, 1995). In approximately 75% of FTMs, testosterone will cause voice pitch to drop to a level sufficient for passability as male even on the telephone (Van Borsel, De Cuypere, Rubens, & Destaerke, 2000).

Clitoral growth begins within the first few months of testosterone initiation and typically plateaus within the first year (Meyer et al., 1986). The degree of enlargement is variable, with a reported range of 3.5-6.0 cm maximal length when stretched (Gooren, n.d.; Meyer et al., 1981; Meyer et al., 1986). Clitoral growth does not appear to be enhanced by topical application of testosterone to the clitoris. Long-term testosterone use causes vaginal and cervical atrophy (Miller, Bedard, Cooter, & Shaul, 1986; Schlatterer et al., 1996), with decreased vaginal secretions and difficult penetration reported by some patients.

In most cases menses stop within 1-6 months (Bromham & Pearson, 1996; Flaherty et al., 2001; Futterweit, 1998; Israel & Tarver, 1997; Meyer et al., 1981; Meyer et al., 1986; Steinbeck, 1997; Tangpricha et al., 2003). If after three months menses have not stopped, the dosage of testosterone may be increased (to the maximum recommended dose) until menses stop or serum free testosterone is within the upper quartile of the normal male range (Table B2, Appendix B). Despite endometrial atrophy, cessation of menses, and reduced fertility there is evidence of ovulation even after several years of testosterone administration (Miller et al., 1986), and testosterone should not be relied upon as a failsafe contraceptive.

There is gradual increased growth, coarseness, and thickness of hairs on the torso and extremities in the first year (Bromham & Pearson, 1996; Kirk & Rothblatt, 1995; Meyer et al., 1981; Schlatterer et al., 1996; Tangpricha et al., 2003). Facial hair increases more slowly, typically taking 1-4 years to reach full growth (Asscheman & Gooren, 1992). Some patients experience male pattern baldness during this later stage of masculinization (Bromham & Pearson, 1996; Feldman & Bockting, 2003; Flaherty et al., 2001; Kirk & Rothblatt, 1995; Tangpricha et al., 2003).

Voice changes, facial hair growth, and male pattern baldness are not reversible, while other changes are reversible (to varying degrees) if hormonal treatment is stopped. Clitoral growth and sterility may or may not be reversible. Reproductive counseling may be advised, particularly for young patients.

Recommended Masculinizing Regimen

Table 3 summarizes our recommendations for a basic regimen for the FTM patient who desires maximum masculinization. The starting dose for patients who are at low risk for adverse effects can be gradually increased to the recommended maximum if needed to achieve the desired changes and to bring free testosterone to the lower half of the male range (Table B2, Appendix B). Once maximum masculinization has been reached (typically changes plateau after two years, although there may still be facial hair growth/male pattern baldness after that time), the dosage can be reduced to an amount sufficient to bring free testosterone to the low-normal male range (Table B2, Appendix B) even prior to oophorectomy. To preserve bone density following oophorectomy, testosterone supplementation should be maintained throughout life (or consider bisphosphonates), and Calcium/Vitamin D supplementation is recommended.

The largest transgender hormone study done to date (van Kesteren et al., 1997) found no increased mortality in androgen-treated FTMs, and concluded that "no serious morbidity was observed which could be related to androgen treatment" (p. 337). However, given the methodological limitations of this study, the long-term risks of androgen therapy in FTMs are unclear. Some reports suggest that androgen use may worsen lipid abnormalities, obstructive sleep apnea, obesity, and acne (Asscheman & Gooren, 1992; Asscheman et al., 1994; Feldman & Bockting, 2003; Flaherty et al., 2001; Futterweit, 1998; Giltay & Gooren, 2000; Goh, Loke, & Ratnam, 1995; Kirk & Rothblatt, 1995; McCredie et al., 1998; Meyer et al., 1986; Steinbeck, 1997; van Kesteren et al., 1997). Increased visceral depot, particularly pronounced in FTMs who gained weight after starting testosterone (Elbers, Asscheman, Seidell, Megens, & Gooren, 1997; Elbers et al., 1999), is a concern as this is associated with increased risk for cardiovascular disease and non-insulin-dependent diabetes mellitus. The aromatization of testosterone to estrogen may increase risk of malignancy in patients with a strong family history of estrogen-dependent cancers (Israel & Tarver, 1997; Moore et al., 2003; Toorians & Gooren, 2001). There are case reports of polycythemia in non-transgender men treated with androgens (Drinka et al., 1995; Viallard et al., 2000), and erythrocytosis may be a concern for FTMs with chronic hypoxemic respiratory disease or those who are at risk of hemachromatosis.

Intramuscular and transdermal androgen preparations minimize hepatic exposure to androgens so have the potential to reduce adverse hepatic effects. Because intramuscular androgen preparations are administered intermittently, some people may notice cyclic variation in effects, such as fatigue and irritability at the end of the injection cycle or aggression and expansive mood at the beginning of the injection cycle. This may be mitigated by injecting weekly rather than every two weeks, or by using a transdermal or oral preparation. Transdermal

TABLE 3. Basic Masculinizing Regimen

Agent	Intramuscular injection (esterified testosterone)		Transdermal gel	Transdermal patch
	Testosterone cypionate	Testosterone enanthate	Testosterone crystals dissolved in gel	
Pre-oophorectomy	25-40 mg[a] every week (or 50-80 mg every two weeks); gradually increase each month until blood testosterone is within normal male range or there are visible changes (typically 50-100 mg every week, or 100-200 mg every 2 weeks)		5-10 g qd; start with 2.5 g qd if there are comorbid conditions that may be exacerbated by testosterone	5-10 mg/24 hours, applied daily; start with 2.5 mg patch if there are comorbid conditions that may be exacerbated by testosterone
Maintenance (after 2 years) or post-oophorectomy	Reduce to level needed to keep serum free testosterone within the lower-middle end of the male reference interval (Table B2). Monitor risk of osteoporosis.			

[a]Ensure patient knows how much to inject–there are 100 mg/ml and 200 mg/ml preparations.

testosterone may be preferred by patients who have difficulty self-injecting, have significant adverse effects related to the injection cycle, or need a slow, even titration (Meyer et al., 2001).

Testosterone increases serum levels of anticoagulants and sulfonylureas, and may interact with corticosteroids.

Alternative Regimens and Agents

Alternative forms of testosterone. Testosterone undecanoate does not have the hepatotoxicity associated with older 17-alkylated forms of oral testosterone (e.g., methyltestosterone) and is considered safe for FTM masculinization, with 160-240 mg po qd recommended by Asscheman and Gooren (1992). It is generally not preferred as it is less effective than IM or transdermal testosterone in suppressing menstruation, with only 50% of patients experiencing menstrual cessation after six months taking oral testosterone (Feldman, 2005; Gooren, n.d.). It is also much more expensive than testosterone esters; in British Columbia testosterone undecanoate costs approximately $120/month (160 mg po qd), compared to approximately $10/month for testosterone esters (150 mg q 2 weeks).

Progestins. Progestins are not typically included in FTM endocrine therapy, but can be used for a short period of time to assist with menstrual cessation. Medroxyprogesterone acetate can be given by IM injection (150 mg every three months) to stop menses either before or concurrent with starting testosterone, stopping the injections after 3-6 months on testosterone (Asscheman & Gooren, 1992; Gooren, 1999; Kirk & Rothblatt, 1995; Schlatterer et al., 1998). One transgender clinic (Dimensions, 2000a) performs a "progestin challenge" (Gambrell, 1982; Valenzuela, Sabatel, Valls, Nieto, & Gonzalez-Gomez, 1993) within 3-6 months of menstrual cessation, and every 2-3 months thereafter until there is no further bleeding, to reduce risk of endometrial hyperplasia.

Gonadotropin-releasing hormone (GnRH) analogues. GnRH-analogues (e.g., leuprolide acetate) have a longer half-life than natural GnRH and after a period of brief overstimulation down-regulate the pituitary, with consequent reduction of follicle-stimulating hormone and LH. This causes a decrease in estrogen levels similar to postmenopausal levels. GnRH analogues are often used with strongly dysphoric young FTMs to delay puberty, but are not commonly used in the treatment of transgender adults as they are expensive and tend to have stronger adverse effects than testosterone. However, they may be used if testosterone or progestins are not tolerated (Asscheman & Gooren, 1992).

Assessment Prior to Initiating FTM Endocrine Therapy

Comprehensive primary care evaluation. A full primary care evaluation (Feldman & Goldberg, 2006) should be completed, with particular attention to weight and risks/history of cardiovascular disease, diabetes/glucose intolerance, dyslipidemia, estrogen-dependent cancer, gynecologic disease (including polycystic ovarian disease), and hepatic disease. If there are additional primary care concerns these should be appropriately investigated; for example, stress testing should be considered for patients at high risk for cardiovascular disease or with any cardiovascular symptoms. When possible, efforts should be made to stabilize and control co-morbid conditions with medication, lifestyle changes, or other suitable interventions prior to initiating hormones. Pregnancy and unstable coronary artery disease are absolute contraindications to androgen use. Patients at risk of becoming pregnant require adequate birth control.

Cigarette smoking is associated with increased risk for cardiovascular disease. We recommend a harm reduction approach that strongly encourages patients to reduce or stop smoking, along with a clear recommendation that their testosterone dosage must be kept low as long as they are smoking.

Baseline evaluation. To assist in monitoring of adverse effects, baseline values should be recorded for lipid profile, fasting glucose (and glycosylated hemoglobin if high risk for diabetes/glucose intolerance), complete blood count, and liver enzymes. Serum free testosterone[2] may be evaluated if there is clinical suspicion of hyperandrogenism or if the patient wants to be informed of changes to serum testosterone levels with androgen therapy.

Written informed consent document. The WPATH *Standards* (Meyer et al., 2001) state that a written informed consent document reflecting a detailed discussion of the anticipated effects and possible risks of hormone therapy must be included as part of the medical record. Sample informed consent forms for FTM endocrine therapy are included as Appendix D.

Monitoring Recommendations Following Initiation of FTM Endocrine Therapy

At minimum patients should be seen every month after initiating treatment or while adjusting medication dosages, then every 3-4 months for the first year, then every 6 months thereafter. The primary focus of monitoring cross-sex hormone use is to assess the degree of masculinization and the possible presence of adverse effects of medication. However, as with monitoring of any long-term medication, monitoring should take place in the context of comprehensive care of all health concerns.

Evaluation of masculinization. Masculinization takes place gradually over a period of years. Observed changes to male pattern hair growth and voice should be noted, and the patient should be asked about changes to menstrual pattern, mood, clitoral growth, libido, and sexual function. Other changes should also be noted.

To avoid a supraphysiological dose of testosterone, serum free testosterone should be checked 2-4 weeks after starting testosterone or after a dose adjustment, and every 6-12 months thereafter. The biochemical goal is to achieve levels within the male reference interval (Table B2, Appendix B). Some clinicians check trough levels for patients using IM testosterone preparations; others prefer midcycle levels.

Monitoring of adverse effects. All exams should include assessment of weight, cardiovascular risk, diabetes risk, and blood pressure. There are case reports of destabilization of bipolar disorder, schizophrenia, and schizoaffective disorder in non-transgender men with the use of testosterone, and clinicians have also found this in FTMs (Feldman, 2005). Mental health should be monitored carefully in FTMs with these conditions for the duration of testosterone therapy.

At minimum, laboratory tests should include the following tests, summarized in Table B2 of Appendix B:

1. Fasting blood glucose: 3 and 6 months after starting testosterone or after a dose adjustment, then annually. Increase frequency and monitor glycosylated hemoglobin if elevated lipids, significant weight gain, elevated fasting glucose levels, personal history of glucose intolerance, or family history of diabetes.
2. Hgb: 3 and 6 months after starting testosterone or after a dose adjustment, then annually.
3. Lipid profile: 3 and 6 months after starting testosterone or after a dose adjustment, then annually; increase frequency if pre-existing high lipid levels or an increase in lipid levels, significant weight gain, personal history of glucose intolerance, or family history of diabetes.
4. Liver enzymes: 3 and 6 months after starting testosterone or after dose increase, then annually.

Ongoing comprehensive primary care. Feldman and Goldberg (2006) provide detailed protocols for primary care of FTMs undergoing endocrinologic masculinization. Cardiovascular risk factors should be aggressively screened for and treated, and osteoporosis assessment should be considered for FTMs who are at risk (age 60 + if taking testosterone for < 5-10 years; age 50 + if taking testosterone for > 5-10 years; earlier for patients who have taken testosterone intermittently, have had oophorectomy, or are otherwise at risk). Primary care of the FTM patient includes screening for all other types of cancer (e.g., lung, colorectal, anal) as for natal females, as well as periodic screening for concerns relating to sexual health, mental health, and substance use.

FTMs should receive regular monitoring by a primary care provider for breast cancer both before and after chest surgery, as chest reconstruction typically does not involve the removal of all breast tissue. If the uterus and cervix are present, regular gynecologic screening is also recommended as part of basic primary care, with total hysterectomy and oophorectomy recommended for patients who cannot tolerate regular pelvic and Pap exams (Feldman & Goldberg, 2006). After androgen-induced cessation of menses, vaginal bleeding should be evaluated as for post-menopausal women.

CONCLUDING REMARKS

Individual tailoring of endocrine regimens to fit the transgender patient's history, risk factors, desired outcomes, and administration preferences holds promise both for maximization of desired effects and minimization of adverse effects. We hope that the recommendations in this document help clinicians feel more confident to determine when endocrine therapy may be appropriate, and to care for patients who are undergoing endocrinologic feminization or masculinization.

NOTES

1. In British Columbia, nurse practitioners can prescribe anti-androgens, estrogen, and progestins but not testosterone (Registered Nurses Association of British Columbia/College of Registered Nurses of British Columbia, 2005).

2. There are varying clinical opinions on the accuracy and reliability of testosterone assays. The values given in this document reflect laboratory practices in British Columbia, Canada, as of early 2005. One lab in British Columbia now offers bio-available testosterone (BAT) as an alternative to free testosterone, and it is possible that BAT may become more widely used in the near future.

REFERENCES

Asscheman, H., & Gooren, L. J. G. (1992). Hormone treatment in transsexuals. *Journal of Psychology & Human Sexuality, 5*(4), 39-54.

Asscheman, H., Gooren, L. J. G., & Eklund, P. L. (1989). Mortality and morbidity in transsexual patients with cross-gender hormone treatment. *Metabolism, 38,* 869-873.

Asscheman, H., Gooren, L. J. G., Megens, J. A. J., Nauta, J., Kloosterboer, H. J., & Eikelboom, F. (1994). Serum testosterone level is the major determinant of the male-female differences in serum levels of high-density lipoprotein (HDL) cholesterol and HDL2 cholesterol. *Metabolism, 43,* 935-939.

Basson, R. J. (2001). Towards optimal hormonal treatment of male to female gender identity disorder. *Journal of Sexual and Reproductive Medicine, 1*(1), 45-51.

Basson, R. J., & Prior, J. C. (1998). Hormonal therapy of gender dysphoria: The male-to-female transsexual. In D. Denny (Ed.), *Current concepts in transgender identity* (pp. 277-296). New York: Garland Publishing.

Bockting, W. O., Knudson, G., & Goldberg, J. M. (2006). Counseling and mental health care for transgender adults and loved ones. *International Journal of Transgenderism, 9*(3/4), 35-82.

Bowman, C., & Goldberg, J. M. (2006). Care of the patient undergoing sex reassignment surgery. *International Journal of Transgenderism, 9*(3/4), 135-165.

Bromham, D., & Pearson, R. (1996). The pharmacological treatment of transsexuals. *British Journal of Sexual Medicine, 23*(5) [no page numbers in file copy].

Buffat, J. (2003). Clinical observations of cross-sex hormonal substitution on behavioural and psychological changes induced in transsexuals. *Sexologies, 12,* 53-55.

Cadario, B. J., & Leathem, A. M. (Eds.) (2003). *Drug information reference* (5th ed.). Vancouver, BC, Canada: BC Drug and Poison Information Centre.

De Sutter, P. (2001). Gender reassignment and assisted reproduction: Present and future reproductive options for transsexual people. *Human Reproduction, 16,* 612-614.

de Vries, A. L. C., Cohen-Kettenis, P. T., & Delemarre-van de Waal, H. (2006). Clinical management of gender dysphoria in adolescents. *International Journal of Transgenderism, 9*(3/4), 83-94.

Dimensions (2000a). *Dimensions treatment guidelines for FTM transition.* San Francisco, CA: Castro-Mission Health Center, San Francisco Department of Public Health. Retrieved January 1, 2005, from http://tghealth-critiques.tripod.com/protoc2.htm

Dimensions (2000b). *Dimensions treatment guidelines for MTF transition.* San Francisco, CA: Castro-Mission Health Center, San Francisco Department of Public Health. Retrieved January 1, 2005, from http://tghealth-critiques.tripod.com/protoc1.htm

Dimensions (2003a). *Informed consent for estrogen therapy for male to female transition.* San Francisco, CA: Castro-Mission Health Center, San Francisco Department of Public Health. Retrieved January 1, 2005, from http://tghealth-critiques.tripod.com/consen3.htm

Dimensions (2003b). *Informed consent for testostorone therapy for female-to-male transition.* San Francisco, CA: Castro-Mission Health Center, San Francisco Department of Public Health. Retrieved January 1, 2005, from http://tghealth-critiques.tripod.com/consen2.htm

Drinka, P. J., Jochen, A. L., Cuisinier, M., Bloom, R., Rudman, I., & Rudman, D. (1995). Polycythemia as a complication of testosterone replacement therapy in nursing home men with low testosterone levels. *Journal of the American Geriatrics Society, 43,* 899-901.

Elbers, J. M. H., Asscheman, H., Seidell, J. C., Megens, J. A. J., & Gooren, L. J. G. (1997). Long-term testosterone administration increases visceral fat in female to male transsexuals. *Journal of Clinical Endocrinology & Metabolism, 82*, 2044-2047.

Elbers, J. M. H., Asscheman, H., Seidell, J. C., & Gooren, L. J. G. (1999). Effects of sex steroid hormones on regional fat depots as assessed by magnetic resonance imaging in transsexuals. *American Journal of Physiology, 276*, E317-E325.

Feldman, J. (2005). *Masculinizing hormone therapy with testosterone 1% topical gel*. Paper presented at the XIX Biennial Symposium of the Harry Benjamin International Gender Dysphoria Association, Bologna, Italy.

Feldman, J., & Bockting, W. O. (2003). Transgender health. *Minnesota Medicine, 86*, 25-32.

Feldman, J., & Goldberg, J. M. (2006). Transgender primary medical care. *International Journal of Transgenderism, 9*(3/4), 3-34.

Flaherty, C., Franicevich, J., Freeman, M., Klein, P., Kohler, L., Lusardi, C., Martinez, L., Monihan, M., Vormohr, J., & Zevin, B. (2001). *Protocols for hormonal reassignment of gender*. San Francisco: San Francisco Department of Public Health. Retrieved January 1, 2005, from http://www.dph.sf.ca.us/chn/HlthCtrs/HlthCtrDocs/TransGendprotocols.pdf

Futterweit, W. (1998). Endocrine therapy of transsexualism and potential complications of long-term treatment. *Archives of Sexual Behavior, 27*, 209-226.

Gambrell, R. D. Jr. (1982). Clinical use of progestins in the menopausal patient: Dosage and duration. *Journal of Reproductive Medicine, 27*, 531-538.

Gay and Lesbian Medical Association (2001). *Healthy People 2010 companion document for lesbian, gay, bisexual, and transgender (LGBT) health*. San Francisco, CA: Gay and Lesbian Medical Association. Retrieved January 1, 2005, from http://www.glma.org/policy/hp2010/index.shtml

Giltay, E. J., & Gooren, L. J. G. (2000). Effects of sex steroid deprivation/administration on hair growth and skin sebum production in transsexual males and females. *Journal of Clinical Endocrinology & Metabolism, 85*, 2913-2921.

Goh, H. H., Loke, D. F., & Ratnam, S. S. (1995). The impact of long-term testosterone replacement therapy on lipid and lipoprotein profiles in women. *Maturitas, 21*, 65-70.

Gooren, L. J. G. (n.d.). Transsexualism: Introduction and general aspects of treatment. Retrieved January 1, 2005, from http://www.xs4all.nl/~txtbreed/gender/gooren.html

Gooren, L. J. G. (1999). Hormonal sex reassignment. *International Journal of Transgenderism, 3*. Retrieved January 1, 2005, from http://www.symposion.com/ijt/ijt990301.htm

Hage, J. J., Bouman, F. G., & Bloem, J. J. A. M. (1992). Surgical depilation in 20 male-to-female transsexuals. *Gender Dysphoria, 1*, 3-8.

Israel, G. E., & Tarver, D. E. I. (1997). *Transgender care: Recommended guidelines, practical information, and personal accounts*. Philadephia, PA: Temple University Press.

Jin, B., Turner, L., Walters, W. A. W., & Handelsman, D. J. (1996). The effects of chronic high dose androgen or estrogen treatment on the human prostate. *Journal of Clinical Endocrinology Metabolism, 81*, 4290-4295.

Kammerer, N., Mason, T., Connors, M., & Durkee, R. (1999). Transgender health and social service needs in the context of HIV risk. *International Journal of Transgenderism, 3*(1 + 2). Retrieved January 1, 2005, from http://www.symposion.com/ijt/hiv_risk/kammerer.htm

Kirk, S., & Rothblatt, M. (1995). *Medical, legal and workplace issues for the transsexual*. Watertown, MA: Together Lifeworks.

Kuiper, B., & Cohen-Kettenis, P. T. (1988). Sex reassignment surgery: a study of 141 Dutch transsexuals. *Archives of Sexual Behavior, 17*, 439-457.

Leavitt, F., Berger, J. C., Hoeppner, J. A., & Northrop, G. (1980). Presurgical adjustment in male transsexuals with and without hormonal treatment. *Journal of Nervous and Mental Disease, 168*, 693-697.

Levy, A., Crown, A., & Reid, R. W. (2003). Endocrine intervention for transsexuals. *Clinical Endocrinology, 59*, 409-418.

Lubbert, H., Leo-Rossberg, I., & Hammerstein, J. (1992). Effects of ethinyl estradiol on semen quality and various hormonal parameters in a eugonadal male. *Fertility and Sterility, 58*, 603-608.

McCredie, R. J., McCrohon, J. A., Turner, L., Griffiths, K. A., Handelsman, D. J., & Celermajer, D. S. (1998). Vascular reactivity is impaired in genetic females taking high-dose androgens. *Journal of the American College of Cardiology, 32*, 1331-1335.

Meyer, W. J., III, Bockting, W. O., Cohen-Kettenis, P. T., Coleman, E., Di Ceglie, D., Devor, H., Gooren, L., Hage, J. J., Kirk, S., Kuiper, B., Laub, D., Lawrence, A., Menard, Y., Monstrey, S., Patton, J., Schaefer, L., Webb, A., & Wheeler, C. C. (2001). *The standards of care for Gender Identity Disorders* (6th ed.). Minneapolis, MN: Harry Benjamin International Gender Dysphoria Association.

Meyer, W. J., III, Finkelstein, J. W., Stuart, C. A., Webb, A., Smith, E. R., Payer, A. F., & Walker, P. A. (1981). Physical and hormonal evaluation of transsexual patients during hormonal therapy. *Archives of Sexual Behavior, 10*, 347-356.

Meyer, W. J., III, Webb, A., Stuart, C. A., Finkelstein, J. W., Lawrence, B., & Walker, P. A. (1986). Physical and hormonal evaluation of transsexual patients: A longitudinal study. *Archives of Sexual Behavior, 15*, 121-138.

Miller, N., Bedard, Y. C., Cooter, N. B., & Shaul, D. L. (1986). Histological changes in the genital tract in transsexual women following androgen therapy. *Histopathology, 10*, 661-669.

Moghetti, P., Tosi, F., Tosti, A., Negri, C., Misciali, C., Perrone, F., Caputo, M., Muggeo, M., & Castello, R. (2000). Comparison of spironolactone, flutamide, and finasteride efficacy in the treatment of hirsutism: A randomized, double blind, placebo-controlled trial. *Journal of Clinical Endocrinology & Metabolism*, *85*, 89-94.

Moore, E., Wisniewski, A., & Dobs, A. (2003). Endocrine treatment of transsexual people: A review of treatment regimens, outcomes, and adverse effects. *Journal of Clinical Endocrinology & Metabolism*, *88*, 3467-3473.

Morgenthaler, M., & Weber, M. (2005). Pathological rupture of the distal biceps tendon after long-term androgen substitution. *Zeitschrift für Orthopädie und Ihre Grenzgebiete*, *137*, 368-370.

Oriel, K. A. (2000). Medical care of transsexual patients. *Journal of the Gay & Lesbian Medical Association*, *4*, 185-194.

Paquet, P., Fumal, I., Piérard-Franchimont, C., & Piérard, G. E. (2002). Long-pulsed ruby laser-assisted hair removal in male-to-female transsexuals. *Journal of Cosmetic Dermatology*, *1*, 8-12.

Prior, J. C., Vigna, Y. M., & Watson, D. (1989). Spironolactone with physiological female steroids for presurgical therapy of male-to-female transsexualism. *Archives of Sexual Behavior*, *18*, 49-57.

Prior, J. C., Vigna, Y. M., Watson, D., Diewold, P., & Robinow, O. (1986). Spironolactone in the presurgical therapy of male to female transsexuals: Philosophy and experience of the Vancouver Gender Dysphoria Clinic. *Journal of Sex Information & Education Council of Canada*, *1*, 1-7.

Registered Nurses Association of British Columbia/College of Registered Nurses of British Columbia (2005). *Scope of practice for nurse practitioners (family): Standards, limits and conditions* (Report No. 424) [Electronic version]. Vancouver, BC: Author.

Reutrakul, S., Ongphiphadhanakul, B., Piaseu, N., Krittiyawong, S., Chanprasertyothin, S., Bunnag, P., & Rajatanavin, R. (1998). The effects of oestrogen exposure on bone mass in male to female transsexuals. *Clinical Endocrinology*, *49*, 811-814.

Rossouw, J. E., Anderson, G. L., Prentice, R. L., LaCroix, A. Z., Kooperberg, C., Stefanick, M. L., Jackson, R. D., Beresford, S. A., Howard, B. V., Johnson, K. C., Kotchen, J. M., & Ockene, J. (2002). Risks and benefits of estrogen plus progestin in healthy postmenopausal women: Principal results From the Women's Health Initiative randomized controlled trial. *Journal of the American Medical Association*, *288*, 321-333.

Scarabin, P. Y., Oger, E., & Plu-Bureau, G. (2003). Differential association of oral and transdermal oestrogen-replacement therapy with venous thromboembolism risk. *Lancet*, *362*, 428-432.

Schlatterer, K., von Werder, K., & Stalla, G. K. (1996). Multistep treatment concept of transsexual patients. *Experimental and Clinical Endocrinology and Diabetes*, *104*, 413-419.

Schlatterer, K., Yassouridis, A., von Werder, K., Poland, D., Kemper, J., & Stalla, G. K. (1998). A follow-up study for estimating the effectiveness of a cross-gender hormone substitution therapy on transsexual patients. *Archives of Sexual Behavior*, *27*, 475-492.

Schroeter, C. A., Groenewegen, J. S., Reineke, T., & Neumann, H. A. M. (2003). Ninety percent permanent hair reduction in transsexual patients. *Annals of Plastic Surgery*, *51*, 243-248.

Shenenberger, D. W., & Utecht, L. M. (2002). Removal of unwanted facial hair. *American Family Physician*, *66*, 1907-1911.

Slabbekoorn, D., Van Goozen, S. H. M., Gooren, L. J. G., & Cohen-Kettenis, P. T. (2001). Effects of cross-sex hormone treatment on emotionality in transsexuals. *International Journal of Transgenderism*, *5*. Retrieved January 1, 2005, from http://www.symposion.com/ijt/ijtvo05no03_02.htm

Sosa, M., Jodar, E., Arbelo, E., Dominguez, C., Saavedra, P., Torres, A., Salido, E., Liminana, J. M., Gomez De Tejada, M. J., & Hernandez, D. (2004). Serum lipids and estrogen receptor gene polymorphisms in male-to-female transsexuals: Effects of estrogen treatment. *European Journal of Internal Medicine*, *15*, 231-237.

Steinbeck, A. (1997). Hormonal medication for transsexuals. *Venereology: Interdisciplinary, International Journal of Sexual Health*, *10*, 175-177.

Strauss, R. H., & Yesalis, C. E. (1991). Anabolic steroids in the athlete. *Annual Review of Medicine*, *42*, 449-457.

Tangpricha, V., Ducharme, S. H., Barber, T. W., & Chipkin, S. R. (2003). Endocrinologic treatment of gender identity disorders. *Endocrine Practice*, *9*, 12-21.

Toorians, A. W., & Gooren, L. J. G. (2001). *Effects of androgen treatment and of androgen-derived estrogens on prolactin (PRL) levels in a female-to-male transsexual with a prolactinoma*. Paper presented at the 17th Biennial Symposium of the Harry Benjamin International Gender Dysphoria Association Symposium, Galveston, TX.

Toorians, A. W., Gooren, L. J. G., & Asscheman, H. (2001). *Venous thrombo-embolism and (oral) estrogen use*. Paper presented at the 17th Biennial Symposium of the Harry Benjamin International Gender Dysphoria Association Symposium, Galveston, TX.

Toorians, A. W., Thomassen, M. C., Zweegman, S., Magdeleyns, E. J., Tans, G., Gooren, L. J. G., & Rosing, J. (2003). Venous thrombosis and changes of hemostatic variables during cross-sex hormone treatment in transsexual people. *Journal of Clinical Endocrinology & Metabolism*, *88*, 5723-5729.

T'Sjoen, G., Rubens, R., De Sutter, P., & Gooren, L. J. G. (2004). Author's response: The endocrine care of transsexual people. *Journal of Clinical Endocrinology & Metabolism*, *89*, 1014-1015.

Valenzuela, P., Sabatel, R. M., Valls, V., Nieto, A., & Gonzalez-Gomez, F. (1993). Progestin challenge test in postmenopausal patients. *International Journal of Gynaecology & Obstetrics*, *43*, 313-316.

Viallard, J. F., Marit, G., Mercie, P., Leng, B., Reiffers, J., & Pellegrin, J. L. (2000). Polycythaemia as a complication of transdermal testosterone therapy. *British Journal of Haematology, 110,* 237-238.

Van Borsel, J., De Cuypere, G., Rubens, R., & Destaerke, B. (2000). Voice problems in female-to-male transsexuals. *International Journal of Language & Communication Disorders, 35,* 427-442.

van Kesteren, P. J. M., Asscheman, H., Megens, J. A. J., & Gooren, L. J. G. (1997). Mortality and morbidity in transsexual subjects treated with cross-sex hormones. *Clinical Endocrinology, 47,* 337-342.

White Holman, C., & Goldberg, J. M. (2006). Social and medical transgender case advocacy. *International Journal of Transgenderism, 9*(3/4), 197-217.

Wysowski, D. K., Freiman, J. P., Tourtelot, J. B., & Horton, M. L. (1993). Fatal and nonfatal hepatotoxicity associated with flutamide. *Annals of Internal Medicine, 118,* 860-864.

doi:10.1300/J485v09n03_06

APPENDIX A. Comparative Costs of Medications Recommended for Adult Transgender Endocrine Therapy

Prices shown in Tables A1 and A2 are in Canadian dollars, and represent the price in British Columbia, Canada as of 2005. The costs shown do not include the dispensing fee set by each pharmacy and billed each time a prescription is refilled; as of 2005, this was an average of $9.25 in BC, although compounding pharmacies may charge significantly more.

TABLE A1. Comparative Prices: Feminizing Agents

Agent	Administration	Dose	2005 BC Price
Estrogen			
17β-estradiol	Transdermal	0.1 mg/24 hours, applied twice per week	~$25/month
	Oral	2 mg qd	~$14/month
Estradiol valerate	Intramuscular injection	30 mg q 2 weeks	~$10/month
Androgen antagonist			
Spironolactone	Oral	300 mg qd	~$22/month
Finasteride	Oral	5.0 mg qd	~$58/month
Progestin			
Micronized progesterone	Oral	300 mg qd	~$87/month
Medroxyprogesterone acetate	Oral	30 mg qd	~$33/month
Combination: norethindrone acetate and 17β-estradiol	Transdermal	140/50 ug	~$26/month

TABLE A2. Comparative Prices: Masculinizing Agents

Agent	Administration	Dose	2005 BC Price
Testosterone esters (cypionate or enanthate)	Intramuscular injection	150 mg q 2 weeks	~$10/month
Testosterone crystals dissolved in gel	Gel	5 g qd	~$120/month
	Patch	5 mg qd	~$120/month

These tables are intended to provide a very approximate sense of price differentials, rather than an estimated cost of a particular regimen. Cost of medications vary considerably from country to country, and may or may not be covered by health insurance. Consult a local pharmacy for a closer estimation of out-of-pocket costs in your area.

APPENDIX B. Summary of Laboratory Investigations

Tables B1 and B2 are minimum timelines. Closer monitoring should be performed for patients at risk for or with co-existing cardiovascular disease, diabetes, hepatic disease, etc.

TABLE B1. Male-to-Female (MTF) Laboratory Summary

Timeline for Laboratory Tests	
Baseline (before starting feminizing endocrine therapy)	Free testosterone, lipid profile, fasting blood glucose (and glycosylated hemoglobin if diabetes or suspected glucose intolerance), liver enzymes, prolactin, electrolytes, urea, creatinine
	Additional tests as clinically indicated (e.g., CBC, coagulation profile)
1 week after starting/changing dose of spironolactone	Serum potassium, urea, creatinine
1 month after starting/changing dose of estrogen	Liver enzymes, lipid profile, fasting glucose
	If taking spironolactone: serum potassium, urea, and creatinine
3 months after starting estrogen	Free testosterone: repeat every 3 months until free testosterone is in target range of < 7.2 pg/mL or 75 pmol/L
	Liver enzymes, lipid profile, fasting glucose, prolactin
	If taking spironolactone: serum potassium, urea, and creatinine
6 months after starting estrogen and every 6 months thereafter if dose is stable	Liver enzymes, fasting glucose
	If taking spironolactone: serum potassium, urea, and creatinine
	Add lipid profile every 12 months (once estrogen dose is stable)
	Add prolactin at 6 months, 12 months, 24 months, and 36 months

Testosterone Reference Ranges[a] *(goal: reduce to low end of normal female range)*			
	Sex	Age range	Value
Free testosterone	F	3-60 years	< 7.5 pmol/L
		over 60 years	< 6.5 pmol/L
Total testosterone	F	over 11 years	< 1.4 nmol/L

[a]Values listed are those used by Vancouver Hospital laboratories, Vancouver, BC, Canada.

TABLE B2. Female-to-Male (FTM) Laboratory Summary

Timeline for Laboratory Tests

Baseline (before starting masculinizing endocrine therapy)	Lipid profile, fasting glucose (and glycosylated hemoglobin if high risk for diabetes/glucose intolerance), complete blood count, and liver enzymes
	Free testosterone if clinical suspicion of hyperandrogenism or if patient wants to know of changes after starting testosterone
2-4 weeks after starting/changing dose	Free testosterone (trough or midcycle if IM)
3 months after starting testosterone	Hgb, fasting blood glucose, lipid profile, liver enzymes
6 months after starting testosterone	Hgb, fasting blood glucose, lipid profile, liver enzymes
	Free testosterone (trough or midcycle if IM)
12 months after starting testosterone and annually thereafter	Hgb, fasting blood glucose, lipid profile, liver enzymes
	Free testosterone (trough or midcycle if IM)

Testosterone Reference Ranges[a]
(goal: elevate to within normal male range)

	Sex	Age Range	Value
Free testosterone	M	20-29 years	32-92 pmol/L
	M	30-39 years	30-87 pmol/L
	M	40-60 years	23-83 pmol/L
	M	over 60 years	22-63 pmol/L
Total testosterone	M	over 15 years	10-38 nmol/L

[a]Values listed are those used by Vancouver Hospital laboratories, Vancouver, BC, Canada.

APPENDIX C. Informed Consent Form for Feminizing Medications
Adapted from Dimensions (2003a)

This form refers to the use of estrogen and/or androgen antagonists (sometimes called "anti-androgens" or "androgen blockers") by persons in the male-to-female spectrum who wish to become feminized to reduce gender dysphoria and facilitate a more feminine gender presentation. While there are risks associated with taking feminizing medications, when appropriately prescribed they can greatly improve mental health and quality of life.

You are asked to initial the statements on this form to show that you understand the benefits, risks, and changes that may occur from taking feminizing medication. If you have any questions or concerns about the information below, please talk with the people involved in your care so you can make fully informed decisions about your treatment. It is your right to seek another opinion if you want additional perspective on any aspect of your care.

Please initial and date each statement.

Feminizing Effects

Patient   Provider   Date

1. _____   _____   __/__/__   I understand that estrogen, androgen antagonists, or a combination of the two may be prescribed to reduce male physical features and feminize my body.

2. _____   _____   __/__/__   I understand that the feminizing effects of estrogen and androgen antagonists can take several months or longer to become noticeable, and that the rate and degree of change can't be predicted.

3. _____   _____   __/__/__   I understand that if I am taking estrogen I will probably develop breasts, and:

   - Breasts may take several years to develop to their full size.
   - Even if estrogen is stopped, the breast tissue that has developed will remain.
   - As soon as breasts start growing, it is recommended to start doing monthly breast self-exam, and to have an annual breast exam by a doctor or nurse.
   - There may be milky nipple discharge (galactorrhea). This can be caused by taking estrogen or by an underlying medical condition. It is advised to check with a doctor to determine the cause.
   - It is not known if taking estrogen increases the risk of breast cancer.

4. _____   _____   __/__/__   I understand that the following changes are generally not permanent (that is, they will likely reverse if I stop taking feminizing medications):

   - Skin may become softer.
   - Muscle mass decreases and there may be a decrease in upper body strength.
   - Body hair growth may become less noticeable and grow more slowly, but it will likely not stop completely even after years on medication.
   - Male pattern baldness may slow down, but will probably not stop completely, and hair that has already been lost will likely not grow back.
   - Fat may redistribute to a more feminine pattern (decreased in abdomen, increased on buttocks/hips/thighs–changing from "apple shape" to "pear shape").

5. _____   _____   __/__/__   I understand that taking feminizing medications will make my testicles produce less testosterone, which can affect my overall sexual function:

   - Sperm may not mature, leading to reduced fertility. The ability to make sperm normally *may or may not* come back even after stopping taking feminizing medication. The options for sperm banking have been explained to me. I understand that I may still be able to make someone pregnant and am aware of birth control options (if applicable).
   - Testicles may shrink by 25-50%. Regular testicular examinations are still recommended.
   - The amount of fluid ejaculated may be reduced.

- There is typically decrease in morning and spontaneous erections.
- Erections may not be firm enough for penetrative sex.
- Libido (sex drive) may decrease.

Patient   Provider   Date

6. _____   _____   __/__/__   I understand that there are some aspects of my body that are not significantly changed by feminizing medications:

- Beard/moustache hair may grow more slowly and be less noticeable, but will not go away.
- Voice pitch will not rise and speech patterns will not become more feminine.
- The laryngeal prominence ("Adam's apple") will not shrink.

Although feminizing medication does not change these features, there are other treatments that may be helpful. If there are any concerns about these issues, referrals can be provided to help explore treatment options.

Risks of Feminizing Medications

7. _____   _____   __/__/__   I understand that the medical effects and safety of feminizing medications are not fully understood, and that there may be long-term risks that are not yet known.

8. _____   _____   __/__/__   I understand that I am strongly advised not to take more medication than I am prescribed, as this increases health risks. I have been informed that taking more than I am prescribed will not make feminization happen more quickly or increase the degree of change: Extra estrogen can be converted to testosterone, which may slow or stop feminization.

9. _____   _____   __/__/__   I understand that feminizing medications can damage the liver, possibly leading to liver disease. I have been advised that I should be monitored for possible liver damage as long as I am taking feminizing medications.

10. _____   _____   __/__/__   I understand that feminizing medications will result in changes that will be noticeable by other people, and that some transgender people in similar circumstances have experienced harassment, discrimination, and violence, while others have lost support of loved ones. I have been advised that referrals can be made for support/counseling if I feel this would be helpful.

Medical Risks Associated with Estrogen

11. _____   _____   __/__/__   I understand that taking estrogen increases the risk of blood clots, which can result in:

- pulmonary embolism (blood clot to the lungs), which may cause permanent lung damage or death
- stroke, which may cause permanent brain damage or death
- heart attack
- chronic leg vein problems

_____   _____   __/__/__   I understand that the risk of blood clots is much worse if I smoke cigarettes, especially if I am over 40. I understand that the danger is so high that I have been advised that I should stop smoking completely if I start taking estrogen. I am aware that I can ask my doctor for advice about options to stop smoking.

12. _____   _____   __/__/__   I understand that taking estrogen can increase deposits of fat around my internal organs, which is associated with increased risk for diabetes and heart disease.

13. _____   _____   __/__/__   I understand that taking estrogen can cause increased blood pressure. I have been advised that if I develop high blood pressure, my doctor will work with me to try to control it by diet, lifestyle changes, and/or medication.

APPENDIX C (continued)

Patient   Provider   Date

14. _____   _____   __/__/__   I have been informed that taking estrogen increases the risk of gallstones. I understand that if I have abdominal pain that is severe or prolonged, it is recommended that I discuss this with my doctor.

15. _____   _____   __/__/__   I have been informed that estrogen can cause nausea and vomiting, similar to morning sickness in pregnant women. I understand that if nausea/vomiting are severe or prolonged, it is recommended that I discuss this with my doctor.

16. _____   _____   __/__/__   I have been informed that estrogen can cause headaches or migraines. I understand that if I am frequently having headaches or migraines, or the pain is unusually severe, it is recommended that I talk with my doctor.

17. _____   _____   __/__/__   I understand that it is not known if taking estrogen increases the risk of non-cancerous tumours of the pituitary gland (prolactinoma). I have been informed that although prolactinoma is typically not life-threatening, it can damage vision and cause headaches. I understand that this will be monitored for at least three years when I start taking estrogen.

18. _____   _____   __/__/__   I have been informed that I am more likely to have dangerous side effects from estrogen if I smoke, am overweight, am over 40 years old, or have a history of blood clots, high blood pressure, or a family history of breast cancer.

19. _____   _____   __/__/__   I have been informed that if I take too much estrogen, my body may convert it into testosterone, which may slow or stop feminization.

Risks Associated with Androgen Antagonists

20. _____   _____   __/__/__   I have been informed that spironolactone affects the balance of water and salts in the kidneys, and that this may:

- increase the amount of urine produced, making it necessary to urinate more frequently
- reduce blood pressure
- increase thirst
- rarely, cause high levels of potassium in the blood, which can cause changes to heart rhythm that may be life-threatening

21. _____   _____   __/__/__   I understand that some androgen antagonists make it more difficult to evaluate the results of PSA (prostate-specific antigen) tests, which can make it more difficult to monitor prostate problems. I have been informed that if I am over 50, I should have my prostate evaluated every year.

Prevention of Medical Complications

22. _____   _____   __/__/__   I agree to take feminizing medications as prescribed and to tell my care provider if I am not happy with the treatment or am experiencing any problems.

23. _____   _____   __/__/__   I understand that the right dose or type of medication prescribed for me may not be the same as for someone else.

24. _____   _____   __/__/__   I understand that physical examinations and blood tests are needed on a regular basis to check for negative side effects of feminizing medications.

Patient   Provider   Date

25. _____   _____   __/__/__   I understand that feminizing medications can interact with other medication (including other sources of hormones), dietary supplements, herbs, alcohol, and street drugs. I understand that being honest with my care provider about what else I am taking will help prevent medical complications that could be life-threatening. I have been informed that I will continue to get medical care no matter what information I share.

26. _____   _____   __/__/__   I understand that some medical conditions make it dangerous to take estrogen or androgen antagonists. I agree that if my doctor suspects I may have one of these conditions, I will be checked for it before the decision to start or continue feminizing medication is made.

27. _____   _____   __/__/__   I understand that I can choose to stop taking feminizing medications at any time, and that it is advised that I do this with the help of my doctor to make sure there are no negative reactions to stopping. I understand that my doctor may suggest I reduce or stop taking feminizing medication, or switch to another type of feminizing medication, if there are severe side effects or health risks that can't be controlled.

My signature below confirms that:

- My doctor has talked with me about the benefits and risks of feminizing medication, the possible or likely consequences of hormone therapy, and potential alternative treatment options.
- I understand the risks that may be involved.
- I understand that this form covers known effects and risks and that there may be long-term effects or risks that are not yet known.
- I have had sufficient opportunity to discuss treatment options with my doctor. All of my questions have been answered to my satisfaction.
- I believe I have adequate knowledge on which to base informed consent to the provision of feminizing medication.

Based on this:

_____ I wish to begin taking estrogen.

_____ I wish to begin taking androgen antagonists (e.g., Spironolactone).

_____ I do not wish to begin taking feminizing medication at this time.

Whatever your current decision is, please talk with your doctor any time you have questions, concerns, or want to re-evaluate your options.

_____   _____

Patient Signature   Date

_____   _____

Prescribing Clinician Signature   Date

APPENDIX D. Informed Consent Form for Testosterone Therapy
Adapted from Dimensions (2003b)

This form refers to the use of testosterone by persons in the female-to-male spectrum who wish to become more masculine to reduce gender dysphoria and facilitate a more masculine gender presentation. While there are risks associated with taking testosterone, when appropriately prescribed it can greatly improve mental health and quality of life.

You are asked to initial the statements on this form to show that you understand the benefits, risks, and changes that may occur from taking testosterone. If you have any questions or concerns about the information below, please talk with the people involved in your care so you can make fully informed decisions about your treatment. It is your right to seek another opinion if you want additional perspective on any aspect of your care.

Please initial and date each statement.

Masculinizing Effects

Patient   Provider   Date

1. _____   _____   __/__/__   I understand that testosterone may be prescribed to reduce female physical characteristics and masculinize my body.

2. _____   _____   __/__/__   I understand that the masculinizing effects of testosterone can take several months or longer to become noticeable, that the rate and degree of change can't be predicted, and that changes may not be complete for 2-5 years after I start testosterone.

3. _____   _____   __/__/__   I understand that the following changes will likely be permanent even if I stop taking testosterone:

   - Lower voice pitch (i.e., voice becoming deeper).
   - Increased growth of hair, with thicker/coarser hairs, on arms, legs, chest, back, and abdomen.
   - Gradual growth of moustache/beard hair.
   - Hair loss at the temples and crown of the head, with the possibility of becoming completely bald.
   - Genital changes *may or may not* be permanent if testosterone is stopped. These include clitoral growth (typically 1-3 cm) and vaginal dryness.

4. _____   _____   __/__/__   I understand that the following changes are usually not permanent (that is, they will likely reverse if I stop taking testosterone):

   - Acne, which may be severe and can cause permanent scarring if not treated.
   - Fat may redistribute to a more masculine pattern (decreased on buttocks/hips/thighs, increased in abdomen–changing from "pear shape" to "apple shape").
   - Increased muscle mass and upper body strength.
   - Increased libido (sex drive).
   - Menstrual periods typically stop within 1-6 months of starting testosterone.

5. _____   _____   __/__/__   I understand that it is not known what the effects of testosterone are on fertility. I have been informed that even if I stop taking testosterone I *may or may not* be able to get pregnant in the future. I understand that even after testosterone stops my menstrual periods it may still be possible for me to get pregnant, and am aware of birth control options (if applicable). I have been informed that I can't take testosterone if I am pregnant.

6. _____   _____   __/__/__   I understand that there are some aspects of my body that will not be changed by testosterone:

   - Breasts may appear slightly smaller due to fat loss, but will not substantially shrink.
   - Although voice pitch will likely drop, other aspects of speech will not become more masculine.
   - Although testosterone does not change these features, there are other treatments that may be helpful. If there are any concerns about these issues, referrals can be provided to help explore treatment options.

Risks of Testosterone

Patient   Provider   Date

7. _____ _____ __/__/__ I understand that the medical effects and safety of testosterone are not fully understood, and that there may be long-term risks that are not yet known.

8. _____ _____ __/__/__ I understand that I am strongly advised not to take more testosterone than I am prescribed, as this increases health risks. I have been informed that taking more than I am prescribed will not make masculinization happen more quickly or increase the degree of change: Extra testosterone can be converted to estrogen, which may slow or stop masculinization.

9. _____ _____ __/__/__ I understand that testosterone can cause changes that increase my risk of heart disease, including:

- decreasing good cholesterol (HDL) and increasing bad cholesterol (LDL)
- increasing blood pressure
- increasing deposits of fat around my internal organs

10. _____ _____ __/__/__ I have been advised that my risks of heart disease are greater if people in my family have had heart disease, if I am overweight, or if I smoke.

11. _____ _____ __/__/__ I have been advised that heart health checkups, including monitoring of my weight and cholesterol levels, should be done periodically as long as I am taking testosterone.

12. _____ _____ __/__/__ I understand that testosterone can damage the liver, possibly leading to liver disease. I have been advised that I should be monitored for possible liver damage as long as I am taking testosterone.

13. _____ _____ __/__/__ I understand that testosterone can increase the red blood cells and hemoglobin, and while the increase is usually only to a normal male range (which does not pose health risks), a high increase can cause potentially life-threatening problems such as stroke and heart attack. I have been advised that my blood should be monitored periodically while I am taking testosterone.

14. _____ _____ __/__/__ I understand that taking testosterone can increase my risk for diabetes by decreasing my body's response to insulin, causing weight gain, and increasing deposits of fat around my internal organs. I have been advised that my fasting blood glucose should be monitored periodically while I am taking testosterone.

15. _____ _____ __/__/__ I understand that testosterone can be converted to estrogen by various tissues in my body, and that it is not known whether this increases the risks of ovarian cancer, breast cancer, or uterine cancer.

16. _____ _____ __/__/__ I understand that taking testosterone can lead to my cervix and the walls of my vagina becoming more fragile, and that this can lead to tears or abrasions that increase the risk of sexually transmitted infections (including HIV) if I have vaginal sex–no matter what the gender of my partner is. I have been advised that frank discussion with my doctor about my sexual practices can help determine how best to prevent and monitor for sexually transmitted infections.

17. _____ _____ __/__/__ I have been informed that testosterone can cause headaches or migraines. I understand that if I am frequently having headaches or migraines, or the pain is unusually severe, it is recommended that I talk with my health care provider.

18. _____ _____ __/__/__ I understand that testosterone can cause emotional changes, including increased irritability, frustration, and anger. I have been advised that my doctor can assist me in finding resources to explore and cope with these changes.

19. _____ _____ __/__/__ I understand that testosterone will result in changes that will be noticeable by other people, and that some transgender people in similar circumstances have experienced harassment, discrimination, and violence, while others have lost support of loved ones. I have been advised that my doctor can assist me in finding advocacy and support resources.

APPENDIX D (continued)

Prevention of Medical Complications

    Patient   Provider   Date

20. _____   _____   __/__/__   I agree to take testosterone as prescribed and to tell my doctor if I am not happy with the treatment or am experiencing any problems.

21. _____   _____   __/__/__   I understand that the right dose or type of medication prescribed for me may not be the same as for someone else.

22. _____   _____   __/__/__   I understand that physical examinations and blood tests are needed on a regular basis to check for negative side effects of testosterone.

23. _____   _____   __/__/__   I understand that testosterone can interact with other medication (including other sources of hormones), dietary supplements, herbs, alcohol, and street drugs. I understand that being honest with my doctor about what else I am taking will help prevent medical complications that could be life-threatening. I have been informed that I will continue to get medical care no matter what information I share.

24. _____   _____   __/__/__   I understand that some medical conditions make it dangerous to take testosterone. I agree that if my doctor suspects I may have one of these conditions, I will be checked for it before the decision to start or continue testosterone is made.

25. _____   _____   __/__/__   I understand that I can choose to stop taking testosterone at any time, and that it is advised that I do this with the help of my doctor to make sure there are no negative reactions to stopping. I understand that my doctor may suggest I reduce or stop taking testosterone if there are severe side effects or health risks that can't be controlled.

My signature below confirms that:

- My doctor has talked with me about the benefits and risks of testosterone, the possible or likely consequences of hormone therapy, and potential alternative treatment options.
- I understand the risks that may be involved.
- I understand that this form covers known effects and risks and that there may be long-term effects or risks that are not yet known.
- I have had sufficient opportunity to discuss treatment options with my doctor. All of my questions have been answered to my satisfaction.
- I believe I have adequate knowledge on which to base informed consent to the provision of testosterone therapy.

Based on this:

_____ I wish to begin taking testosterone.

_____ I do not wish to begin taking testosterone at this time.

Whatever your current decision is, please talk with your doctor any time you have questions, concerns, or want to re-evaluate your options.

_____   _____
Patient Signature   Date

_____   _____
Prescribing Clinician Signature   Date

Care of the Patient Undergoing Sex Reassignment Surgery

Cameron Bowman, MD, FRCSC

Joshua M. Goldberg

SUMMARY. Sex reassignment surgery (SRS) has proven to be an effective intervention for the patient with gender dysphoria. As with any surgery, the quality of care provided before, during, and after SRS has a significant impact on patient outcomes. This article is intended to help primary care providers who are already familiar with routine transgender care to understand the specialized processes involved in SRS. Topics include guidelines for the recommendation of SRS, feminizing and masculinizing surgical procedures, suggested timelines for various interventions, expected course and recovery, risks and complications, and revisional surgery that may be required. doi:10.1300/ J485v09n03_07 *[Article copies available for a fee from The Haworth Document Delivery Service: 1-800- HAWORTH. E-mail address: <docdelivery@haworthpress.com> Website: <http://www.HaworthPress.com> © 2006 by The Haworth Press, Inc. All rights reserved.]*

KEYWORDS. Transgender, transsexual, gender dysphoria, sex reassignment surgery

Sex reassignment surgery (SRS) has proven to be an effective intervention for the patient with gender dysphoria. Patient satisfaction following SRS is high (Lawrence, 2003; Michel, Ansseau, Legros, Pitchot, & Mormont, 2002), and reduction of gender dysphoria following SRS has psychological and social benefits (Pfäfflin & Junge, 1998; Mate-Kole, Freschi, & Robin, 1990). As with any surgery, the quality of care provided before, during, and after SRS has a significant impact on patient outcomes (Pfäfflin, 1992).

This article is intended to help primary care providers who are already familiar with basic transgender medical care (Feldman & Goldberg, 2006) to understand the specialized processes involved in SRS. Topics include guidelines for the recommendation of SRS, feminizing and masculinizing surgical procedures, suggested timelines for various interventions, expected course and recovery, risks and complications, and revisional surgery that may be required.

These guidelines are not intended to cover the details of operative techniques, nor can they

Cameron Bowman, MD, FRCSC, is affiliated with the Division of Plastic Surgery, Department of Surgery, University of British Columbia, Vancouver, BC, Canada. Joshua M. Goldberg is Education Consultant of the Transgender Health Program, Vancouver, BC, Canada.

Address correspondence to: Dr. Cameron Bowman, #1000-1200 Burrard Street, Vancouver, BC, Canada V6Z 2C7.

This manuscript was created for the Trans Care Project, a joint initiative of Transcend Transgender Support & Education Society and Vancouver Coastal Health's Transgender Health Program, with funding from the Canadian Rainbow Health Coalition. The authors thank Trevor Corneil, Stan Monstrey, and Kathy Wrath for their comments on an earlier draft, Donna Lindenberg for creating the illustrations, and Olivia Ashbee, A. J. Simpson, and Rodney Hunt for research assistance.

[Haworth co-indexing entry note]: "Care of the Patient Undergoing Sex Reassignment Surgery." Bowman, Cameron, and Joshua M. Goldberg. Co-published simultaneously in *International Journal of Transgenderism* (The Haworth Medical Press, an imprint of The Haworth Press, Inc.) Vol. 9, No. 3/4, 2006, pp. 135-165; and: *Guidelines for Transgender Care* (ed: Walter O. Bockting, and Joshua M. Goldberg) The Haworth Medical Press, an imprint of The Haworth Press, Inc., 2006, pp. 135-165. Single or multiple copies of this article are available for a fee from The Haworth Document Delivery Service [1-800-HAWORTH, 9:00 a.m. - 5:00 p.m. (EST). E-mail address: docdelivery@haworthpress. com].

cover every risk, sequella, or complication that might arise. Rather, this article is intended to provide a general orientation for the family physician or nurse whose patient is undergoing SRS. Information written specifically for transgender patients, their loved ones, and clinicians unfamiliar with medical terminology (e.g., counselors) is available as an online supplement (Simpson & Goldberg, 2006a; Simpson & Goldberg, 2006b).

SRS is a multidisciplinary endeavour drawing on plastic surgery, urology, gynecology, reproductive endocrinology, and otolaryngology. Some SRS procedures (e.g., breast augmentation, mastectomy, hysterectomy, and oophorectomy) involve relatively minor modification of surgical procedures routinely performed for the non-transgender population. For optimal results, the surgeon should be familiar with trans-specific modification to standard techniques, and according aftercare considerations. While post-operative care following these procedures is usually straightforward and complications are typically easily managed by the primary care provider, surgical consultation may be required.

Genital reassignment surgery is a more complex procedure with multiple trans-specific considerations. Consultation with an experienced surgeon is advised when questions surrounding these complex constructive procedures arise.

GUIDELINES FOR THE RECOMMENDATION OF SRS

For any type of surgery, all patients must meet general criteria. The patient must (a) be physically fit and psychologically prepared for surgery, (b) have a good understanding of the interventions to be performed, and realistic goals and expectations of the surgery, and (c) have given their informed consent for the procedures. As part of informed consent, the patient should be informed of, and understand, any alternative procedures; risks and complications of the interventions must be reviewed and understood.

With some types of surgery (including but not limited to SRS), detailed protocols are used to ensure that surgical treatment is appropriate

and that the patient is a suitable candidate. The Harry Benjamin International Gender Dysphoria Association (HBIGDA) *Standards of Care* (Meyer et al., 2001) provide such guidance in relation to SRS.

SRS and the WPATH Standards of Care

The WPATH *Standards of Care* discuss psychological and physical assessment of the patient prior to surgery, recommend criteria for SRS eligibility and readiness, and outline minimum standards for surgeon competence. Each topic is discussed below.

Evaluation by Mental Health Professional(s) Prior to SRS

The WPATH *Standards of Care* state that prior to chest/breast surgery, at least one mental health professional with specialized training in transgender health should evaluate the patient's eligibility and readiness for SRS. Evaluation by two mental health professionals is required prior to gonadal removal or genital surgery. Qualifications for surgical assessors and guidelines for psychological assessment prior to surgery are discussed by Bockting and colleagues (2006).

The mental health professional(s) will provide a letter of documentation outlining the eligibility criteria that have been met and the rationale for recommending SRS. *Eligibility* refers to the minimum criteria that anyone seeking these medical interventions must meet, and *readiness* refers to the client being mentally ready for the procedure. Readiness does not imply that the client must no longer have any mental health concerns; rather, sufficient stability needs to be in place to both make an informed decision and to be adequately prepared to deal with the physical, emotional, and social consequences of the decision. Table 1 summarizes the eligibility and readiness criteria in the WPATH *Standards of Care*.

Evaluation by mental health professionals is not required for other types of SRS (e.g., facial feminizing surgery, voice pitch-elevating surgery), but as with any type of surgery the surgeon may ask for the patient to be evaluated by a mental health clinician if there are concerns about co-existing mental health problems or

TABLE 1. Summary of The World Professional Association for Transgender Health's *Standards of Care: Eligibility and Readiness Criteria* (Meyer et al., 2001)

Eligibility	Readiness
Chest or Breast Surgery	
1. Able to give informed consent	1. Consolidation of gender identity
2. Informed of anticipated effects and risks	2. Improved or continuing mental stability
3. Completion of 3 months of "real life experience" OR have been in psychotherapy for duration specified by a mental health professional (usually minimum of 3 months)	
4. FTM chest surgery may be done as first step, alone or with hormones; MTF breast augmentation may be done after 18 months on hormones (to allow time for hormonal breast development)	
Genital Surgery, Hysterectomy, and Oophorectomy	
1. Able to give informed consent	1. Consolidation of gender identity
2. On hormones for at least 12 months (if needing and medically able to take hormones)	2. Improved or continuing mental stability
3. At least 1 year "real life experience"	
4. Completion of any psychotherapy required by the mental health professional	
5. Informed of cost, hospitalization, complications, aftercare, and surgeon options	

insufficient competency to make medical decisions.

In addition to evaluation by mental health professionals, the WPATH *Standards* state that to fulfill professional responsibility to the patient "the surgeon must understand the diagnosis that has led to the recommendation for genital surgery" (Meyer et al., 2001, p. 19). The WPATH *Standards* state that the surgeon should speak at length with the patient to be satisfied that the patient is likely to benefit from the procedures, and should seek to establish a working relationship with the other health care professionals who are involved in the patient's physical and mental health care. This includes coordination of pre- and post-operative care with the patient's primary care provider.

Physical Assessment Prior to Surgery

Assessment of physical health and investigation of any medical conditions of concern are standard pre-operative procedures. Prior to SRS, assessment should include evaluation of the effects of endocrine therapy on the liver and other organ systems. The WPATH *Standards of Care* explicitly state that it is unethical to deny SRS solely on the basis of HIV or Hepatitis B/C seropositivity (Meyer et al., 2001). Decisions about SRS suitability should be made based on a comprehensive evaluation of the patient's overall health, not on seropositivity alone (Israel & Tarver, 1997; Kirk, 1999).

Surgeon Competence

In addition to Board-certification as a urologist, gynecologist, plastic surgeon or general surgeon, documented supervised training with a more experienced SRS surgeon is required. Surgeons are expected to attend professional meetings where new techniques are presented.

Ideally, the surgeon will be knowledgeable about more than one of the surgical techniques that may be used to facilitate choice of the technique best suited to the patient's individual needs. If the surgeon is skilled in a single technique, the patient should be so informed, and those who do not want or are unsuitable for this procedure should be referred to another surgeon.

Regret Following SRS

With any irreversible medical procedure there is a risk of patient dissatisfaction, and primary care providers are often concerned that their transgender patients will experience regret following SRS. To address this concern it is helpful to understand (a) the incidence and causes of post-surgical regret, and (b) protective measures in place to help prevent regret following SRS.

Temporary concerns are relatively common after any surgery, and in both the transsexual and non-transsexual literature typically relate to post-operative pain, surgical complications, discrepancy between hoped-for results and actual results, and initial difficulty adjusting to the impact of surgery on immediate relationships (Michel et al., 2002). Dissatisfaction, disappointment, doubt, or other psychological difficulties that represent normal adjustment and resolve (spontaneously or with psychotherapeutic assistance) in the first year after surgery are distinguished from a persistent wish that surgery had not been pursued.

Persistent regret is more rare following surgery, and may (for reversible surgeries) be accompanied by a request for surgical reversal. In studies of non-transsexual individuals who reported regret following a variety of surgical procedures–including surgical sterilization (Jamieson et al., 2002; Miller, Shain, & Pasta, 1991; Rosenfeld, Taskin, Kafkashli, Rosenfeld, & Chuong, 1998; Rubinstein, Benjamin, & Kleinkopf, 1979; Vemer et al., 1986), mastectomy (Anderson, 2001; Borgen et al., 1998; Lantz et al., 2005; Montgomery et al., 1999; Payne, Biggs, Tran, Borgen, & Massie, 2000; Taucher, Gnant, & Jakesz, 2003), breast reconstruction (Harcourt & Rumsey, 2001; Montgomery et al., 1999), breast augmentation (Coon, Burris, Coleman, & Lemon, 2002; Roberts, Wells, & Walden, 1999; Tweed, 2003), oophorectomy (Elit, Esplen, Butler, & Narod, 2001), orchiectomy (Clark, Wray, & Ashton, 2001), limb salvage surgery (Eiser, Darlington, Strike, & Grimer, 2001), gastric banding (Victorzon & Tolonen, 2001), and colpocleisis (Wheeler et al., 2005)–the regret rate ranged from < 1% to 23%. The reported reasons for regret included adverse physical effects of surgery, loss of physical functioning, poor aesthetic result, failure to achieve desired effect, lack of support available before and after surgery, change in intimate relationship, psychological issues not recognized prior to surgery, and incongruence between patient preferences regarding decision involvement and their actual level of involvement.

Persistent regret among post-operative transsexuals has been studied since the early 1960s. The most comprehensive meta-review done to date (Pfäfflin & Junge, 1998) analyzed 74 follow-up studies and 8 reviews of outcome studies published between 1961 and 1991, for a total of 1000-1600 male-to-female (MTF) and 400-550 female-to-male (FTM) patients. Pfäfflin and Junge concluded that in this 30 year period, less than 1% of FTMs and 1.0-1.5% of MTFs experienced persistent regret following SRS. Studies published since 1991 (Cohen-Kettenis & Van Goozen, 1997; Landen, Walinder, Hambert, & Lundstrom, 1998; Lawrence, 2003; Pfäfflin, 1992; Rakic, Starcevic, Maric, & Kelin, 1996; Rehman, Lazer, Benet, Schaefer, & Melman, 1999; Smith, Van Goozen, Kuiper, & Cohen-Kettenis, 2005) report lower rates of regret for both MTFs and FTMs, likely due to improved quality of psychological and surgical care for individuals undergoing SRS in the last 15 years.

Numerous studies have explored clinical practices that may help in the prevention of regret following SRS, and negative prognostic factors. There are three key factors in persistent regret following SRS: (a) incorrect diagnosis of gender dysphoria or of co-existing psychopathology, (b) poor quality of surgical intervention, and (c) lack of ability to live in the desired gender role (Kuiper & Cohen-Kettenis, 1998; Michel et al., 2002; Pfäfflin, 1992). The latter issue is influenced by numerous psychosocial issues, including lack of support by loved ones, psychological dysfunction, fluctuating gender identity, and insufficient professional support during treatment (Kuiper & Cohen-Kettenis, 1998; Landen et al., 1998; Smith et al., 2005). None are considered absolute contraindications for SRS, but all are considered risk factors that warrant careful clinical attention. The WPATH *Standards of Care* (Meyer et al., 2001) require "real life experience" (RLE) in the desired gender role as part of the pre-surgical evaluative process prior to genital surgery or gonadal removal. The RLE provides an opportunity to evaluate the impact of transition on the patient's support network (loved ones, friends, etc.), and the impact of the stresses of transition on the patient's psychological resilience.

Inaccurate diagnosis of gender dysphoria or co-existing psychopathology and poor quality of the surgical intervention relate to clinical competence for mental health professionals and surgeons involved in transsexual care. As discussed previously, the WPATH *Standards of Care* (Meyer et al., 2001) outline competency requirements for clinicians involved in SRS, and WPATH also provides opportunities for scientific interchange among professionals through its biennial conferences, publications, and email discussion lists.

While psychotherapy is not an absolute requirement for SRS, supportive professional and peer counseling can be helpful with preparation and adjustment, and should be accessible to all patients before and after surgery. The primary care provider can assist by discussing patient awareness of resources and, where needed, facilitating referrals to trans-experienced professionals.

FEMINIZING SURGERY (MALE-TO-FEMALE)

Surgical Procedures

Augmentation Mammaplasty (Breast Augmentation)

Feminizing hormonal therapy often effects some breast development. However, this is not always sufficient for the MTF patient to live comfortably. In these cases surgical augmentation may be recommended. Breast augmentation is a common procedure which is performed by the plastic surgeon. It will usually be delayed until after hormonal therapy has been undertaken for a period of 18 months to allow time for maximal hormonal breast development. Breast augmentation is therefore sometimes performed simultaneously with vaginoplasty.

As shown in Figure 1, breast augmentation is most often performed using saline-filled implants placed sub-muscularly via an incision

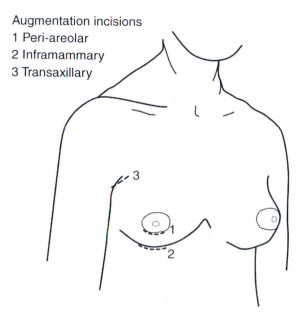

FIGURE 1. Location of incisions for MTF augmentation mammaplasty.

Augmentation incisions
1 Peri-areolar
2 Inframammary
3 Transaxillary

under the breast (near the inframammary fold) or around the areola. Although the technique is essentially the same as augmentation mammaplasty in non-transgender women, there are important anatomical differences in male and female chests that guide modification for the MTF transsexual. Compared to non-transgender women, the breast envelope of the MTF patient is often undeveloped and tight and there may be less lipomatous tissue (Kanhai, Hage, Asscheman, & Mulder, 1999). A staged approach involving initial tissue expansion, as in reconstruction following mastectomy, is sometimes used for optimal results (Greenwald & Stadelmann, 2001).

As discussed by Dahl and colleagues (2006), there is no clinical consensus on the best way to promote nipple and breast development in transgender women. Results vary, but in general, the nipple-areola complex appears under-developed and lateralized even after years of hormone treatment. Even after two years of feminizing hormones MTF breast development typically corresponds to the conical shape seen in young adolescents, without the ptosis normally seen as a result of aging. The patient should be made aware that implants cannot perfectly imitate adult breasts. In particular, the age-related changes seen in non-transgender women and cleavage between the breasts is very difficult to create (Kanhai et al., 1999).

MTF Genital Reconstruction

Vaginoplasty

The term vaginoplasty includes several procedures which transform the male external genitalia into female genitalia. The goals of vaginoplasty include: (a) creation of a sensate and aesthetically acceptable vulva–including clitoris, labia minora and majora, and vaginal introitus; (b) shortening of the urethra, with creation of a urethral opening that allows a downward urinary stream; (c) creation of a stable and sensate neovagina with adequate dimensions for penetrative sexual intercourse, ideally lined with moist, elastic, hairless epithelium; (d) elimination of erectile tissue, to avoid narrowing of the introitus and protrusion of the urethral meatus/clitoris during sexual arousal; and (e) preservation of orgasmic capability (Karim, Hage, & Mulder, 1996; Krege, Bex, Lummen, & Rubben, 2001; Laub, Laub, & Biber, 1988; Perovic, Stanojevic, & Djordjevic, 2000; Schrang, 1997).

Vaginoplasty includes orchiectomy, creation of a vaginal cavity and neoclitoris, labiaplasty,

and penile dissection with partial penectomy. It is usually performed by the plastic surgeon in a single operative setting, although some surgeons prefer to perform labiaplasty and clitoroplasty as a second surgery following healing of the initial vaginoplasty.

The penile inversion technique is most commonly used to create the neovagina (Hage, 1995; Karim et al., 1996; Laub et al., 1988; Monstrey, Hoebeke, et al., 2001; Perovic et al., 2000; Takata & Meltzer, 2000). In this technique the majority of skin from the shaft of the penis is inverted and used to line the inner walls of the neovagina. In some cases, extra skin is required to line the inner vagina. This is usually harvested from the patient's lower abdomen, or scrotal skin grafts may be used (Eldh, 1993; Monstrey, Hoebeke et al., 2001; Takata & Meltzer, 2000). Use of a segment of the colon–rectosigmoid pedicled transplant–is the third choice if penile inversion or skin grafts from other locations fail (Hage, 1995; Karim et al., 1996; Kim et al., 2003; Maas, Eijsbouts, Hage, & Cuesta, 1999; Monstrey, Hoebeke et al., 2001). A portion of the horizontal part of the urethra is preserved and used to fashion the female urethra and surrounding tissue. As shown in Figure 2, the neovagina is positioned posterior to the prostate, which is untouched.

FIGURE 2. MTF vaginoplasty.

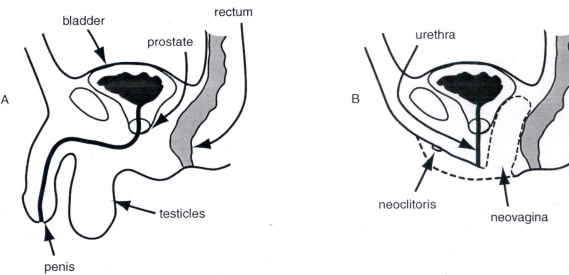

Adapted from: Hage, J.J. (1995). Medical requirements and consequences of sex reassignment surgery. *Medicine, Surgery and the Law*, 35(1), 17-24.

Labia minora are constructed from prepuce or penile skin, and labia majora are constructed from scrotal skin (Eldh, 1993; Krege et al. 2001; Laub et al., 1988; Perovic et al., 2000; Rubin, 1993). In the sensate pedicled clitoroplasty technique, a small portion of the glans is preserved by maintaining attachments to its nerve and blood supply (Eldh, 1993; Giraldo et al., 2004; Perovic et al., 2000; Rehman & Melman, 1999; Rubin, 1993; Tiewtranon, Chokerungvaranon, Jindarak, & Wannachamras, 2001). This then functions as the neoclitoris. Revisions may be performed after the vaginoplasty to refine the appearance of the clitoris, labia, or the superior aspect of the labia majora (anterior commisure). This is discussed further in the section on revisions.

Orchiectomy Without Vaginoplasty

Orchiectomy as a single procedure may be sought by patients who would like to reduce the risks and side effects of feminizing hormones by lowering the dosage needed to oppose endogenous testosterone (Herzog & Santucci, 2002; Reid, 1996; Rubin, 1993). Typically the testes are removed with preservation of scrotal skin in case vaginoplasty/labiaplasty are sought in the future (Israel & Tarver, 1997), but there is risk of shrinkage or damage of the skin. Accordingly, some surgeons recommend against orchiectomy as a separate procedure for the patient who wishes to pursue vaginoplasty at a later date; others feel the benefits of early orchiectomy outweigh the potential risks (Reid, 1996).

Penectomy Without Vaginoplasty

Some MTF patients seek penectomy without vaginoplasty (also known as "nullification") as a less invasive alternative when vaginal penetration is not desired by the patient. A shallow vaginal dimple is created that does not require dilation (as in vaginoplasty), and a new urethral opening is created to allow the patient to urinate in a sitting position. As penile tissue is typically used in vaginoplasty, penectomy as a separate procedure is not recommended if the patient wishes to pursue vaginoplasty at a later date.

Facial Feminizing Surgery

Drawing on techniques from soft tissue plastic surgery, maxillofacial surgery, and reconstructive surgery, facial feminizing surgery techniques were pioneered by maxillofacial surgeon Douglas Ousterhout in the USA (Ousterhout, 1987, 1997, 2003) and are now widely available. Facial feminizing surgery involves the use of one or more procedures to reduce stereotypically masculine features and impart more conventionally feminine features to the patient's head and neck region (Becking, Tuinzing, Hage, & Gooren, 1996; Conrad & Yoskovitch, 2003; Hage, 1995; Hage, Vossen, & Becking, 1997; Monstrey, Hoebeke et al., 2001; Wolfort, Dejerine, Ramos, & Parry, 1990). Facial feminizing surgery procedures include, but are not limited to: removal of supraorbital bossing ("brow bossing") and orbital rim contouring, brow elevation, rhinoplasty, ear pinning, augmentation of the lip vermilion area, cheek augmentation, widening of the zygomatic complex, chin/jaw reduction, clockwise rotation of the bimaxillary complex, and reduction laryngochondroplasty (also known as "tracheal shave" or "Adam's apple reduction").

Voice Pitch-Elevating Surgery

Surgical alteration of the laryngeal framework and/or vocal cords is sought by some transsexual women who have not been able to sufficiently elevate pitch through speech therapy alone (Brown, Perry, Cheesman, & Pring, 2000; Donald, 1982; Isshiki, Taira, & Tanabe, 1983; Kunachak, Prakunhungsit, & Sujjalak, 2000; Neumann, Welzel, Gonnermann, & Wolfradt, 2002a, 2002b; Oates & Dacakis, 1997; Wagner, Fugain, Monneron-Girard, Cordier, & Chabolle, 2003; Yang, Palmer, Murray, Meltzer, & Cohen, 2002). Techniques, risks/complications, and outcome data are discussed by Davies and Goldberg (2006).

Other Feminizing Surgical Procedures

Other surgical procedures to reduce masculine features and approximate a female habitus include suction-assisted lipoplasty of the waist and augmentation of the hips or buttocks (Hage,

1995; Ousterhout, 1997, 2003). Hair transplantation may also be desired (Ousterhout, 2003). As these are not trans-specific procedures, they are not discussed in this article; post-operative care protocols are the same as for the non-transgender population.

Removal of the eleventh and twelfth rib is sought by some MTFs to create a more defined waist. This surgery is not recommended as potential complications include damage to lower chest wall rigidity and impairment of lower lung inflation (Israel & Tarver, 1997).

Injection of free (gelatinous) silicone is extremely hazardous. Use of free silicone is not legal in many countries, including Canada and the USA, but may be performed by non-medical personnel (Israel & Tarver, 1997; Schmid, Tzur, Leshko, & Krieger, 2005). Any MTF patient who has undergone free silicone injection as part of breast augmentation or contouring of hips, buttocks, or the face should be referred for immediate medical evaluation, as effects of free silicone injection include severe disfigurement, neurological impairment, pulmonary disease (including embolism), and death (Chastre et al., 1983; Coulaud et al., 1983; Duong, Schonfeld, Yungbluth, & Slotten, 1998; Farina et al., 1997; Fox, Geyer, Husain, la-Latta, & Grossman, 2004; Gaber, 2004; Schmid et al., 2005).

Suggested Timelines and Sequencing

Vaginoplasty is a shorter and less complex intervention than phalloplasty. As such, it is safe–and even desirable–to perform both breast augmentation and vaginoplasty within the same operative setting (Kanhai, Hage, Asscheman, & Mulder, 1999; Ratnam & Lim, 1982). Doing so minimizes the risks associated with general anesthesia. However, the surgeries may also be performed separately.

With the exception of tracheal shaves, most facial feminizing surgical procedures may be performed safely at least 3 months before or after the vaginoplasty, provided there are no complications. If forehead surgery and rhinoplasty are both sought, it is recommended they be performed together (Ousterhout, 2003). Electrolysis treatment should be stopped completely at least 2 weeks prior to facial surgery and should

not be resumed sooner than 3 months following chin or jaw surgery (Ousterhout, 2003).

Pitch-elevating surgery should be performed last in the sequence of feminizing surgeries as some types of pitch-elevating surgery narrow the trachea, making endotracheal intubation more difficult. Endotracheal intubation may also destabilize recently altered vocal cords (Monstrey, Hoebeke et al., 2001).

Expected Course and Recovery

Pre-Operative

Following receipt of letters of recommendation and an initial interview with the surgeon to determine appropriateness of SRS, the MTF patient will meet with the surgical team. A history and physical examination will be performed. It is helpful if the general practitioner provides a letter reviewing the pertinent past medical history of the patient. A discussion outlining the patient's goals will be undertaken and a timeframe for the various interventions will be established following the guidelines of the surgical team and the WPATH *Standards of Care* (Meyer et al., 2001). The specific procedures will be outlined with the patient, including the possible need for harvesting extra skin to line the neovagina as well as the expected course and recovery period. Risks and complications will be reviewed. To prevent intra-vaginal hair growth from use of hair-bearing grafts (scrotal skin, base of penis), patients undergoing vaginoplasty will be provided with referral information for clinicians with experience in MTF genital electrolysis.

The effects of smoking on skin quality, wound healing, and vascularity will be discussed and patients will be strongly encouraged to stop smoking. Smoking cessation resources will be identified.

In conjunction with the prescribing physician, feminizing endocrine therapy is stopped 2 to 4 weeks pre-operatively (depending on the specific medication and its route of administration). Medications affecting the coagulation cascade must be stopped 7 to 10 days prior to surgery. Prior consultation with an appropriate physician is required in the case of complicating medical factors.

Peri-Operative

The patient undergoing breast augmentation as a single surgery will be admitted and, in most cases, be discharged home the same day as surgery. Patients will be instructed not to eat or drink after midnight the night prior to surgery. While in hospital, patients will have routine monitoring by the nursing and surgical staff and residents. Pain management is usually straightforward, allowing for early discharge home with oral analgesics. Antibiotics are usually given in hospital.

In the case of a vaginoplasty, patients are admitted the day prior to surgery. They will undergo a "bowel prep"–including phosphosoda and antibiotics–to cleanse the bowel of particulate matter, and will take nothing by mouth after midnight. Blood will be drawn and an electrocardiogram will be obtained. Occasionally, a chest x-ray is taken. Patients will undergo pre-operative shaving prior to their surgery.

The course in hospital will average 6 to 8 days and the patient will remain on bedrest restriction for much of this time. Patients may use PCA (patient controlled analgesia) and will typically remain on parenteral anti-coagulants and antibiotics until the patient is mobile. A prosthesis will be placed into the neovagina at the time of surgery and will be left in place for 5 days to ensure the penile skin flap (and any additional graft used) will be well apposed to the inner vaginal walls in maximum dimensions. After this, the prosthetic device and Foley catheter will be removed and the patient will be instructed in the routine care of the neovagina. For the next several weeks the prosthesis will be left in place much of the time, being removed only occasionally for routine douching.

Peri-operative recovery from facial feminizing surgery depends on the specific techniques used, particularly the degree of bone revision versus soft tissue work. Minor procedures may be performed on an outpatient basis with same-day discharge; more extensive bone reconstruction will likely be done on an inpatient basis with discharge the following day (Ousterhout, 2003).

Post-Operative

MTF Augmentation Mammaplasty

Patients who have undergone a breast augmentation will wear an underwire bra and leave their dressings intact for 3 days following surgery. After this, the gauze dressings may be removed but the steri-strips along the incision lines should be left in place. The patient may then shower, taking care to avoid soaking the incisions. The steri-strips should be gently patted dry and will fall off on their own in 7 to 10 days.

It is normal for incisions to be erythematous, but this erythema should not extend or progress to more than 1 to 2 cm from the incision. It is also normal to see or feel the suture knot at the end of the incision line. These superficial suture knots can be a nuisance; however, they are not a cause for concern. If they work their way to the surface (usually around 3 weeks) they can be clipped free. Bruising and swelling is expected and is not a cause for concern unless there is an unusually large amount of swelling (mass) on one side. Feelings of sharp shooting pain, burning sensations, and/or general discomfort are common during the healing process and will eventually disappear.

Patients are usually comfortable 1 to 2 days following the procedure and often back to their daily routine in 1 to 2 weeks. However, strenuous activity should be avoided for 3 to 4 weeks. Patients will be instructed in implant displacement breast massage which should be started 3 to 5 days following surgery, if tolerated.

MTF Genital Reconstruction

Patients who have undergone a vaginoplasty will begin to feel more comfortable during the second post-operative week. The prosthesis will be left in place, only being removed for routine cleaning once per day initially. The amount of time the prosthesis is left out will gradually be increased over the next 8 weeks, as per the written protocol that will be given to the patient. After this time, the prosthesis should be used once per day if the patient is not engaging in regular sexual vaginal penetration. Daily dilation is necessary to prevent vaginal stricture; insufficient dilation can lead to loss of vaginal depth and width.

The patient will be asked to follow up in the clinic in the week following vaginoplasty, and then periodically after that. She will have a physical examination, including a manual pelvic exam to ensure viability of the skin flap and patency of the neovagina. The neoclitoris is inspected for viability and sensation. The quality of wound healing is assessed (dehiscence, infection, or hypertrophic scarring). In addition, bowel and bladder function is queried. If skin grafts are required, full thickness grafts may be taken above the pubic area or the flank area at both sides. There will most likely be a transverse incision just above the pubic region, with steri-strips in place. Graft donor sites should be inspected at the first visit with the primary care provider for the absence of infection and wound healing problems.

Following vaginoplasty the MTF patient is still at risk for prostate cancer, as the prostate is not removed (Feldman & Goldberg, 2006). The patient should be made aware of this risk and informed of screening recommendations.

MTF Facial Feminizing Surgery

Post-operative recovery from facial feminizing surgery depends on the specific procedure–particularly the degree of bony work versus soft tissue work–and techniques used. The following protocols are used by Dr. Douglas Ousterhout, the originator of facial feminizing surgery (Ousterhout, 2003).

Forehead surgery. Following scalp advancement, brow elevation, removal of supraorbital bossing, or orbital rim contouring, dressings can be removed the day following surgery. Gentle washing of the hair can then commence, with care taken not to wet any supporting dressings used for simultaneous nose or chin surgery. Pain medication and antibiotics will be prescribed. Swelling and bruising around the eyes typically resolve within 10 to 12 days following surgery. Patients are typically able to return to work within 7 days following surgery, but it is not advisable to perform any activities that require exertion until 2 weeks after surgery. Sutures and staples used to close scalp incisions are usually removed within 8 days following surgery.

Cheek augmentation. Pain medication and antibiotics will be prescribed. Temporary numbness and swelling may interfere with speaking, smiling, yawning and chewing for the first 1 to 3 days following surgery and it is advisable to avoid foods requiring substantial biting or chewing for the first 2 weeks. Swelling typi-cally completely resolves within 2 weeks following surgery. The teeth can be cleaned as normal, with care not to disturb the incision line if the implant has been placed through the mouth.

Rhinoplasty. Internal nasal packing typically remains for 1 to 2 days to support nasal tissues during the early phase of healing. There will be an external cast on the nose for 8 days following surgery; care must be taken not to wet this dressing when bathing. Pain medication will be prescribed. Eccyhmosis around the nose and eyes typically fades within 2 weeks of surgery. If glasses are required, special instructions will be given as the nasal pads that support glasses cannot touch the nose until one month after surgery. Activities that involve exertion should not be performed until 1 month after surgery.

Chin reduction. Chin reduction usually requires significant bony work so recovery can take 4 to 5 weeks, with swelling remaining beneath the mandible for 3 to 4 months. The patient can typically return to light work within 5 to 6 days of surgery.

Jaw reduction. The face is typically moderately swollen and bruised following jaw reduction. Swelling gradually resolves over 10 to 14 weeks and the surgical results are often not apparent until the new contour has resolved 3 to 4 months after surgery. The patient can typically return to work within 10 to 14 days of surgery.

Lip augmentation. Most postoperative swelling following augmentation of the vermilion area of the upper/lower lip resolves within 10 to 14 days of surgery.

Risks and Complications of MTF SRS

General risks related to operative procedures include deep vein thrombosis, pulmonary embolism, and death. Obviously, these are very serious complications and surgeons, anesthetists, and nurses take various measures to reduce associated risk. These include intravenous hydration, active monitoring, the use of compression stockings and/or pneumatic compression devices, judicious anticoagulation, and early mobilization. Once home, patients should stay well-hydrated and should not remain in bed for extended periods. Tender, warm, or swollen legs; chest pain; or continued dizzy spells should be investigated in the hospital emergency room. If a patient experiences sudden shortness of breath, emergency medical assistance should be sought.

There are additional risks and complications specific to each surgical feminization procedure or group of procedures commonly performed together. These are discussed below.

MTF Augmentation Mammaplasty

Risks associated with augmentation mammaplasty include wound infection; post-operative bleeding/hematoma; capsular contracture–thickening and contracture of scar tissue which naturally forms around the breast implant; asymmetry of breast size, shape, or position; asymmetry of the nipple-areola complex; and implant failure, infection, or extrusion (Kanhai et al., 1999; Leslie, Buscome, & Davenport, 2000; Ratnam & Lim, 1982). Scar management, including massage and sun avoidance, will be discussed with the patient; hypertrophic scarring is possible due to intrinsic or extrinsic factors. Decreased sensation to the nipple-areola complex is common and usually resolves spontaneously within a few weeks. Partial or permanent loss of nipple or skin sensation may occur. There may be visible and palpable wrinkling of the skin over the implant, particularly if breast development has been minimal after hormone treatment or the patient is thin. Management of complications relating to MTF augmentation mammaplasty is discussed in Table 2.

MTF Genital Reconstruction

Risks of MTF genital reconstruction using the penile inversion method include infection; post-operative bleeding/hematoma; recto-vaginal fistula; partial or complete flap necrosis; vaginal or urethral stricture or stenosis; prolapse of the neovagina; and unsatisfactory size/shape of the neovagina, clitoris, or labia (Crichton, 1993; Eldh, 1993; Greenwald & Stadelmann, 2001; Krege et al., 2001; Liguori, Trombetta, Buttazzi, & Belgrano, 2001; Rubin, 1993; Takata & Meltzer, 2000). Scar management will be discussed with the patient; hypertrophic scarring is possible due to intrinsic or extrinsic factors. If the patient has not undergone epilation of the donor site prior to

vaginoplasty, the use of hair-bearing tissue to create the neovagina may result in intravaginal hair growth (Israel & Tarver, 1997; Takata & Meltzer, 2000). Management of complications relating to MTF genital reconstruction is discussed in Table 3.

Partial or complete flap necrosis leading to loss of the clitoris is a devastating but fortunately rare complication (Krege et al., 2001; Takata & Meltzer, 2000). Vascular compromise would most likely occur in the early post-operative period. By the time the patient is discharged home the risk of total flap failure is quite low.

Decreased erogenous sensation is a potential risk of vaginoplasty. However, sexual outcomes are generally good. At followup (mean 4.2 years after surgery) of 71 MTFs who underwent vaginoplasty at Gent University Hospital between 1998 and 1999, erogenous sensation was present in all but one patient (98.6%), and 94% of patients reported achieving orgasm at least occasionally (Monstrey, Hoebeke, et al., 2001). Other studies report orgasmic capability among 63% to 92% of MTFs following vaginoplasty (Kim et al., 2003; Krege et al., 2001; Lawrence, 2005; Rakic et al., 1996; Rehman et al., 1999; Rubin, 1993). A study of 14 MTFs found that although self-reported orgasmic capacity decreased following vaginoplasty, reported frequency of sex increased by 75% and sexual satisfaction remained high (Lief & Hubschman, 1993).

Occasionally the neo-vagina will not be long enough or will contract in size. This is usually the result of inadequate dilating. Stretching with progressively larger dilators may be sufficient; in some cases surgical correction is required.

MTF Facial Feminizing Surgery

Risks of facial feminizing surgery include infection of the wound or implants, transient numbness due to edema, numbness due to nerve damage (potentially permanent), and dissatisfaction with the aesthetic results (Ousterhout, 2003). Following rhinoplasty there may be a mild scleral hemorrhage and edema around the nose which typically resolves spontaneously after several weeks. Prophylactic antibiotics may be

TABLE 2. Management of Complications Following MTF Augmentation Mammaplasty

Complication	Signs and symptoms	Treatment
Post-operative bleeding or hematoma	Expanding painful mass on one side	Expanding hematoma will need to be evacuated, and the bleeding stopped, in the operating room. In most cases the implant can be saved and replaced at that time.
Infection	Blanching erythema which spreads beyond the incisional margins, combined with tenderness, fever, malaise, and leukocytosis	Small infections can be treated with course of antibiotics. Abscesses often need to be drained in the operating room or under ultrasonic guidance. The surgeon should be consulted for treatment of persistent infections caused by multidrug-resistant organisms. Infection within the breast implant pocket necessitates removal of the implant; after the infection is treated, a new implant can be placed at a later date.
Seroma	Gradual and progressive swelling of the breast due to fluid accumulation	Seromas usually resolve spontaneously with time. Aspiration may be required by the surgeon (one or more times).
Wound healing problems	Most often small dehiscences due to stitch rupture or minor infection	If minor, treat with basic wound care such as dressing changes and antibiotic ointment. If the incision line is progressively opening such that the wound is gaping, contact the surgeon.
Asymmetry	Asymmetrical breast size, shape, or position, or asymmetrical positioning of the nipple-areola complex	Revisional surgery after re-evaluation, following resolution of swelling and implant settling (4 to 6 months).
Capsular contracture	Excessive firmness of the breasts and shape distortion, shortly after surgery or many years after, on one or both sides	Surgical removal of thickened capsule, with implant replacement or removal.
Implant extrusion	Exposure of implant caused by infection, wound healing problems, or lack of tissue coverage	Removal of the implant and replacement at a later date.
Implant failure	Sudden change in size or shape of breast	Removal and replacement of the damaged implant.
Hypertrophic scarring	Thick, raised, red scars	Discuss prevention measures, including sun avoidance and massage. Severe scarring may require surgical revision.

prescribed to prevent infection; implant infection necessitates removal.

Revisional Surgery

Surgical revisions may be required to improve aesthetic or functional result. The most common revisions following breast augmentation are (a) replacement of an implant, (b) exchanging implants for those of a different size, (c) exchanging implants for those of a different type, (d) placing the implants in a slightly different location, and (e) scar revisions. The most common revisions following vaginoplasty include (a) clitoroplasty–adjusting the size, shape, location, or hooding of the neo-

TABLE 3. Management of Complications Following MTF Genital Reconstruction

Complication	Signs and symptoms	Treatment
Post-operative bleeding or hematoma	Ongoing bleeding and swelling at the operative site immediately following surgery	Management by hospital staff.
	Bleeding in first few weeks (typically following dilation)	Minor bleeding after dilation can be controlled by applying pressure to the site. The surgeon should be consulted if there is recurrent bleeding.
	Persistent bloody or purulent discharge with dilation	Weekly application of silver nitrate to areas of granulation tissue until area re-epithelializes. A uterine or bone curette may be used to scrap areas with profuse granulation.
Infection	Progressive pain and blanching erythema which spreads beyond the incisional margins, combined with tenderness, fever, malaise, and leukocytosis	Small infections can be treated with a course of antibiotics. Abscesses often need to be drained in the operating room or under ultrasonic guidance. The surgeon should be consulted for treatment of persistent infections caused by multidrug-resistant organisms.
Wound healing problems	Most often small dehiscences due to stitch rupture or minor infection	If minor, treat with basic wound care, including dressing changes and antibiotic ointment. If incision line is progressively opening such that the wound is gaping, contact the surgeon.
Recto-vaginal fistula	Gas or feces passing from the vagina due to communication between neovagina and rectum; fistula confirmed by speculum examination or contrast X-ray study	Surgical repair.
Partial or complete flap necrosis (loss of clitoris)	Usually presents early with non-blanching erythema or mottling of the skin, which progressively becomes darker and nonviable. Does not usually happen after discharge from hospital	Immediate contact with surgeon is required.
Vaginal stricture or stenosis	Pain or difficulty with vaginal penetration	Prevent by lifelong daily patient dilation. Surgeon should be consulted to dicuss treatment. Options range from progressive dilation to surgical revision.
Urethral stricture or stenosis	Dysuria, difficulty voiding, diminished urine stream, increased time and effort required for urination	If immediately following removal of Foley catheter, replace catheter for 2-3 more days until swelling around meatus subsides and patient can void spontaneously. For late stenosis, consult with surgeon—if minor, dilation with a Foley catheter may suffice; if major, surgical revision may be necessary.
Swelling or irregularities of urethral meatus	Urine spraying, rather than voiding in a steady stream	Usually resolves spontaneously within a few months after surgery, as swelling subsides. Surgical repair may be needed in severe cases.

TABLE 3 (continued)

Complication	Signs and symptoms	Treatment
Prolapse of the neovagina	"Falling out" sensation, dyspareunia	Surgical repair.
Intravaginal hair growth	Vaginal irritation or discharge, with hair visible on examination with speculum	Prevent by epilation of donor site prior to vaginoplasty. Mechanical removal of intravaginal hair after surgery may only be partially effective.
Hypertrophic scarring	Thick, raised, red scars	Severe scarring may require surgical revision.

clitoris, (b) labiaplasty–adjusting the size or shape of the labia minora or majora, (c) commisuroplasty–narrowing the anterior commisure, or superior aspect of the labia majora, and (d) deepening or widening the neovagina (Meltzer, 2001; Monstrey, Hoebeke, et al., 2001; Rubin, 1993; Wilson, 2002).

MASCULINIZING SURGERY (FEMALE-TO-MALE)

Surgical Procedures

FTM Chest Surgery

Chest surgery reduces dysphoria relating to breasts and allows the FTM patient to live more easily in the male gender role, improving psychological and social functioning (Hage, 1995; Hage & Bloem, 1995; Monstrey, Hoebeke et al., 2001). Chest surgery may be the sole surgical step in gender transition (Meyer et al., 2001).

Subcutaneous Mastectomy

The mastectomy procedure (performed by the plastic surgeon) should achieve more than just a flat chest: ideally, the subcutaneous mastectomy results in a chest which has an aesthetically pleasing male contour, is fully sensate, and has minimal scarring (Gilbert & Gilbert, n.d.; Hage, 1995; Hage & van Kesteren, 1995). The procedure consists of removal of most of the breast tissue, removal of excess skin, and removal of the inframammary fold (Hage &

Bloem, 1995; Hage & van Kesteren, 1995). Sparing of the nipple and areola is possible if the nipple-areolar complex is appropriately sized and shaped, but often reduction and repositioning of the nipple-areolar complex is required to approximate male nipples. Revisional surgery is often required (Hage & Bloem, 1995).

The choice of technique must be appropriately selected for the patient's breast size and skin quality. Small breasts with good skin elasticity may be removed with a minimum of incisions and subsequent scarring. A periareolar (or "keyhole") approach, illustrated in Figure 3a, is most often utilized in these instances (Hage & Bloem, 1995; Monstrey, Selvaggi et al., 2001). Moderately sized breasts (B cup) with good skin elasticity can most often be removed with a concentric incision which gathers skin and leaves a scar completely around the areola, illustrated in Figure 3b (Colic & Colic, 2000; Gilbert & Gilbert, n.d.). Large breasts or moderately-sized breasts with poor elasticity will require more incisions to remove excess skin (Hage & Bloem, 1995; Monstrey, Selvaggi et al., 2001). Very large or pendulous breasts require a full mastectomy, which includes removal of the nipple and free grafting of the nipple-areolar complex to the appropriate new location (Gilbert & Gilbert, n.d.; Monstrey, Selvaggi et al., 2001). This technique, illustrated in Figure 3c, will impact nipple sensation significantly but may be the only option for large or inelastic breasts. Skin which is inelastic–often due to years of breast binding–can adversely affect the outcome, and will influence

FIGURE 3a. FTM chest surgery: Keyhole approach for smaller breasts.

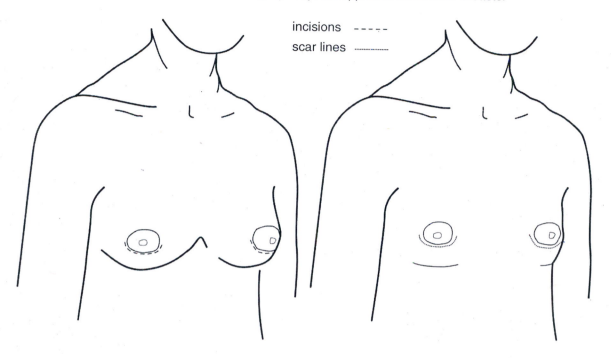

FIGURE 3b. FTM chest surgery: Concentric incision ("pursestring") approach.

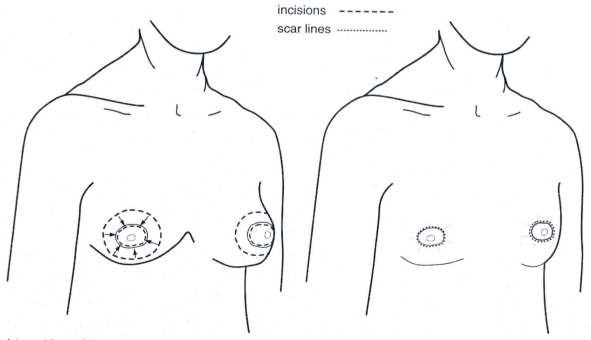

Adapted from: Gilbert, D.A., & Gilbert, D.M. (n.d.) Chest contouring in the female transgender patient. Unpublished manuscript.

FIGURE 3c. FTM chest surgery: Full mastectomy with grafting of free nipple.

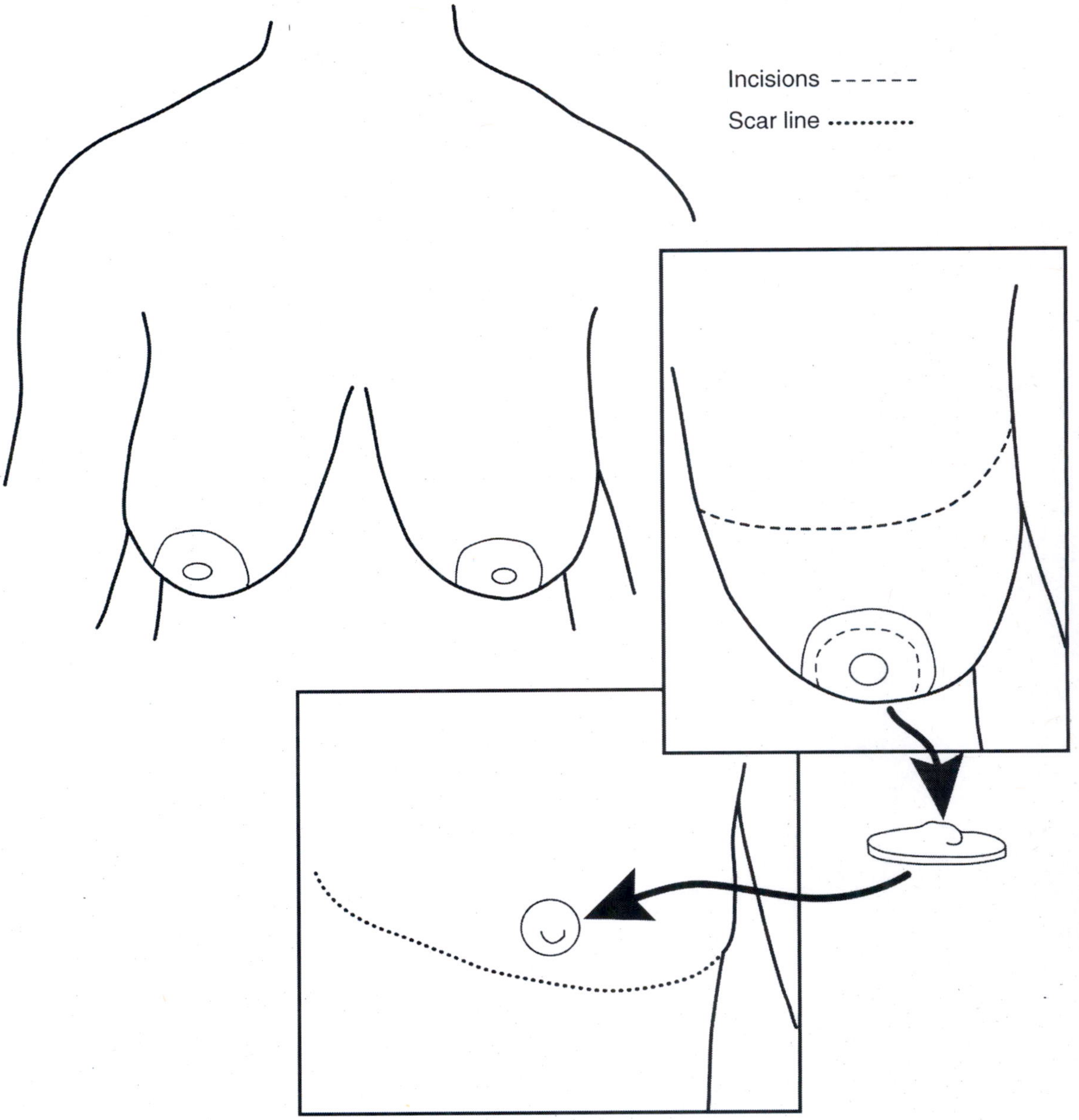

Incisions - - - - - -
Scar line ··········

and limit the surgeon's choice of technique (Hage & Bloem, 1995).

Breast Reduction

Some FTM patients will choose a breast reduction in lieu of a subcutaneous mastectomy. Prior reduction affects options for reconstruction so should be approached cautiously for the patient who wants a full reconstruction in the future.

Hysterectomy and Oophorectomy

Hysterectomy and oophorectomy may be sought to reduce gender dysphoria relating to the presence of the uterus and fallopian tubes, to treat pre-existing gynecological problems, to prevent menstrual bleeding in the patient who cannot tolerate testosterone, or to obviate the necessity for regular Pap testing in the severely dysphoric patient who cannot tolerate vaginal examination (by removal of the cervix in a total hysterectomy). While there are no data on the risks of long-term testosterone use, there are concerns about the potential risk of ovarian and uterine cancer, and preventive hysterectomy and oophorectomy are recommended by some clinicians (Feldman & Goldberg, 2006). Oophorectomy also allows the reduction of testosterone dosage, and hence associated health risks and side effects. In the FTM patient bilateral oophorectomy is typically accompanied by bilateral removal of the fallopian tubes (salpingectomy).

Hysterectomy and oophorectomy are gynecological procedures which can usually be performed by minimally invasive laparoscopic surgery (Ergeneli, Duran, Ozcan, & Erdogan, 1999; Gerli et al., 2001; Saridogan & Cutner, 2004). If the patient intends to pursue phalloplasty, laparoscopic incision is preferred to spare abdominal flaps that may be required for revisions (Ergeneli et al., 1999; Hage, 1995). Vaginal hysterectomy may be difficult in the FTM patient who has no history of vaginal sexual penetration, particularly if there is vaginal atrophy relating to long-term testosterone administration (Gerli et al., 2001; Saridogan & Cutter, 2004).

Some patients may have vaginectomy performed concurrent with a vaginal or abdominal hysterectomy. If urethral extension is sought as part of future genital reconstruction vaginectomy should not be performed prior to urethroplasty, as vaginal mucosa is used to lengthen the urethra (Chesson et al., 1996; Hage, Bouman, & Bloem, 1993b).

FTM Genital Reconstruction

Vaginectomy and Urethral Lengthening

These procedures are usually performed by the urologist and are a requisite part of a phalloplasty, but optional in metaidoioplasty (described below). All vaginal mucosa is excised and the levator ani muscles are approximated to help obliterate the previous vaginal cavity. Vaginal mucosa is then typically recruited to lengthen the urethra which will carry urine through the neophallus in a metaidoioplasty or a phalloplasty (Hage, Bouman, & Bloem, 1993a; Hage, Torenbeek, Bouman, & Bloem, 1993). Alternatives to vaginal mucosa

reported in the literature include bladder mucosa grafts and buccal mucosa grafts (Hage, Bouman, & Bloem, 1993b; Levine & Elterman, 1998; Ralph, 1999; Rohrmann & Jakse, 2003).

Metaidoioplasty

Metaidoioplasty (sometimes spelled "metaidioplasty" or "metoidioplasty"), a less complex procedure than phalloplasty, results in a small sensate phallus that may allow for urination while standing (Hage, 1996). The hormonally enlarged clitoris, which is analogous to and functions as the glans penis, is released from its surrounding tissues (Perovic & Djordjevic, 2003). A flap of skin from the labia minora is then "wrapped around" the stalk to add bulk, resulting in a small phallus which has erogenous sensation (Takata & Meltzer, 2000). As described in the preceding paragraph, the fixed part of the urethra can be extended and incorporated into the microphallus by recruiting tissue from the vaginal mucosa (Hage, 1996; Perovic & Djordjevic, 2003). This will produce a microphallus which can transmit urine to its distal end under the neoglans.

Since the clitoris is intervened upon to a lesser degree than in phalloplasty, the metaidoioplasty likely results in greater preservation of erogenous sensation than in phalloplasty. However, the microphallus created by metaidoioplasty is typically not large enough for sexual penetration, and does not appear adult in size (Hage, 1996, Monstrey, Hoebeke, et al., 2001; Takata & Meltzer, 2000). Hage (1996) estimated the size of the microphallus to be between half the size of the patient's little finger and the patient's thumb; others report an average of 5.7 cm (range 4-10 cm) for the microphallus created by metaidoioplasty (Perovic & Djordjevic, 2003). Despite the limits of size and sexual function, metaidoioplasty is an option for those FTM patients who do not want to undergo the lengthy phalloplasty procedure with its higher rate of complications and donor site morbidity.

Phalloplasty

The goals of phalloplasty are (a) creation of a sensate and aesthetically acceptable penis with sufficient length and bulk to be viable for penetrative sexual intercourse (with the aid of a prosthetic erectile device), (b) extension of the urethra to the tip of the penis to allow voiding while standing, (c) preservation of orgasmic capability, and (d) minimal scarring, disfigurement, and functional loss in the donor area (Chesson et al., 1996; Gilbert, Gilbert, Jordan, Schlossberg, & Chesson, 1998; Gilbert, Schlossberg, & Jordan, 1995; Hage, 1995, 1999; Hage, Bloem, & Suliman, 1993; Jordan, 2002; Khouri & Casoli, 1997; Santanelli, 2000). Phalloplasty is a long and complex microsurgical procedure that requires free tissue transfer to create the neophallus (Chang & Hwang, 1986; Chesson et al., 1996; Gilbert et al., 1998; Gottlieb & Levine, 1993; Hage & de Graaf, 1993; Monstrey, Hoebeke, et al., 2001; Rohrmann & Jakse, 2003; Takata & Meltzer, 2000). The flap is usually harvested from the forearm (Chang & Hwang, 1986; Gilbert et al., 1998; Khouri & Casoli, 1997; Veselý, Kucera, Hrbaty, Stupka, & Rezai, 1999), although use of flaps from the fibula, dorsalis pedis, tensor fasciae latae, groin, deltoid, anterolateral thigh, and lateral arm have also been reported in the literature (Hage, Bloem, & Suliman, 1993; Hage, Winters, & Van Lieshout, 1996; Khouri & Casoli, 1997; Mutaf, 2000; Santanelli & Scuderi, 2000; Sengezer & Sadove, 1993). As illustrated in Figure 4, a small segment of the ulnar forearm is rolled into a tube to form the urethra. This is then rolled within a larger piece of the forearm (including fat and skin) to form a "tube within a tube." The procedure results in an adult male-size phallus which transmits urine.

Ideally, the phallus will also carry general and erogenous sensation by coaptation of nerves–including the dorsal nerve of the clitoris–to its base. The native clitoris is not removed but is de-epithelialized and covered by the base of the phallus to preserve erogenous sensation (Monstrey, Hoebeke, et al., 2001).

It typically takes 1 year to ensure anatomic and functional stability of the neophallus. After this time, an erectile prosthesis may be placed (Chesson et al., 1996; Hage, Bloem, & Bouman, 1993; Hoebeke, De Cuypere, Ceulemans, & Monstrey, 2003; Mulcahy, 2003). Tattooing of the neoglans may also be performed as a later procedure to help create a visible demarcation between the penile shaft and the glans (Hage, de

Graaf, Bouman, & Bloem, 1993; Monstrey, Hoebeke, et al., 2001).

Differences in male and female anatomy make it more complex to create a de novo phallus in the FTM than to reconstruct a neophallus in the non-transgender male. FTM phalloplasty involves removal of a significant amount of tissue from the forearm and subsequent grafting of this donor site with skin from the thigh (Gilbert et al., 1995; Monstrey, Hoebeke et al., 2001). In addition, dissection of groin vessels and nerves is necessary, and a vein graft from the leg is often required. Thus, multiple surgical sites are produced, all carrying inherent risks for the patient. The procedure produces a large conspicuous scar on the patient's forearm and includes an extended hospital stay of approximately 10 to 14 days. Phalloplasty is an option for those FTM patients who would accept a large donor scar and potential reduction in erogenous sensation in exchange for the construction of a functional adult male phallus.

Scrotoplasty

In a survey of gender clinic FTM patients (N = 200), 96% expressed the desire for a scrotum, compared to 52% requesting phalloplasty (Hage, Bout, Bloem, & Megens, 1993). A scrotum not only provides aesthetic satisfaction to the patient but also facilitates life in the male role by more closely approximating male appearance in underwear and swim trunks.

Performed by the urologist or plastic surgeon, the scrotoplasty recruits tissue from the labia majora to create a neoscrotal pouch which is appropriately situated over the obliterated introitus (Chesson et al., 1996; Gottlieb & Levine, 1993; Greenwald & Stadelmann, 2001; Hage, 1992; Perovic & Djordjevic, 2003; Sengezer & Sadove, 1993). After stability is ensured, testicular implants may be placed. Although the skin is initially tight, over time the weight of the prosthesis stretches the redraped labial skin to create a more natural appearance (Hage, Bouman, & Bloem, 1993c).

Other Masculinizing Surgeries

Various procedures may be performed by the plastic surgeon to reduce stereotypical feminine characteristics and approximate mascu-

FIGURE 4. FTM phalloplasty.

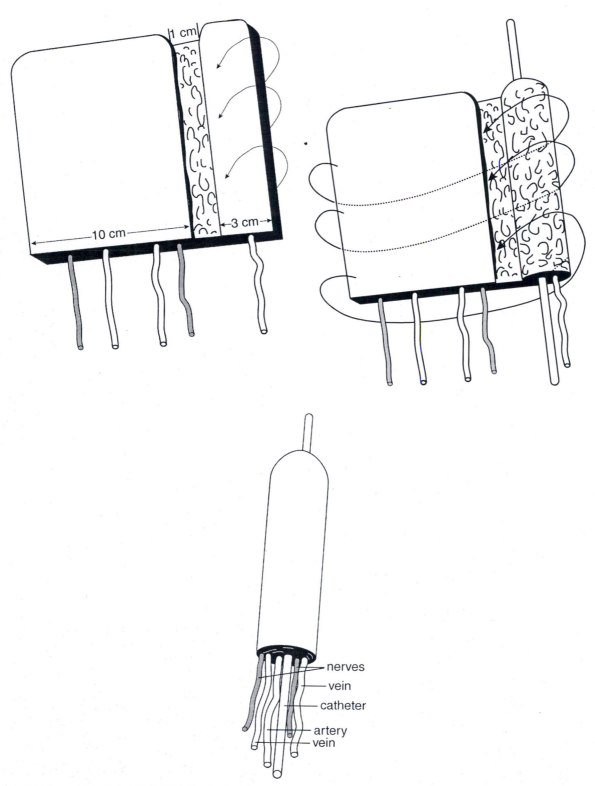

Adapted from: Mulcahy, J.J. (2003). Penile implants in constructed neophallus. *International Journal of Impotence Research*, 15, 5129-131.

line facial features and male habitus. Little has been written about these procedures in transsexuals and it is difficult to find surgeons experienced in their execution. These procedures include, but are not limited to: rhinoplasty; chin/jaw implantation; liposuction to reduce fat in the hips, thighs, and buttocks; and calf or pectoral implantation (Chesson et al., 1996; Hage, 1995; Meyer et al., 2001; Monstrey, Hoebeke et al., 2001).

Suggested Timelines and Sequencing

SRS in the FTM who desires both top and bottom constructive procedures is more complex than in the MTF patient. This is mainly due to the larger number of surgical interventions involved for FTMs. "Bottom surgery" in particular consists of multiple procedures, usually performed by different surgical teams. Included in these procedures are the hysterectomy and oophorectomy (gynecologist), vaginectomy and lengthening of the fixed part of the urethra (urologist), scrotoplasty (urologist or plastic surgeon), and metaidoioplasty (urologist) or phalloplasty (plastic surgeon).

In general, every general anesthesia carries risk for any patient. For this reason, specific procedures are often combined into a single operative setting. Many combinations have been tried, including performing almost all the procedures in a single operative setting (Monstrey, Hoebeke et al., 2001). However, this approach has been found to produce increased morbidity for the patient, and as such, the following regimen is commonly utilized.

Chest Surgery (Possibly with Hysterectomy and Oophorectomy)

Chest surgery is typically the first intervention performed. The hysterectomy and oophorectomy may be performed within the same operative setting (Greenwald & Stadelmann, 2001; Hage, 1995); alternatively, hysterectomy may be performed later if chest surgery is done early in transition, before the one year "real life experience" required for hysterectomy has been completed (Meyer et al., 2001). Some surgical teams perform hysterectomy and oophorectomy at the same time as genital reconstruction (Monstrey, Hoebeke et al., 2001).

Genital Surgery (Possibly with Hysterectomy and Oophorectomy)

After a minimum of 4 to 6 months the second intervention may be undertaken as long as the eligibility and readiness requirements in the WPATH *Standards of Care* (Meyer et al., 2001) have been met. This is the longest operation and typically includes the vaginectomy, urethral lengthening, scrotoplasty, and phalloplasty or metaidoioplasty; some surgical teams prefer to separate genital surgery into two steps, with combined hysterectomy and oophorectomy, vaginectomy, and urethral lengthening performed separate from phalloplasty or metaidoioplasty (Benet & Melman, 1999; Gilbert et al., 1998; Hage, Bouman, de Graaf, & Bloem, 1993). If the patient chooses a metaidoioplasty, this can usually be performed by a single surgeon and requires less operative time. In the case of a phalloplasty, the urological and plastic surgical teams work simultaneously to minimize the length of the general anesthesia. The choice of a metaidoioplasty does not negate a phalloplasty later on.

Tattooing of the Neoglans

Tattooing of the neoglans may be safely performed 6 to 8 months following the phalloplasty. Ideally, it will be done before the return of full sensation to the phallus (Monstrey, Hoebeke et al., 2001).

Implant Placement

If he chooses, the patient may have testicular implants and, in the case of a phalloplasty, an erectile prosthesis may be placed (Greenwald & Stadelmann, 2001, Hoebeke et al., 2003; Hage, Bloem, & Bouman, 1993). These implants are placed in a single setting, a minimum of 1 year after the second intervention. This ensures stability of wound healing and functionality.

Facial Masculinization Surgery

Facial masculinizing surgical procedures may be performed safely at least 3 months before or after the regimen above, provided there are no complications in any of the previous surgeries. Depending on the nature of the complications, further surgery should ideally be postponed until the patient has fully recovered.

Expected Course and Recovery

Pre-Operative

Following receipt of letters of recommendation and an initial interview with the surgeon to: determine appropriateness of SRS, the FTM patient will meet with the surgical team and a history and physical examination will be performed. It is helpful if the primary care provider provides a letter reviewing the pertinent past medical history of the patient. A discussion outlining the patient's goals will be undertaken and a timeframe for the various interventions will be established following the guidelines of the surgical team and the WPATH *Standards of Care* (Meyer et al., 2001). The specific procedures will be outlined with the patient, including the expected course and recovery times. Risks and complications will be reviewed.

The effects of smoking on skin quality, wound healing, and vascularity are discussed, where appropriate, and patients are strongly encouraged to stop smoking. This is an absolute requirement if a free flap phalloplasty will be performed in the future (Chesson et al., 1996). Smoking cessation resources will be identified if desired.

In conjunction with the prescribing physician and depending on the specific medication and its route of administration, masculinizing endocrine therapy may be stopped 2 to 4 weeks pre-operatively. Medications affecting the coagulation cascade must be stopped 7 to 10 days prior to surgery. Prior consultation with an appropriate physician is required in the case of complicating medical factors.

The ulnar side of the arm is usually chosen for the urethral reconstruction as there is less hair growth. In the case of the patient who has particularly hairy forearms due to hormonal therapy, epilation prior to surgery may be necessary to prevent hair growth in the neourethra. Excess hair is believed to promote bacterial colonization and calculus formation (Fang et al., 1999; Khouri & Casoli, 1997; Mutaf, 2000; Ralph, 1999) and some surgeons therefore require electrolysis to be completed at least 3 months prior to phalloplasty (Gilbert et al., 1995; Hage, Bouman, & Bloem, 1993b). Epilation may also be desired by the patient to reduce hair on skin that will be used to create the shaft of the penis; it is certainly less awkward to have this done before rather than after the phalloplasty procedure.

Peri-Operative

FTM Chest Surgery

The patient undergoing chest surgery will typically be admitted the same day as surgery and, in most cases, be discharged the same day (for breast reduction or mastectomy using the periareolar or concentric incision, without hysterectomy or oophorectomy) or the following day (if full mastectomy with nipple grafts have been performed, or if the patient has undergone simultaneous hysterectomy and oophorectomy). Patients will be instructed not to eat or drink after midnight the night prior to surgery. While in hospital, patients will have routine monitoring by the nursing and surgical staff and residents. Pain management is usually straightforward, allowing for early discharge home with oral analgesics. Antibiotics are usually prescribed.

FTM Genital Reconstruction

The patient undergoing metaidoioplasty is typically admitted the same day as surgery. If urethral lengthening is not simultaneously performed, the patient will in most cases be discharged the following day. The patient who undergoes urethral extension as part of the procedure will have a suprapubic catheter placed at the time of the operation; this is usually removed during the first week. The patient will remain in hospital until the urologist is satisfied with the patency of the neourethra, typically 5 to 10 days.

In the case of a phalloplasty, patients are admitted the day prior to surgery. They will undergo a "bowel prep"–including phosphosoda and antibiotics–and will take nothing by mouth after midnight. Blood will be drawn and an electrocardiogram will be obtained. Occasionally, a chest x-ray is taken. Patients will undergo pre-operative shaving prior to their surgery. The course in hospital will average 10 to 14 days and the patient will remain on bedrest for most of this time. The phallus will be closely monitored every hour for the first 2 days by the nursing and surgical staff, as any compromise in the vascularity of the phallus may necessitate a prompt return to the operating room. A suprapubic catheter is placed at the time of the operation and this is usually removed during the first week; the Foley catheter will remain in place for 2 to 3 weeks. Patients will use patient-controlled analgesia and remain on intravenous blood thinners and antibiotics for 5 days. The skin-grafted forearm will be wrapped under occlusive dressings for 5 days.

Post-Operative

FTM Chest Surgery

Patients who have undergone a subcutaneous mastectomy will continue to wear a tensor bandage around the chest for a period of 1 month. Homecare nursing will be arranged to help empty and monitor drains in the operative sites; the drains will be removed by the plastic surgeon during a clinic visit 3 to 7 days following surgery. Antibiotics continue until the drains are removed.

Steri-strips will be placed along the suture lines. Patients may shower 3 days following surgery. The steri-strips should be gently patted dry and will fall off on their own in 7 to 10 days.

It is normal for incisions to be erythematous, but this erythema should not extend or progress to more than 1 to 2 cm from the incision. It is also normal to see or feel the suture knot at the end of the incision line. These superficial suture knots can be a nuisance; however, they are not a cause for concern. If they work their way to the surface (usually around 3 weeks) they can be clipped free. Bruising and swelling is expected and is not a cause for concern unless there is an unusually large amount of swelling. Patients are usually comfortable 1 or 2 days following the procedure and often back to their daily routine in 1 to 2 weeks. However, strenuous activity should be avoided for 4 weeks.

Following chest surgery the FTM patient must still be screened for breast cancer, as all glandular tissue may not be completely removed (Feldman & Goldberg, 2006). The patient should be made aware of this risk and informed of screening recommendations.

FTM Genital Reconstruction

The patient will follow-up with the plastic surgeon and urologist frequently in the early post-operative period. Typically, the patient will have two outpatient appointments 5 to 7 days after discharge from the hospital. The Foley catheter will be removed in the clinic and antibiotics will continue until this time. The neophallus and neoscrotum should be inspected periodically; if phalloplasty was performed, the forearm with its split thickness skin graft (STSG), the donor thigh (source of the STSG), and the donor calf (source of the vein graft) should also be examined on a regular basis.

The neophallus is inspected for quality of wound healing–including dehiscence, infection, or hypertrophic scarring–ability to void, and presence of urinary fistulae or stricture (typically a late finding). In the patient who has undergone phalloplasty, vascularity of the neophallus will be evaluated by checking the color, temperature, turgor, pulse, and capillary refill of the neophallus, along with quality of wound healing and sensation and function in the donor forearm. The skin graft donor site will be dressed with a sheet of gauze which becomes incorporated into the ensuing eschar (scab). It may be gradually trimmed away as it lifts up from its edges over the following 1 to 2 weeks.

Occasionally, an arterial-venous fistula (AVF) is created within the neophallus during phalloplasty. This is a connection, intentionally made, between the main artery and vein. A palpable "thrill," or vibration, will be present at the distal end of the neophallus. AVFs may close spontaneously, or may be disconnected in a minor procedure performed in the clinic several weeks after the phalloplasty.

Risks and Complications of FTM SRS

General risks related to operative procedures include deep vein thrombosis, pulmonary embolism, and death. Obviously, these are very serious complications and surgeons, anesthetists and nurses take various measures to reduce associated risk. These include intravenous hydration, active monitoring, the use of compression stockings and/or pneumatic compression devices, judicious anticoagulation, and early mobilization. Once home, patients should stay well-hydrated and should not remain in bed for extended periods. Tender, warm, or swollen legs; chest pain; or continued dizzy spells should be investigated in the emergency room. If a patient experiences sudden shortness of breath, emergency medical assistance should be sought.

There are additional risks and complications specific to each surgical masculinization procedure or group of procedures commonly performed together. These are discussed below.

Subcutaneous Mastectomy or Breast Reduction

Risks associated with subcutaneous mastectomy and breast reduction include infection, post-operative bleeding/hematoma, seroma, mastectomy flap necrosis, nipple necrosis with loss of the nipple, contour abnormalities, and nipple asymmetry (Hage & Bloem, 1995). Scar management, including massage and sun avoidance, will be discussed with the patient; hypertrophic scarring is possible due to intrinsic or extrinsic factors. Decreased sensation to the chest wall and nipple-areola complex is common and usually resolves spontaneously within a few months (Hage & Bloem, 1995). Patients who have undergone the free nipple graft technique initially will have insensate nipples, which may or may not regain some degree of sensation. Management of complications relating to chest surgery is discussed in Table 4.

Hysterectomy and Oophorectomy

This is a routine gynecologic procedure. Complications and risks are no different in the FTM patient than the non-transgender patient.

FTM Genital Reconstruction

Risks associated with FTM genital reconstruction regardless of procedure include infection, post-operative bleeding/hematoma, seroma, and hypertrophic scar formation. Management of complications relating to FTM genital reconstruction is discussed in Table 5.

Laceration of the rectum is an uncommon complication of vaginectomy or vaginal hysterectomy (Hoffman, Lynch, Lockhart, & Knapp, 1999). Urethral fistula or stricture is common following urethral lengthening in either metaidioplasty or phalloplasty (Fang et al., 1999; Khouri & Casoli, 1997; Levine & Elterman, 1998; Monstrey, Hoebeke et al., 2001; Ralph, 1999; Rohrmann & Jakse, 2003; Takata & Meltzer, 2000). Additional risks of phalloplasty include partial or complete flap necrosis, compromised sensation and function of the hand and wrist of the donor arm, dissatisfaction with the size or shape of the neophallus, or dissatisfaction with the aesthetic appearance of donor sites (Benet & Melman, 1999; Chesson et al., 1996; Fang et al., 1999; Greenwald & Stadelmann, 2001; Hage, 1995, 1996; Hage, Bouman, & Bloem, 1993c; Monstrey, Hoebeke, et al., 2001; Takata & Meltzer, 2000). The poor aesthetic result of the donor forearm is one of the disadvantages of the current phalloplasty method (Gottlieb & Levine, 1993; Hage, Bloem, & Suliman, 1993). Implant extrusion, infection, or failure may occur after scrotoplasty or penile prosthetic placement (Gilbert, Jordan, Devine, & Winslow, 1992; Hage 1997; Hage, Bloem, & Bouman, 1993; Hage, Bouman, & Bloem, 1993c; Hage & de Graaf, 1993; Hoebeke et al., 2003; Khouri & Casoli, 1997; Khouri, Young, & Casoli, 1998).

Decreased sensation at all sites is common and usually resolves spontaneously within a few weeks to months. Following phalloplasty the neophallus will be insensate for the first several months, with sensation gradually progressing from base to tip throughout the following year. Decreased sensation in the grafted forearm may be significant, but usually improves over time as small nerves branch into the skin graft; however, sensation will never fully return. Decreased erogenous sensation is a potential risk of metaidoioplasty and phalloplasty (Hage, Bouman, de Graaf et al., 1993), but sexual satisfaction can remain even in the presence of decreased tactile and erogenous sensation, and orgasmic capability is reported by most patients (Fang et al., 1999; Gottlieb & Levine, 1993; Khouri et al., 1998; Lief & Hubschman, 1993).

TABLE 4. Management of Complications Following FTM Chest Surgery

Complication	Signs and symptoms	Treatment
Post-operative bleeding or hematoma	Expanding painful mass on one side of the chest wall, often with increased bloody output in the drain	Evacuation in the operating room.
Infection	Progressive pain and blanching erythema which spreads beyond the incisional margins, combined with fever, malaise and leukocytosis	Small infections can be treated with course of antibiotics. Abscesses often need to be drained in the operating room or under ultrasonic guidance. The surgeon should be consulted for treatment of persistent infections caused by multidrug-resistant organisms.
Seroma	Similar to hematoma, but usually occurs after the drain has been removed	Aspiration may be required by the primary care provider or the surgeon (one or more times).
Wound healing problems	Most often small dehiscences due to stitch rupture or minor infection	If minor, treat with basic wound care, including dressing changes and antibiotic ointment. If incision line is progressively opening such that the wound is gaping, contact the surgeon.
Mastectomy flap necrosis	Usually presents early with non-blanching erythema or mottling of the skin, which progressively becomes darker and non-viable	Treat small necrotic areas with basic wound care, such as dressing changes. For larger areas of flap loss, follow and dress regularly; grafting may be required at a later date.
Nipple necrosis (loss of nipple)	Typically presents early with progressive darkening of the nipple and areola, or absence of capillary refill; if free nipple graft, loss would not be detected until 5 days after surgery when occlusive dressings are taken down by the surgeon	If nipple necrosis occurs in the immediate post-operative period (within hours), attempt to save nipple by loosening dressings or removing stitches; if unsuccessful, surgeon may remove nipple and replace as free graft. If the necrosis is not detected immediately, the non-viable nipple would likely need to be debrided, with future nipple reconstruction using local flaps or tattooing techniques.
Contour abnormalities	Asymmetrical appearance after resolution of post-operative swelling (8-12 weeks)	Major asymmetries may be addressed with revisional liposuction.
Nipple asymmetry	Asymmetrical size or location of nipples after resolution of post-operative swelling (at least 3 months following surgery)	Revisional surgery.
Hypertrophic scarring	Thick, raised, red scars	Discuss prevention measures, including sun avoidance and massage. Severe scarring may require surgical revision.

Partial necrosis of the neophallus occurs occasionally, most often in the early post-operative phase. By the time the patient is discharged home he will have undergone skin grafting, or will be undergoing a wound care regimen appropriate for the circumstance. Complete flap loss is a devastating complication which, fortunately, is a rare ocurrence. Again, vascular compromise of the flap would most likely occur in the early post-operative period. By the time

TABLE 5. Management of Complications Following FTM Genital Reconstruction

Complication	Signs and symptoms	Treatment
Post-operative bleeding or hematoma (all sites)	Usually presents with ongoing bleeding and swelling of the phallus or donor forearm while patient is still in hospital; intra-abdominal (or retro-peritoneal) hematomas also may occur in the early post-operative period	Evacuation in the operating room.
Infection (all sites)	Progressive pain and blanching erythema which spreads beyond the incisional margins, combined with fever, malaise and leukocytosis	Small infections can be treated with course of antibiotics. Abscesses often need to be drained in the operating room or under ultrasonic guidance. The surgeon should be consulted for treatment of persistent infections caused by multidrug-resistant organisms.
Seroma (recipient site)	Surgeon must differentiate a seroma from a urinary fistula	Aspiration by the surgeon.
Wound healing problems (all sites)	Most often small dehiscences due to stitch rupture or minor infection	If minor, treat with basic wound care, including dressing changes and antibiotic ointment. If incision line is progressively opening such that the wound is gaping, contact the surgeon.
Partial or complete flap necrosis (loss of phallus)	Usually presents early with non-blanching erythema or mottling of the skin, which progressively becomes darker and non-viable; unusual after discharge from the hospital	Immediate contact with surgeon is required.
Compromised sensation and/or function of hand and wrist (donor arm)	Compromised hand or wrist function is common after phalloplasty but typically resolves within a few weeks; permanent numbness in the hand or wrist of the donor forearm is rare	Approximately 5% of patients require prolonged physiotherapy to recover fully.
Urethral fistula	Urine flow from location other than urethral opening: occurs in up to 45% of phalloplasties	The surgeon should be notified and the fistula should be monitored and kept clean. Most urethral fistulae are self-resolving. A fistula which does not resolve within 2-3 weeks will likely require revisional surgery by a urologist.
Urethral stricture	Progressive inability to void; may be accompanied by fistulae	Dilation by urologist under local anesthesia. A deep stricture at the junction of the native and neo-urethra may require revision in the operating room.
Implant infection, extrusion, or failure	Increased warmth or drainage from the incisions following implantation, visible extrusion of testicular prostheses or erectile prosthesis, inflammation or change in size or shape	Surgical removal with later replacement.

TABLE 5 (continued)

Complication	Signs and symptoms	Treatment
Mechanical failure of hydraulic erectile prosthesis	Erectile dysfunction	Mechanical repair, or surgical removal with later replacement
Hypertrophic scarring (all sites)	Thick, raised, red scars	Severe scarring may require surgical revision

the patient is discharged home the risk of total flap failure is quite low.

Revisional Surgery

Performing an aesthetically pleasing subcutaneous mastectomy in the biological female who desires a male chest can be a challenging operation. It differs from mastectomy for breast disease or as a prophylactic measure, since the goals are very different: The aim of chest surgery in the FTM is not just to remove all of the breast tissue, but also to recontour the chest to create a masculine appearance (Gilbert & Gilbert, n.d.). The procedure is also usually more difficult than a gynecomastia correction since the FTM transsexual often has considerably more breast volume and a greater degree of ptosis to contend with. Moreover, the common practice of "breast binding" severely impacts the quality of breast skin (Hage & van Kesteren, 1995), which is a major factor in choosing the correct surgical procedure. As such, subcutaneous mastectomy in the FTM patient has a fairly high rate of revisional surgery associated with it; revisions are needed by 33-45% of patients (Selvaggi et al., 2005). Patients with larger breasts or poor skin quality have a higher chance of requiring revisional surgery. Typical chest surgery revisions include, but are not limited to (a) liposuction to improve contour abnormalities, (b) scar revisions, (c) excision of skin excess, wrinkling or puckering, and (d) adjustment of nipple-areola complex position or size (Colic & Colic, 2000).

Revisional surgery after phalloplasty is less common as an isolated procedure. However, since many patients choose to have testicular implants and/or erectile prostheses placed later, it is simple to perform minor revisions, such as revision of the coronal rim, at the same time.

Revisions may also be necessary to correct urinary dysfunction, a common complication of urethral lengthening.

CONCLUSION

The primary care provider plays an important role in preparation of the patient for surgery and in evaluation following discharge from hospital. While minor complications after routine procedures can typically be managed by the trans-experienced primary care provider, due to the unique and complex nature of SRS, consultation with the original surgeon is advised whenever there are concerns about care.

REFERENCES

Anderson, B. O. (2001). Prophylactic surgery to reduce breast cancer risk: A brief literature review. *The Breast Journal, 7,* 321-330.

Becking, A. G., Tuinzing, D. B., Hage, J. J., & Gooren, L. J. G. (1996). Facial corrections in male to female transsexuals: A preliminary report on 16 patients. *Journal of Oral and Maxillofacial Surgery, 54,* 413-418.

Benet, A. E. & Melman, A. (1999). Gender dysphoria and creation of the neo-phallus. In W. J. G. Hellstrom (Ed.), *Handbook of Sexual Dysfunction* (pp. 102-105). Lawrence, KS: American Society of Andrology.

Bockting, W. O., Knudson, G., & Goldberg, J. M. (2006). Counseling and mental health care for transgender adults and loved ones. *International Journal of Transgenderism, 9*(3/4).

Borgen, P. I., Hill, A. D., Tran, K. N., Van Zee, K. J., Massie, M. J., Payne, D., & Biggs, C. G. (1998). Patient regrets after bilateral prophylactic mastectomy. *Annals of Surgical Oncology, 5,* 603-606.

Brown, M., Perry, A., Cheesman, A. D., & Pring, T. (2000). Pitch change in male-to-female transsexuals: has phonosurgery a role to play? *International Journal of Language and Communication Disorders, 35,* 129-136.

Chang, T. S., & Hwang, W. Y. (1986). Forearm flap in one-stage reconstruction of the penis. *Plastic and Reconstructive Surgery, 74,* 251-258.

Chastre, J., Basset, F., Viau, F., Dournovo, P., Bouchama, A., Akesbi, A., & Gilbert, C. (1983). Acute pneumonitis after subcutaneous injections of silicone in transsexual men. *New England Journal of Medicine, 308,* 764-767.

Chesson, R. R., Gilbert, D. A., Jordan, G. H., Schlossberg, S. M., Ramsey, G. T., & Gilbert, D. M. (1996). The role of colpocleisis with urethral lengthening in transsexual phalloplasty. *American Journal of Obstetrics and Gynecology, 175,* 1443-1449.

Clark, J. A., Wray, N. P., & Ashton, C. M. (2001). Living with treatment decisions: Regrets and quality of life among men treated for metastatic prostate cancer. *Journal of Clinical Oncology, 19,* 72-80.

Cohen-Kettenis, P. T., & Van Goozen, S. H. M. (1997). Sex reassignment of adolescent transsexuals: A follow-up study. *Journal of the American Academy of Child and Adolescent Psychiatry, 36,* 263-271.

Colic, M. M., & Colic, M. M. (2000). Circumareolar mastectomy in female-to-male transsexuals and large gynecomastias: A personal approach. *Aesthetic Plastic Surgery, 24,* 450-454.

Conrad, K., & Yoskovitch, A. (2003). Endoscopically facilitated reduction laryngochondroplasty. *Archives of Facial Plastic Surgery, 5,* 345-348.

Coon, S. K., Burris, R., Coleman, E. A., & Lemon, S. J. (2002). An analysis of telephone interview data collected in 1992 from 820 women who reported problems with their breast implants to the Food and Drug Administration. *Plastic and Reconstructive Surgery, 109,* 2043-2051.

Coulaud, J. M., Labrousse, J., Carli, P., Galliot, M., Vilde, F., & Lissac, J. (1983). Adult respiratory distress syndrome and silicone injection. *Toxicological European Research/Recherche Européenne en Toxicologie, 5,* 171-174.

Crichton, D. (1993). Gender reassignment surgery for male primary transsexuals. *South African Medical Journal, 83,* 347-349.

Dahl, M., Feldman, J., Goldberg, J. M., & Jaberi, A. (2006). Physical aspects of transgender endocrine therapy. *International Journal of Transgenderism, 9*(3/4), 111-134.

Davies, S., & Goldberg, J. M. (2006). Clinical aspects of transgender speech feminization and masculinization. *International Journal of Transgenderism, 9*(3/4), 167-196.

Donald, P. J. (1982). Voice change surgery in the transsexual. *Head and Neck Surgery, 4,* 433-437.

Duong, T., Schonfeld, A. J., Yungbluth, M., & Slotten, R. (1998). Acute pneumopathy in a nonsurgical transsexual. *Chest, 113,* 1127-1129.

Eiser, C., Darlington, A.-S. E., Stride, C. B., & Grimer, R. (2001). Quality of life implications as a consequence of surgery: Limb salvage, primary and secondary amputation. *Sarcoma, 5,* 189-195.

Eldh, J. (1993). Construction of a neovagina with preservation of the glans penis as a clitoris in male transsexuals. *Plastic and Reconstructive Surgery, 91,* 895-900.

Elit, L., Esplen, M. J., Butler, K., & Narod, S. (2001). Quality of life and psychosexual adjustment after prophylactic oophorectomy for a family history of ovarian cancer. *Familial Cancer, 1,* 149-156.

Ergeneli, M. H., Duran, E. H., Ozcan, G., & Erdogan, M. (1999). Vaginectomy and laparoscopically assisted vaginal hysterectomy as adjunctive surgery for female-to-male transsexual reassignment: Preliminary report. *European Journal of Obstetrics, Gynecology, and Reproductive Biology, 87,* 35-37.

Fang, R. H., Kao, Y. S., Ma, S., & Lin, J. T. (1999). Phalloplasty in female-to-male transsexuals using free radial osteocutaneous flap: A series of 22 cases. *British Journal of Plastic Surgery, 52,* 217-222.

Farina, L. A., Palacio, V., Salles, M., Fernandez-Villanueva, D., Vidal, B., & Menendez, P. (1997). Scrotal granuloma caused by oil migrating from the hip in 2 transsexual males (scrotal sclerosing lipogranuloma). *Archivos Espanoles de Urologia, 50,* 51-53.

Feldman, J., & Goldberg, J. M. (2006). Transgender primary medical care. *International Journal of Transgenderism, 9*(3/4), 3-34.

Fox, L. P., Geyer, A. S., Husain, S., la-Latta, P., & Grossman, M. E. (2004). Mycobacterium abscessus cellulitis and multifocal abscesses of the breasts in a transsexual from illicit intramammary injections of silicone. *Journal of the American Academy of Dermatology, 50,* 450-454.

Gaber, Y. (2004). Secondary lymphoedema of the lower leg as an unusual side-effect of a liquid silicone injection in the hips and buttocks. *Dermatology, 208,* 342-344.

Gerli, S., Rossetti, D., Pacifici, A., Aviles, E., Dominici, C., Mattei, A., & Di Renzo, G. C. (2001). Hysterectomy for the transsexual. *Journal of the American Association of Gynecologic Laparoscopists, 8,* 613-614.

Gilbert, D. A., & Gilbert, D. M. (n.d.). Chest contouring in the female transgender patient. Unpublished manuscript.

Gilbert, D. A., Gilbert, D. M., Jordan, G. H., Schlossberg, S. M., & Chesson, R. R. (1998). Ulnar forearm free flap for phallic construction in transsexuals. In R. M. Ehrlich, G. J. Alter, & R. Zorab (Eds.), *Reconstructive and plastic surgery of the external genitalia: Adult and pediatric* (pp. 319-326). Philadelphia, PA: Saunders.

Gilbert, D. A., Jordan, G. H., Devine, C. J., Jr., & Winslow, B. H. (1992). Microsurgical forearm "cricket bat-transformer" phalloplasty. *Plastic and Reconstructive Surgery, 90,* 711-716.

Gilbert, D. A., Schlossberg, S. M., & Jordan, G. H. (1995). Ulnar forearm phallic construction and penile reconstruction. *Microsurgery, 16,* 314-321.

Giraldo, F., Esteva, I., Bergero, T., Cano, G., Gonzalez, C., Salinas, P., Rivada, E., Lara, J. S., & Soriguer, F. (2004). Corona glans clitoroplasty and urethropreputial vestibuloplasty in male-to-female transsexuals: The vulval aesthetic refinement by the Andalusia Gender Team. *Plastic and Reconstructive Surgery, 114*, 1543-1550.

Gottlieb, L. J., & Levine, L. A. (1993). A new design for the radial forearm free-flap phallic construction. *Plastic and Reconstructive Surgery, 92*, 276-283.

Greenwald, D., & Stadelmann, W. (2001). Gender reassignment. *eMedicine Journal, 2*. Retrieved January 1, 2005, from http://www.emedicine.com/plastic/topic434.htm.

Hage, J. J. (1992). *From peniplastica totalis to reassignment surgery of the external genitalia in female-to-male transsexuals.* Amsterdam: Vrije University Press.

Hage, J. J. (1995). Medical requirements and consequences of sex reassignment surgery. *Medicine, Science and the Law, 35*, 17-24.

Hage, J. J. (1996). Metaidoioplasty: An alternative phalloplasty technique in transsexuals. *Plastic and Reconstructive Surgery, 97*, 161-167.

Hage, J. J. (1997). Dynaflex prosthesis in total phalloplasty. *Plastic and Reconstructive Surgery, 99*, 479-485.

Hage, J. J. (1999). Surgical formation of the glans in phalloplasty. In R. M. Ehrlich, G. J. Alter, & R. Zorab (Eds.), *Reconstructive and plastic surgery of the external genitalia: Adult and pediatric* (pp. 361-364). Philadelphia, PA: Saunders.

Hage, J. J., & Bloem, J. J. A. M. (1995). Chest wall contouring for female-to-male transsexuals: Amsterdam experience. *Annals of Plastic Surgery, 34*, 59-66.

Hage, J. J., Bloem, J. J. A. M., & Bouman, F. G. (1993). Obtaining rigidity in the neophallus of female-to-male transsexuals: A review of the literature. *Annals of Plastic Surgery, 30*, 327-333.

Hage, J. J., Bloem, J. J. A. M., & Suliman, H. M. (1993). Review of the literature on techniques for phalloplasty with emphasis on the applicability in female-to-male transsexuals. *Journal of Urology, 150*, 1093-1098.

Hage, J. J., Bouman, F. G., & Bloem, J. J. A. M. (1993a). Construction of the fixed part of the neourethra in female-to-male transsexuals: Experience in 53 patients. *Plastic and Reconstructive Surgery, 91*, 904-910.

Hage, J. J., Bouman, F. G., & Bloem, J. J. A. M. (1993b). Preconstruction of the pars pendulans urethrae for phalloplasty in female-to-male transsexuals. *Plastic and Reconstructive Surgery, 91*, 1303-1307.

Hage, J. J., Bouman, F. G., & Bloem, J. J. A. M. (1993c). Constructing a scrotum in female-to-male transsexuals. *Plastic and Reconstructive Surgery, 91*, 914-921.

Hage, J. J., Bouman, F. G., de Graaf, F. H., & Bloem, J. J. A. M. (1993). Construction of the neophallus in female-to-male transsexuals: The Amsterdam experience. *Journal of Urology, 149*, 1463-1468.

Hage, J. J., Bout, C. A., Bloem, J. J. A. M., & Megens, J. A. (1993). Phalloplasty in female-to-male transsexu-als: What do our patients ask for? *Annals of Plastic Surgery, 30*, 323-326.

Hage, J. J., & de Graaf, F. H. (1993). Addressing the ideal requirements by free flap phalloplasty: Some reflections on refinements of technique. *Microsurgery, 14*, 592-598.

Hage, J. J., de Graaf, F. H., Bouman, F. G., & Bloem, J. J. A. M. (1993). Sculpturing the glans in phalloplasty. *Plastic and Reconstructive Surgery, 92*, 157-161.

Hage, J. J., Torenbeek, R., Bouman, F. G., & Bloem, J. J. A. M. (1993). The anatomic basis of the anterior vaginal flap used for neourethra construction in female-to-male transsexuals. *Plastic and Reconstructive Surgery, 92*, 102-108.

Hage, J. J., & van Kesteren, P. J. (1995). Chest-wall contouring in female-to-male transsexuals: Basic considerations and review of the literature. *Plastic and Reconstructive Surgery, 96*, 386-391.

Hage, J. J., Vossen, M., & Becking, A. G. (1997). Rhinoplasty as part of gender-confirming surgery in male transsexuals: basic considerations and clinical experience. *Annals of Plastic Surgery, 39*, 266-271.

Hage, J. J., Winters, H. A. H., & Van Lieshout, J. (1996). Fibula free flap phalloplasty: Modifications and recommendations. *Microsurgery, 17*, 358-365.

Harcourt, D., & Rumsey, N. (2001). Psychological aspects of breast reconstruction: A review of the literature. *Journal of Advanced Nursing, 35*, 477-487.

Herzog, M. E., & Santucci, R. A. (2002). Incisionless in-office castration using a veterinary castration device (Burdizzo clamp). *Urology, 59*, 946.

Hoebeke, P., De Cuypere, G., Ceulemans, P., & Monstrey, S. (2003). Obtaining rigidity in total phalloplasty: experience with 35 patients. *Journal of Urology, 169*, 221-223.

Hoffman, M. S., Lynch, C., Lockhart, J., & Knapp, R. (1999). Injury of the rectum during vaginal surgery. *American Journal of Obstetrics and Gynecology, 181*, 274-277.

Israel, G. E., & Tarver, D. E. I., II. (1997). *Transgender care: Recommended guidelines, practical information, and personal accounts.* Philadephia, PA: Temple University Press.

Isshiki, N., Taira, T., & Tanabe, M. (1983). Surgical alteration of the vocal pitch. *Journal of Otolaryngology, 12*, 335-340.

Jamieson, D. J., Kaufman, S. C., Costello, C., Hillis, S. D., Marchbanks, P. A., & Peterson, H. B. (2002). A comparison of women's regret after vasectomy versus tubal sterilization. *Obstetrics & Gynecology, 99*, 1073-1079.

Jordan, G. H. (2002). Total phallic construction, option to gender reassignment. *Advances in Experimental Medicine and Biology, 511*, 275-280.

Kanhai, R. C. J., Hage, J. J., Asscheman, H., & Mulder, J. W. (1999). Augmentation mammaplasty in male-to-female transsexuals. *Plastic and Reconstructive Surgery, 104*, 542-549.

Karim, R. B., Hage, J. J., & Mulder, J. W. (1996). Neovaginoplasty in male transsexuals: Review of surgical techniques and recommendations regarding eligibility. *Annals of Plastic Surgery, 37,* 669-675.

Khouri, R. K., & Casoli, V. M. (1997). Reconstruction of the penis. In S. J. Aston, R. W. Beasley, & C. H. M. Thorne (Eds.), *Grubb and Smith's Plastic Surgery* (5th ed., pp. 1111-1119). Philadelphia, PA: Lippincott-Raven Publishers.

Khouri, R. K., Young, V. L., & Casoli, V. M. (1998). Long-term results of total penile reconstruction with a prefabricated lateral arm free flap. *Journal of Urology, 160,* 383-388.

Kim, S. K., Park, H. H., Lee, K. C., Park, J. M., Kim, J. T., & Kim, M. C. (2003). Long-term results in patients after rectosigmoid vaginoplasty. *Plastic and Reconstructive Surgery, 112,* 143-151.

Kirk, S. (1999). Guidelines for selecting HIV positive patients for genital reconstructive surgery. *International Journal of Transgenderism, 3*(1 + 2). Retrieved January 1, 2005, from http://www.symposion.com/ijt/hiv_risk/kirk.htm.

Krege, S., Bex, A., Lummen, G., & Rubben, H. (2001). Male-to-female transsexualism: A technique, results and long-term follow-up in 66 patients. *BJU International, 88,* 396-402.

Kuiper, A. J., & Cohen-Kettenis, P. T. (1998). Gender role reversal among postoperative transsexuals. *International Journal of Transgenderism, 2*(3). Retrieved January 1, 2005, from http://www.symposion.com/ijt/ijtc0502.htm.

Kunachak, S., Prakunhungsit, S., & Sujjalak, K. (2000). Thyroid cartilage and vocal fold reduction: a new phonosurgical method for male-to-female transsexuals. *Annals of Otology, Rhinology and Laryngology, 109,* 1082-1086.

Landen, M., Walinder, J., Hambert, G., & Lundstrom, B. (1998). Factors predictive of regret in sex reassignment. *Acta Psychiatrica Scandinavica, 97,* 284-289.

Lantz, P. M., Janz, N. K., Fagerlin, A., Schwartz, K., Liu, L., Lakhani, I., Salem, B., & Katz, S. J. (2005). Satisfaction with surgery outcomes and the decision process in a population-based sample of women with breast cancer. *Health Services Research, 40,* 745-767.

Laub, D. R., Laub, D. R., II., & Biber, S. (1988). Vaginoplasty for gender confirmation. *Clinics in Plastic Surgery, 15,* 463-470.

Lawrence, A. A. (2003). Factors associated with satisfaction or regret following male-to-female sex reassignment surgery. *Archives of Sexual Behavior, 32,* 299-315.

Lawrence, A. A. (2005). Sexuality before and after male-to-female sex reassignment surgery. *Archives of Sexual Behavior, 34,* 147-166.

Lenaghan, R., Wilson, N., Lucas, C. E., & Ledgerwood, A. M. (1997). The role of rectosigmoid neocolporrhaphy. *Surgery, 122,* 856-860.

Leslie, K., Buscombe, J., & Davenport, A. (2000). Implant infection in a transsexual with renal failure. *Nephrology Dialysis Transplantation, 15,* 436-437.

Levine, L. A., & Elterman, L. (1998). Urethroplasty following total phallic reconstruction. *Journal of Urology, 160,* 378-382.

Lief, H. I. & Hubschman, L. (1993). Orgasm in the postoperative transsexual. *Archives of Sexual Behavior, 22,* 145-155.

Liguori, G., Trombetta, C., Buttazzi, L., & Belgrano, E. (2001). Acute peritonitis due to introital stenosis and perforation of a bowel neovagina in a transsexual. *Obstetrics and Gynecology, 97,* 828-829.

Maas, S. M., Eijsbouts, Q. A., Hage, J. J., & Cuesta, M. A. (1999). Laparoscopic rectosigmoid colpopoiesis: Does it benefit our transsexual patients? *Plastic and Reconstructive Surgery, 103,* 518-524.

Mate-Kole, C., Freschi, M., & Robin, A. (1990). A controlled study of psychological and social changes after surgical gender reassignment in selected male transsexuals. *British Journal of Psychiatry, 157,* 261-264.

Meltzer, T. R. (2001). *Aesthetic refinements to the secondary labioplasty.* Paper presented at the 17th Biennial Symposium of the Harry Benjamin Gender Dysphoria Association, Galveston, TX.

Meyer, W. J., III, Bockting, W. O., Cohen-Kettenis, P. T., Coleman, E., Di Ceglie, D., Devor, H., Gooren, L., Hage, J. J., Kirk, S., Kuiper, B., Laub, D., Lawrence, A., Menard, Y., Monstrey, S., Patton, J., Schaefer, L., Webb, A., & Wheeler, C. C. (2001). *The standards of care for Gender Identity Disorders* (6th ed.). Minneapolis, MN: Harry Benjamin International Gender Dysphoria Association.

Michel, A., Ansseau, M., Legros, J. J., Pitchot, W., & Mormont, C. (2002). The transsexual: What about the future? *European Psychiatry, 17,* 353-362.

Miller, W. B., Shain, R. N., & Pasta, D. J. (1991). The pre- and poststerilization predictors of poststerilization regret in husbands and wives. *Journal of Nervous and Mental Disease, 179,* 602-608.

Monstrey, S., Hoebeke, P., Dhont, M., De Cuypere, G., Rubens, R., Moerman, M., Hamdi, M., Van Landuyt, K., & Blondeel, P. (2001). Surgical therapy in transsexual patients: A multi-disciplinary approach. *Acta Chirurgica Belgica, 101,* 200-209.

Monstrey, S., Selvaggi, G., Van Landuyt, K., Blondeel, P., Hamdi, M., & Hoebeke, P. (2001). *Subcutaneous mastectomy in female-to-male transsexuals.* Paper presented at the 17th Biennial Symposium of the Harry Benjamin Gender Dysphoria Association, Galveston, TX.

Montgomery, L. L., Tran, K. N., Heelan, M. C., Van Zee, K. J., Massie, M. J., Payne, D. K. et al. (1999). Issues of regret in women with contralateral prophylactic mastectomies. *Annals of Surgical Oncology, 6,* 546-552.

Mulcahy, J. J. (2003). Use of penile implants in the constructed neophallus. *International Journal of Impotence Research, 15*, S129-S131.

Mutaf, M. (2000). A new surgical procedure for phallic reconstruction: Istanbul flap. *Plastic and Reconstructive Surgery, 105*, 1361-1370.

Neumann, K., Welzel, C., Gonnermann, U., & Wolfradt, U. (2002a). Cricothyroidopexy in male-to-female transsexuals: Modification Type IV. *International Journal of Transgenderism, 6*(3). Retrieved January 1, 2005, from http://www.symposion.com/ijt/ijtvo06no03_03.htm

Neumann, K., Welzel, C., Gonnermann, U., & Wolfradt, U. (2002b). Satisfaction of MtF transsexuals with operative voice therapy: A questionnaire-based preliminary study. *International Journal of Transgenderism, 6*(4). Retrieved January 1, 2005, from http://www.symposion.com/ijt/ ijtvo06no04_02.htm

Oates, J. M., & Dacakis, G. (1997). Voice change in transsexuals. *Venereology: Interdisciplinary, International Journal of Sexual Health, 10*, 178-187.

Ousterhout, D. K. (1987). Feminization of the forehead: contour changing to improve female aesthetics. *Plastic and Reconstructive Surgery, 79*, 701-713.

Ousterhout, D. K. (1997). Facial surgery for the transsexual. In G. E. Israel & D. E. I. Tarver, II. (Eds.), *Transgender care: Recommended guidelines, practical information and personal accounts* (pp. 225-228). Philadelphia, PA: Temple University Press.

Ousterhout, D. K. (2003). *Feminization of the transsexual (except for SRS)*. San Francisco: Author.

Payne, D. K., Biggs, C., Tran, K. N., Borgen, P. I., & Massie, M. J. (2000). Women's regrets after bilateral prophylactic mastectomy. *Annals of Surgical Oncology, 7*, 150-154.

Perovic, S. V., & Djordjevic, M. L. (2003). Metoidioplasty: A variant of phalloplasty in female transsexuals. *BJU International, 92*, 981-985.

Perovic, S. V., Stanojevic, D. S., & Djordjevic, M. L. (2000). Vaginoplasty in male transsexuals using penile skin and a urethral flap. *BJU International, 86*, 843-850.

Pfäfflin, F. (1992). Regrets after sex reassignment surgery. In W. O. Bockting & E. Coleman (Eds.), *Gender dysphoria: Interdisciplinary approaches in clinical management* (pp. 69-85). Binghamton, NY: The Haworth Press, Inc.

Pfäfflin, F., & Junge, A. (1998). *Sex reassignment - Thirty years of international follow-up studies; SRS: A comprehensive review, 1961-1991* (R. B. Jacobson & A. B. Meier, Trans.). Düsseldorf, Germany: Symposion Publishing. (Original work published 1992.)

Rakic, Z., Starcevic, V., Maric, J., & Kelin, K. (1996). The outcome of sex reassignment surgery in Belgrade: 32 patients of both sexes. *Archives of Sexual Behavior, 25*, 515-525.

Ralph, D. J. (1999). Urethral complications in phalloplasty. *Boys' Own-UK, 30*, 16-18. Retrieved January 1, 2005, from http://www.transgenderzone.com/library/pr/fulltext/32.htm.

Ratnam, S. S., & Lim, S. M. (1982). Augmentation mammoplasty for the male transsexual. *Singapore Medical Journal, 23*, 107-109.

Rehman, J., Lazer, S., Benet, A. E., Schaefer, L. C., & Melman, A. (1999). The reported sex and surgery satisfactions of 28 postoperative male-to-female transsexual patients. *Archives of Sexual Behavior, 28*, 71-89.

Rehman, J., & Melman, A. (1999). Formation of neoclitoris from glans penis by reduction glansplasty with preservation of neurovascular bundle in male-to-female gender surgery: Functional and cosmetic outcome. *Journal of Urology, 161*, 200-206.

Reid, R. W. (1996). *Orchidectomy as a first stage towards gender reassignment: A positive option*. Paper presented at Gendys '96: The Fourth International Gender Dysphoria Conference, Manchester, England.

Roberts, C. S., Wells, K. E., & Walden, K. (1999). Toward understanding women who request removal of silicone breast implants. *Breast Journal, 5*, 246.

Rohrmann, D., & Jakse, G. (2003). Urethroplasty in female-to-male transsexuals. *European Urology, 44*, 611-614.

Rosenfeld, B. L., Taskin, O., Kafkashli, A., Rosenfeld, M. L., & Chuong, C. J. (1998). Sequelae of postpartum sterilization. *Archives of Gynecology and Obstetrics, 261*, 183-187.

Rubin, S. O. (1993). Sex-reassignment surgery male-to-female: Review, own results and report of a new technique using the glans penis as a pseudoclitoris. *Scandinavian Journal of Urology and Nephrology Supplementum, 154*, 1-28.

Rubinstein, L. M., Benjamin, L., & Kleinkopf, V. (1979). Menstrual patterns and women's attitudes following sterilization by Falope rings. *Fertility and Sterility, 31*, 641-646.

Santanelli, F., & Scuderi, N. (2000). Neophalloplasty in female-to-male transsexuals with the island tensor fasciae latae flap. *Plastic and Reconstructive Surgery, 105*, 1990-1996.

Saridogan, E., & Cutner, A. (2004). The use of McCartney tube during total laparoscopic hysterectomy for gender reassignment: A report of two cases. *BJOG: an International Journal of Obstetrics and Gynecology, 111*, 277-278.

Schmid, A., Tzur, A., Leshko, L., & Krieger, B. P. (2005). Silicone embolism syndrome: A case report, review of the literature, and comparison with fat embolism syndrome. *Chest, 127*, 2276-2281.

Schrang, E. A. (1997). Genital reassignment surgery: A source of happiness for my patients. In G. E. Israel & D. E. I. Tarver, II. (Eds.), *Transgender care: Recommended guidelines, practical information and personal accounts* (pp. 236-240). Philadelphia, PA: Temple University Press.

Selvaggi, G., Ceulemans, P., De Cuypere, G., Van Landuyt, K., Blondeel, P., Hamdi, M., Bowman, C.,

& Monstrey, S. (2005). *Subcutaneous mastectomy in the FTM transsexual: An algorithm for choosing the best technique.* Manuscript submitted for publication.

Sengezer, M., & Sadove, R. C. (1993). Scrotal construction by expansion of labia majora in biological female transsexuals. *Annals of Plastic Surgery, 31,* 372-376.

Simpson, A. J., & Goldberg, J. M. (2006a). *Surgery: A guide for FTMs.* Vancouver, BC: Vancouver Coastal Health Authority. Available online at http://www.vch.ca/transhealth/resources/library/tcpdocs/consumer/surgery-FTM.pdf

Simpson, A. J., & Goldberg, J. M. (2006b). *Surgery: A guide for MTFs.* Vancouver, BC: Vancouver Coastal Health Authority. Available online at http://www.vch.ca/transhealth/resources/library/tcpdocs/consumer/surgery-MTF.pdf

Smith, Y. L. S., Van Goozen, S. H. M., Kuiper, A. J., & Cohen-Kettenis, P. T. (2005). Sex reassignment: Outcomes and predictors of treatment for adolescent and adult transsexuals. *Psychological Medicine, 35,* 89-99.

Takata, L. L., & Meltzer, T. R. (2000). Procedures, postoperative care, and potential complications of gender reassignment surgery for the primary care physician. *Primary Psychiatry, 7,* 74-78.

Taucher, S., Gnant, M., & Jakesz, R. (2003). Preventive mastectomy in patients at breast cancer risk due to genetic alterations in the BRCA1 and BRCA2 gene. *Langenbecks Archives of Surgery, 388,* 3-8.

Tiewtranon, P., Chokerungvaranon, P., Jindarak, S., & Wannachamras, S. (2001). *Sensate pedicled neoclitoris in the neovaginoplasty for 250 male transsexuals.* Paper presented at the 17th Biennial Symposium of the Harry Benjamin Gender Dysphoria Association, Galveston, TX.

Tweed, A. (2003). *Health care utilization among women who have undergone breast implant surgery.* Vancouver, BC: British Columbia Centre of Excellence in Women's Health.

Vemer, H. M., Colla, P., Schoot, B. C., Willemsen, W. N., Bierkens, P. B., & Rolland, R. (1986). Regret after sterilization in women. *Nederlands Tijdschrift voor Geneeskunde, 130,* 410-413.

Veselý, J., Kucera, J., Hrbaty, J., Stupka, I., & Rezai, A. (1999). Our standard method of reconstruction of the penis and urethra in female to male transsexuals. *Acta Chirurgiae Plasticae, 41,* 39-42.

Victorzon, M., & Tolonen, P. (2001). Bariatric Analysis and Reporting Outcome System (BAROS) following laparoscopic adjustable gastric banding in Finland. *Obesity Surgery, 11,* 740-743.

Wagner, I., Fugain, C., Monneron-Girard, L., Cordier, B., & Chabolle, F. (2003). Pitch-raising surgery in fourteen male-to-female transsexuals. *Laryngoscope, 113,* 1157-1165.

Wilson, N. (2002). The aesthetic vulva: Perineal cosmesis in the male-to-female transsexual. *International Journal of Transgenderism, 6*(4). Retrieved January 1, 2005, from http://www.symposion.com/ijt/ijtvo06no04_01.htm

Wheeler, T. L., II., Richter, H. E., Varner, R. E., Burgio, K. L., Redden, D. T., Goode, P. S., & Chen, C. G. (2005). *Regret, satisfaction and symptom improvement: Analysis of the impact of colpocleisis for the management of severe pelvic organ prolapse.* Poster presented at the 31st Annual Scientific Meeting of the Society of Gynecologic Surgeons, Rancho Mirage, CA.

Wolfort, F. G., Dejerine, E. S., Ramos, D. J., & Parry, R. G. (1990). Chondrolaryngoplasty for appearance. *Plastic and Reconstructive Surgery, 86,* 464-469.

Yang, C. Y., Palmer, A. D., Murray, K. D., Meltzer, T. R., & Cohen, J. I. (2002). Cricothyroid approximation to elevate vocal pitch in male-to-female transsexuals: Results of surgery. *Annals of Otology, Rhinology and Laryngology, 111,* 477-485.

doi:10.1300/J485v09n03_07

Clinical Aspects of Transgender Speech Feminization and Masculinization

Shelagh Davies, MSc, RSLP-C
Joshua M. Goldberg

SUMMARY. Societal norms of speech, voice, and non-verbal communication are often strongly gendered. For transgender individuals who experience a mismatch between existing communication behaviours and felt sense of self, changes to the gendered aspects of communication can help reduce gender dysphoria, improving mental health and quality of life. While peer resources are often beneficial in changing overall appearance and presentation, speech and voice modification is best facilitated by a trans-competent speech professional. In this article we review clinical research relating to transgender speech and voice change and discuss clinical protocols for trans-specific assessment, treatment, and outcome evaluation. doi:10.1300/J485v09n03_08 *[Article copies available for a fee from The Haworth Document Delivery Service: 1-800-HAWORTH. E-mail address: <docdelivery@haworthpress.com> Website: <http://www.HaworthPress.com> © 2006 by The Haworth Press, Inc. All rights reserved.]*

KEYWORDS. Transgender, speech, voice, gender transition, gender dysphoria

Transgender individuals may require assistance to feminize or masculinize speech, voice, and non-verbal communication. Changes to the gendered aspects of communication can help reduce gender dysphoria and facilitate gender presentation that is consistent with the felt sense of self, resulting in improved mental health and quality of life. With all parameters of communication, the goal is to allow the outside–speech, voice, and movement–to reflect what the client feels inside. While peer support resources can be highly beneficial in changing overall appearance and presentation, speech and voice modification is best facilitated by a

Shelagh Davies, MSc, is a Registered Speech-Language Pathologist (Canada), Speech/Voice Consultant of the Transgender Health Program and Clinical Instructor in School of Speech and Audiological Sciences, University of British Columbia, Vancouver, BC, Canada. Joshua M. Goldberg is Education Consultant of the Transgender Health Program, Vancouver, BC, Canada.

Address correspondence to: Shelagh Davies, c/o Transgender Health Program, 301-1290 Hornby Street, Vancouver, BC, Canada V6Z 1W2 (E-mail: sd@shelaghdavies.com).

This manuscript was created for the Trans Care Project, a joint initiative of Transcend Transgender Support & Education Society and Vancouver Coastal Health's Transgender Health Program, with funding from the Canadian Rainbow Health Coalition. The authors thank Fionna Bayley, Katharine Blaker, Georgia Dacakis, and Murray Morrison for their comments on an earlier draft, and Donna Lindenberg, Olivia Ashbee, A. J. Simpson, and Rodney Hunt for research assistance.

[Haworth co-indexing entry note]: "Clinical Aspects of Transgender Speech Feminization and Masculinizatione." Davies, Shelagh, and Joshua M. Goldberg. Co-published simultaneously in *International Journal of Transgenderism* (The Haworth Medical Press, an imprint of The Haworth Press, Inc.) Vol. 9, No. 3/4, 2006, pp. 167-196; and: *Guidelines for Transgender Care* (ed: Walter O. Bockting, and Joshua M. Goldberg) The Haworth Medical Press, an imprint of The Haworth Press, Inc., 2006, pp. 167-196. Single or multiple copies of this article are available for a fee from The Haworth Document Delivery Service [1-800-HAWORTH, 9:00 a.m. - 5:00 p.m. (EST). E-mail address: docdelivery@haworthpress.com].

doi:10.1300/J485v09n03_08

trans-competent speech professional who can provide a comprehensive evaluation, design an effective treatment program, and help prevent vocal problems that may arise from changes to habitual fundamental frequency or voice quality.

As with other transgender care, we recommend that speech services be offered in the context of a complete approach to transgender health that includes comprehensive primary care and a coordinated approach to psychological and social issues. Speech services must be individualized based on the individual's goals, the risks and benefits of treatment options, and consideration of social and economic issues.

THE IMPORTANCE OF SPEECH AND VOICE SERVICES IN TRANSGENDER CARE

Although studies assessing transgender speech needs have thus far involved only small numbers of participants, the results suggest that congruency of speech and gender identity is important to transgender individuals in both the male-to-female (MTF) and female-to-male (FTM) continuum.[1] For example, in a survey of a broad range of transgender individuals (N = 179)–including crossdressers and others who did not identify as transsexual–23% of respondents reported a current need for speech therapy (Goldberg, Matte, MacMillan, & Hudspith, 2003). In studies of MTF transsexuals, feminization of communication was rated extremely important by 73% of 11 participants in one study (Wollitzer, 1994), and as "very important" by over half of 28 respondents in another study (Neumann, Welzel, Gonnermann, & Wolfradt, 2002b). A study of FTM transsexuals reported that 88% of 16 participants considered masculinization of communication as important or more important than sex reassignment surgery (Van Borsel, De Cuypere, Rubens, & Destaerke, 2000).

In speech, voice, and transgender health literature, speech feminization is widely recognized as an important element of transgender care for MTFs (Andrews, 1999; Becklund-Freidenberg, 2002; Byrne, Dacakis, & Douglas, 2003; Dacakis, 2002; de Bruin, Coerts, & Greven, 2000; Gold, 1999; Hooper, 1985; King, Lindstedt,

Jensen, & Law, 1999; Neumann & Welzel, 2004; Neumann, Welzel, Gonnermann, & Wolfradt, 2002a; Oates & Dacakis, 1983, 1997; Pausewang-Gelfer & Schofield, 2000; Van Borsel, De Cuypere, & Van den Berghe, 2001; Wiltshire, 1995; Wollitzer, 1994). Speech masculinization for FTMs has not been as well studied (Oates & Dacakis, 1997; Soderpalm, Larsson, & Almquist, 2004; Van Borsel et al., 2000). Generally, the literature surveyed stated that testosterone therapy always results in drop in pitch sufficient to allow FTMs to live as men (Andrews, 1999; de Bruin et al., 2000; Gold, 1999; King et al., 1999; Oates & Dacakis, 1997; Petty, 2004; Soderpalm et al., 2004; Yang, Palmer, Murray, Meltzer, & Cohen, 2002). However, this is not empirically supported. A study of FTMs who had taken testosterone for at least one year (N = 16) found that 25% were sometimes perceived as female on the phone, with 31% expressing interest in therapy to further masculinize speech (Van Borsel et al., 2000). The speech needs of FTMs who do not take testosterone were not discussed in any of the literature surveyed.

There is great variation in the extent to which speech changes are undertaken or desired by transgender individuals. Some transgender persons who desire changes to speech and voice seek maximum feminization or masculinization, while others experience relief with a more androgynous presentation. Some transgender individuals seek to develop two speech patterns (one more masculine, one more feminine) either because they identify as bi-gendered or because external pressures relating to family, employment, cultural community, or other concerns prevent living full-time in a way that is consistent with felt sense of self. Most current transgender speech protocols do not support bi-modal speech as a treatment goal, based on the belief that to effect maximal change it is necessary to have a consistent single speech pattern. Switching back and forth between two speech and voice patterns may be too difficult for some clients, and inconsistent use decreases practice opportunities to acquire the new speech and voice pattern. However, the human capacity to learn and speak more than two languages, develop a specific accent for an acting role, and develop a singing voice that is different than speaking voice suggests it may be possible to develop bi-gender speech and voice. We encourage clinicians to be open to this possibility and not to routinely exclude clients who have two speech patterns as the treatment goal. We recommend that speech services be made available to the full spectrum of the transgender community.

EVIDENCE-BASED PRACTICE IN TRANSGENDER SPEECH AND VOICE CHANGE

The practice recommendations in this article are based on published literature specific to transgender speech, supplemental interviews with four expert clinicians, and the authors' professional experience. As research in this field is limited, some of our recommendations are based on current practices or theoretical rationale where the literature is inconclusive or absent.

In our review of the literature we found a paucity of evidence in the area of transgender speech, particularly in clinical practice. Early clinical research reported single subject case studies (Bralley, Bull, Gore, & Edgerton, 1978; Hooper, 1985; Kalra, 1977; Kaye, Bortz, & Toumi, 1993; Mount & Salmon, 1988; Yardley, 1976); more recently small group studies have reported outcomes of speech therapy (Byrne et al., 2003; Dacakis, 2000; Neumann et al., 2002b; Soderpalm et al., 2004) and pitch-elevating surgery (Brown, Perry, Cheesman, & Pring, 2000; de Jong, 2003; Gross, 1999; Kunachak, Prakunhungsit, & Sujjalak, 2000; Neumann et al., 2002b; Wagner, Fugain, Monneron-Girard, Cordier, & Chabolle, 2003; Yang et al., 2002). However, further research is needed to evaluate specific techniques and protocols.

In the literature and in our discussions with clinicians we noted that decisions about practice protocols were often significantly impacted by budget constraints, the logistics of the clinical setting (e.g., university-based student clinics running from September to April), and protocols necessary for conscientious research but not necessary in regular clinical practice. While there are administrative and logistical realities that need to be considered, we felt it was important to base our recommendations on what we felt to be optimal practice from a *clini-*

cal perspective, based on the evidence currently available.

In North America, many clinicians providing transgender speech services do so in the private practice setting, and data from clients in these settings are rarely published. To assist in greater understanding of transgender speech issues and further development of practice protocols, we encourage clinicians in both university and private practice settings to ask transgender clients for permission to share anonymized assessment data with other speech professionals. As with all research, it is important that transgender clients' involvement in research be fully voluntary–i.e., services should not be contingent on agreement to publish outcome data.

The clinical process of feminization or masculinization of speech and the voice is predicated on the concept that there are "feminine" speech and voice norms and "masculine" speech and voice norms. Within linguistics there is generally recognition that norms of "feminine" and "masculine" discourse and language are socially determined phenomena that vary across cultures, regions, and historical periods. There is less understanding of the ways that voice may also be shaped by social influences (Delph-Janiurek, 1999). This is most obviously problematic in studies which assert universal "female" and "male" speech and voice characteristics based solely on study of English-language speakers, but in reviewing the literature we were also concerned by assumptions of homogeneity relating to age, culture, class, region, and social context between speaker and listener. While there is obvious value in considering existing empirical evidence relating to gender perceptions and attributions in development of speech feminization and masculinization protocols, we believe it is misleading to interpret the existing data relating to gender norms and voice as universally normative. In reviewing research findings we include discussion of the limits of these findings.

CORE COMPETENCIES OF THE SPEECH PROFESSIONAL IN TRANSGENDER CARE

While speech professionals do not need to be experts in every realm of transgender care to work with transgender clients, the clinician providing speech feminization or masculinization services is expected to have basic trans-competence. Trans-competency in clinical services involves both the ability to interact in a respectful way with transgender individuals–sometimes termed *cultural competence* (Kohnert, Kennedy, Glaze, Kan, & Carney, 2003; Núñez, 2000)–and also clinical knowledge and skill relating to (a) speech and voice science, and (b) trans-specific assessment, treatment, and outcome evaluation (Goldberg, 2006).

Cultural competence in transgender speech and voice change refers to the capacity to provide respectful and relevant services to a diverse range of clients. In addition to general skill working with clients from a variety of cultural, ethnic, class, and age groups, the clinician is expected to be familiar with transgender terminology, diversity of gender identity and expression, the processes involved in gender transition, and trans-specific psychosocial issues that shape clients' goals and treatment options (Goldberg & Lindenberg, 2001). The clinician should also be aware of basic protocols such as use of the client's preferred gender pronoun and name in verbal interactions and written records.

Clinical competence in transgender speech and voice change requires a solid foundation in theory relating to adult speech and voice production, speech and voice disorders, speech and voice treatment techniques, and other elements of speech and voice science. We recommend that the speech clinician working with transgender individuals have at least two years clinical experience assessing and treating typical adult speech and voice disorders prior to working with transgender individuals, as the clinical processes of speech and voice feminization or masculinization require a high degree of clinical sophistication.

There are few opportunities to obtain training in speech and voice feminization or masculinization, and many clinicians learn as they work with transgender clients. This article is intended to help clinicians who already have both trans-awareness and experience in speech and voice work to become more familiar with gender differences in speech and voice; the effects of hormones and hormone therapy on speech and voice; treatment options to feminize or masculinize the voice; and trans-specific protocols for assessment, treatment, evaluation, and followup.

Some transgender individuals seek speech services not to feminize or masculinize communication, but rather to address voice quality issues (such as hoarseness or raspiness following pitch-altering surgery), loss of singing range following changes to habitual speaking pitch range, or feelings of disconnection from the voice resulting from rapid hormonal or surgical changes. While clinicians working with transgender clients on these issues should be familiar with relevant trans-specific physical and psychosocial issues, the same clinical protocols generally used to deal with these concerns in other clients can successfully be used with transgender clients–i.e., no special trans-specific clinical protocols are needed. This article focuses on clinical protocols that are unique to speech feminization or masculinization, an area that (unless associated with vocal pathology) is considered trans-specific.

TRANS-SPECIFIC PRACTICE PROTOCOLS

Trans-Specific Speech Assessment

The first step in transgender speech treatment is a thorough assessment to guide the development of a therapeutic evaluation and treatment plan. The following section discusses recommendations relating to establishment of therapeutic rapport, recording of client history and objectives, evaluation of speech parameters, assessment of potential for change, determination of therapeutic goals, discussion of therapeutic options, and preparation for change. The additional evaluation required prior to pitch-elevating surgery is discussed in the section on surgical treatment protocols.

Building Therapeutic Rapport

The relationship between client and clinician begins with the first interactions. In initial sessions, the clinician is not only assessing the client, the client is also assessing the knowledge and supportiveness of the clinician. A relationship grounded in mutual respect, trust, and genuine care for the client's well-being facilitates open communication and encourages active engagement in therapy; conversely, it can be difficult to build therapeutic rapport if conflicts arise in initial sessions. Many transgender individuals have had negative experiences with ill-informed or unempathetic health professionals, and there may be wariness about entering unreservedly into a relationship around communication–which is, by its nature, highly personal.

Because the assessment process sets the stage for all future interaction, it is extremely important to make the client feel respected and safe, and to create a feeling of positive anticipation for the therapy process. Issues that speech professionals need to consider in the intake process include storage of information, privacy issues in setting appointment times, client name preference, use of the client's preferred pronouns, and therapist bias and judgments about transgenderism (King et al., 1999).

Recording Relevant History

Client history should include information about both trans-specific concerns and also general issues that are known to impact therapeutic options and potential outcomes. While some transgender individuals are very comfortable talking about their history, others are more private. In some cases it may be appropriate to revisit sensitive questions after therapeutic rapport is well established, or to lead with general questions unrelated to trans-specific issues. As with the general population, some clients respond well to informal intake (e.g., the question "What brings you to see me?" may elicit a great deal of information); in other cases a more structured interview process or intake form may be beneficial. Sample intake forms are available as an online supplement at http://www.vch.ca/transhealth/resources/library/tcpdocs/guidelines-speech.pdf.

As with any client presenting for speech services, initial intake should include a general medical history, with particular attention to history of nose or throat complaints, respiratory ailments, hearing difficulties, voice disorders (including problems stemming from self-directed attempt to modify voice or heavy use of voice), or any other conditions that could impact speech (de Bruin et al., 2000; Pausewang-

Gelfer, 1999; Soderpalm et al., 2004). To assist in coordination of care, other health professionals involved in the client's general and trans-specific care should be noted (Soderpalm et al., 2004). Clients who present with difficulty swallowing, a dysphonic voice, or other symptoms that may indicate voice disorder–such as vocal fatigue, loss of range, or throat discomfort–should be referred for laryngological examination (Hearing, Speech & Deafness Center, 2005). All current medications, including feminizing or masculinizing hormones, should be recorded.

History of behaviours that may negatively impact speech, such as smoking (tobacco, cocaine, marijuana, etc.) and drinking alcohol should be explored (de Bruin et al., 2000; Pausewang-Gelfer, 1999). Because the stigma associated with substance use makes it difficult to get accurate information about current patterns of use, it may be useful to ask if a client "has ever . . ." rather than asking about current behaviour at the original intake; this can be revisited as part of treatment planning.

History of behaviours that may positively impact speech should also be explored. For example, it may be useful to inquire about personal, professional, and recreational use of voice (e.g., involvement in singing or acting) to determine whether previous training could be tapped during therapy. Previous attempts to feminize or masculinize speech should be investigated, including techniques used, duration of self- or professionally-directed therapy, and the client's subjective feelings about the outcome (Andrews, 1999; Dacakis, 2002; Pausewang-Gelfer, 1999; Perez, 2004).

Trans-specific history should include information about other feminization or masculinization treatments that may affect speech–such as testosterone therapy in FTMs or facial feminization surgery in MTFs–and any noted impact on speech following these treatments (Andrews, 1999; King et al., 1999; Pausewang-Gelfer, 1999; Soderpalm et al., 2004). It is not necessary to inquire specifically about trans-specific treatments that are unlikely to directly impact speech, such as history of chest, breast, or genital surgery. Relevant areas to explore include: (a) consideration of the impact of any planned surgeries on the timing of speech therapy, (b) any factors relating to transition that the client feels are important in terms of motivation and timing of speech therapy–for example, wish to have speech change complete by a specific date to facilitate job change–and (c) any medical or psychosocial issues that the client feels may affect ability to engage in speech change (e.g., some transgender people report changes to concentration and emotional lability as a side effect of hormone regimens).

Evaluating Current Speech Parameters Associated with Gender

Thoroughly assessing the client's speech gives a baseline against which to measure change and provides information about which changes would be most useful (Andrews & Schmidt, 1997; Kaye et al., 1993; King et al., 1999). While voice parameters such as fundamental frequency and speaking frequency range can be measured objectively, many speech characteristics associated with gender, such as melody and vocal timbre, cannot be objectively quantified. A complete clinical impression should include the clinician's objective and subjective findings, and also the client's subjective assessment (Andrews & Schmidt, 1997; Byrne et al., 2003; Coleman, 1983; Dacakis, 2002; de Bruin et al., 2000; Gold, 1999; Mikos & Pausewang-Gelfer, 2001; Oates & Dacakis, 1997; Pausewang-Gelfer, 1999; Pausewang-Gelfer & Schofield, 2000; Wollitzer, 1994).

Following standard practice in an evaluation of speech and voice, audio recordings of the client's performance across a variety of tasks such as reading, picture description, and conversation should be made. These recordings assist the client and clinician in analyzing current communication patterns, setting goals for therapy, and determining a baseline against which to measure change. With the client's permission, the audio recordings may also be used as a resource to train student speech professionals.

If the clinician has access to digital technology and the client feels comfortable being videotaped, the assessment session can be taped and the footage then reviewed with the client. This may be a useful way of evaluating non-verbal communication features such as gestures, movement, and facial expressions. However, many clients find it intrusive, intimi-

dating, and embarrassing to be videotaped, and particularly to watch and discuss the tape with the clinician. We recommend using videotape only if the client is comfortable with this and there is strong clinician-client rapport.

To gather objective data in an assessment, a computer program that measures fundamental frequency, intensity, and vowel formants is necessary. Kay Elemetrics' Computer Speech Lab 4300 and "Dr. Speech" (Tiger DRS Inc.) were mentioned in the literature surveyed (Dacakis, 2002; Mount & Salmon, 1988; Soderpalm et al., 2004). Free software programs that measure fundamental frequency may be downloaded from the internet and can be useful for practice by clients who have computer access.

Client's Subjective Assessment

Because the client's goals for speech feminization or masculinization relate directly to both self-perception and feelings about the perceptions of others, it is important to understand the client's perspective and expectations in both of these areas (Andrews, 1999; Dacakis, 2002; Oates & Dacakis, 1997; Pausewang-Gelfer, 1999; Soderpalm et al., 2004). This may be done through informal discussion and/or formal measures such as standardized questionnaire.

If informal interview is the only tool used, to facilitate later assessment we recommend that the clinician use the same questions in pre- and post-evaluation. For example, the clinician could ask the client to describe three situations involving speaking that the client is dissatisfied with, and three things the client would like to change about the way she or he speaks in these situations.

A standard speech questionnaire like the Vocal Handicap Index or Voice Symptom Scale (Wilson et al., 2004) can be modified to include trans-specific concerns. The Transgender Self-Evaluation Questionnaire, developed by the lead author, is available online at http://www.vch.ca/transhealth/resources/library/tcpdocs/guidelines-speech.pdf; the La Trobe Communication Questionnaire (Byrne et al., 2003) is an example in the published literature.

Whether informal or formal assessment tools are used, it can be informative to ask clients to rate identity, self-perceived behaviour, appearance, and speech on a masculinity/femininity and male/female scale. This allows the clinician to gain a clearer picture of the client's identity and also aids in discussion of the client's feelings about possible discrepancies between gender identity and gender expression (Soderpalm et al., 2004).

Concern about others' perceptions often relates to *passability*–being perceived by others as a man or a woman. The desire to pass is a complex feeling that may be influenced by the client's self-defined gender; community norms; beliefs and expectations of friends, family, co-workers, community peers, or others who are close to the client; internalized transphobia; degree of social support; and experiences of mistreatment (as individuals who are visibly transgender are often more vulnerable to harassment, discrimination, and violence). Because norms relating to social interactions and speech are context-dependent, it is important to know the context for speech that the client is particularly concerned about, such as employment or social relationships (Becklund-Freidenberg, 2002). As the client begins changing speech and voice patterns, reactions of those close to the client (e.g. family, friends, co-workers, community peers) should be discussed (Andrews, 1999; Dacakis, 2002; Oates & Dacakis, 1983; Pausewang-Gelfer, 1999). For clients concerned with passability, the reactions of strangers are important and these should be recorded either through informal estimate or formal means such as a diary.

While some transgender individuals may seek speech services because they have difficulty passing on the telephone or in face-to-face communication, others are more concerned about reducing a perceived discrepancy between speech and identity. Assessing self-perception relates to the fit that clients feel between their current speech and their felt sense of gender–i.e., how the client feels hearing herself or himself talk. The question of how well speech fits with the client's perception of self may be easy for the client to answer right away, or it may come over time with experimentation, practice, and observation of role models. Both the literature and the clinicians we interviewed discussed the importance of a "good fit" between the speech and the client rather than at-

tempting to conform to an external stereotype of femininity or masculinity (Becklund-Freidenberg, 2002; Oates & Dacakis, 1997). Finding this good fit requires introspection on the client's part and an informed opinion about what is possible.

Clinician's Evaluation

Pitch. While there are several factors that together determine attributions of gender to a speaker, studies suggest that fundamental frequency (F_0) is primary in perception of a speaker as male or female (Byrne et al., 2003; Coleman, 1983; Günzburger, 1993; Wollitzer, 1994). Normative data for male and female F_0 vary across languages and dialects (Elert & Hammarberg, 1991; Graddol & Swann, 1989; Rose, 1991; Tom, 2004). Among English-language speakers, the mean F_0 for non-transgender men and women overlaps from 145-165 Hz (Oates & Dacakis, 1997). Studies of English-speaking transsexual women report that bringing F_0 into this range of overlap may not be sufficient, by itself, to shift the gender perception of listeners. For example, transsexual women with F_0 of 145-160 Hz (i.e., within the "gender-neutral" range for English speakers) are usually judged as male (Spencer, 1988; Wolfe, Ratusnik, Smith, & Northrop, 1990). The primacy of F_0 in perception of a speaker's gender in languages other than English was not discussed in the literature we reviewed.

Speech analysis software such as Kay Elemetrics can be used to measure the average speaking pitch and pitch range across several tasks (Dacakis, 2002; Mount & Salmon, 1988; Soderpalm et al., 2004). Data should be recorded in both hertz and semitones to facilitate clinical evaluation, using one of the readily available conversion tables (Hirano, 1981). The visual display of a software analysis program can provide valuable information for a client about habitual and target average speaking pitches, particularly in the context of discussion about typical male and female speaking pitch ranges in the client's primary language.

In addition to noting fundamental frequency and frequency range, it is useful to note if the pitch is higher (for MTFs) or lower (for FTMs) in a less complex task like reading than in spontaneous conversation. If so, the client may already be consciously or unconsciously attempting voice feminization or masculinization.

Although anatomy determines the upper and lower limits of an individual's pitch range, there is evidence that F_0 is largely dependent on social context (Hasegawa & Hata, 1995). Ideally, speaking pitch would be evaluated by collecting data in naturalistic situations common in the client's day-to-day life, and also with a variety of conversational partners. While this wider baseline would be informative, it may be impractical or prohibitively expensive to gather data in a public setting.

Intonation. Intonation (sometimes termed "inflection") is also considered important in gender perception, particularly when F_0 is in the "gender-neutral" range of overlap between male and female norms (Becklund-Freidenberg, 2002; Pausewang-Gelfer & Schofield, 2000; Spencer, 1988; Wolfe et al., 1990). In English, women tend to be more variable in intonation than men, generally using more upward glides and avoiding downward glides and level intonation patterns (Challoner, 2000; de Bruin et al., 2000; Gold, 1999; Oates & Dacakis, 1997; Wolfe et al., 1990; Wollitzer, 1994); as intonation varies significantly across languages, this should not be considered a universal norm.

Intonation patterns should be recorded using speech analysis software at the same time that frequency is recorded. The visual display recording can then be viewed with the client, to illustrate patterns associated with gender–for example, repeated and dramatic decrease in pitch at the end of a sentence is typically considered a male speech pattern among English speakers, while variability in intonation is considered a more typically female pattern among English speakers. Exaggerated intonation shifts may be observed in some transgender women trying to mimic non-transgender women (Wollitzer, 1994), and if present these should be pointed out to the client.

It is also useful to make clinical judgments about inflections during speech. Conversation or a sample of reading can be recorded, then played back with both the client and the clinician listening to the vocal inflections. During the subsequent discussion the clinician can assess the acuity of the client's perceptions. If the client is unable to hear what the clinician perceives to be important, the clinician can then give guidance such as, "Listen to how your voice stays flat when you say . . ." or "Listen to how your voice moves around when you say that. That is what we are looking for."

Resonance. In the literature surveyed, the term *resonance* was used to describe three distinct aspects of speech: (a) the effects of the vocal tract on the sound produced by the larynx (formant frequencies), (b) the vocal quality that corresponds to the perception of vibrations in various parts of the body, or (c) the function of the nose as a resonator. There is empirical evidence that vowel formant frequencies significantly influence the perception of English-language speakers as male or female (Coleman, 1983; Mikos & Pausewang-Gelfer, 2001; Pausewang-Gelfer & Mikos, 2005). Measuring the "corner vowels" /i/, /u/, and /a/ may be particularly useful in assessing transgender speech (Mount & Salmon, 1988; Spencer, 1988), as these vowels represent the maximal range of formant frequencies in vowel productions in many languages (Titze, 1997).

Among English-language speakers, vowel formant frequency is estimated at 20% lower in adult men than adult women (Coleman, 1983; Dacakis, 2002; Oates & Dacakis, 1983). The reasons for this are not clear, but a study of physiologically matched English, Hindi, and Mandarin male and female speakers ($N = 40$) concluded that differences in format frequencies are due primarily to cultural and linguistic factors rather than sex-based anatomical differences (Andrianopolous, Darrow, & Chen, 2001).

The role of the other types of "resonance" is less certain. Singers often refer to "chest resonance" as the full, rich sound that is produced in lower notes and accompanied by a feeling of the voice vibrating in the chest; "head resonance" describes a brighter, forward sound that accompanies sensations of the voice ringing or resonating in the mouth, nose, sinuses, or upper part of the head. While some authors suggest that among English-language speakers "chest resonance" is associated with male speech while "head resonance" is associated with female speech (de Bruin et al., 2000; Gold, 1999; Kujawski, 2003; Oates & Dacakis, 1997), there is no empirical evidence that increasing the subjective feeling of "head resonance" or decreasing the subjective feeling of "chest resonance" increases the perception of MTF speakers as female (Dacakis, 2002). Further study is necessary to see if using these perceptions in training voice production produces difference in vowel formant frequencies.

Vocal intensity. Vocal intensity–the loudness of speech–may be measured with a sound level meter. In North America, the meter is usually placed 30 cm from the lips; at this distance, norms are 68-76 dBA for adult males and 68-74 dBA for adult females (Koschkee & Rammage, 1997). Despite the evidence that there is little sex-mediated difference in the loudness of actual speech, in some regions it is a common stereotype that women tend to speak more softly than men, and some clinicians include this speech parameter in assessment and treatment planning (Andrews, 1999; Dacakis, 2002; de Bruin et al., 2000; Günzburger, 1993; Oates & Dacakis, 1983). We recommend objectively measuring intensity if the client reports it as a problem or if the clinician subjectively feels it may be an issue.

Some transgender individuals who are self-conscious about speech may adopt insufficient vocal intensity in an attempt to avoid public attention, or MTFs may speak quietly to try to "soften" the voice (Dacakis, 2002). This can result in difficulty maintaining desired speech characteristics in situations where a higher vocal intensity is needed to counter high environmental noise or to convey intensity of emotion.

Voice quality. In English, most measures of voice quality are not consistently associated with categorization of voice as masculine or feminine (Andrews & Schmidt, 1997). However, "breathiness" is considered a feminine trait among English-language speakers (Becklund-Freidenberg, 2002; Dacakis, 2002; Gold, 1999; Oates & Dacakis, 1997; Wollitzer, 1994).

Voice quality is typically measured subjectively according to the speech professional's acoustic impression, possibly with the use of perceptual rating scales such as the Perceptual Voice Profile (Oates & Russell, 1997). Jitter and shimmer data may be collected by a software acoustic analysis package to support the clinical impression, but these parameters can be hard to measure accurately, requiring a very quiet space, rigid protocols, and finely calibrated equipment. The client should be referred for a laryngological examination if the voice is judged to be dysphonic.

Articulation. Subjective impression may be made about the quality of articulatory productions. In the literature reviewed, several authors observed that among English-language speakers women tend to articulate more clearly than men but in a light manner, men tend to make harder articulatory contacts and "punch out" their words, men tend to drop final phonemes (e.g., "walkin" instead of "walking"), and men tend to reduce or alter the production of some speech sounds such as voiced "th" (Andrews, 1999; Gold, 1999; Oates & Dacakis, 1983, 1997). The literature includes subjective observations about habitual lip, tongue and jaw positions, without agreement about correlation with gender associations (Günzburger, 1993; Oates & Dacakis, 1983, 1997).

Durational characteristics. Depending on the durational characteristics of the client's primary language, it may be useful for the clinician to observe whether the client sustains voicing through speech sounds, words, and phrases, or uses a more staccato speech style where words and phrases are produced more separately. It has been suggested that in European languages women typically have a longer mean duration of voicing during phrases and isolated words, and linger on occasional vowel sounds (Andrews, 1999; Günzburger, 1993).

Language and discourse. While there are strong social stereotypes about gender norms and language (e.g., use of slang, size modifiers, and tag questions), gender-associated norms of language and discourse are so dependent on an ever-shifting social context that findings from studies done in past decades may not be reflective of current patterns and trends (Becklund-Freidenberg, 2002; Oates & Dacakis, 1983). Additionally, there is strong interplay between gendered language norms and norms relating to culture, class, sexual orientation, and age (Graddol & Swann, 1989; Linville, 1998; Moran, McCloskey, & Cady, 1995; Morris & Brown, 1994), so norms appropriate for one client would not be appropriate for another. If there are habits relating to modifiers, qualifiers, indirect versus direct speaking style, or other elements of language that the client finds discomforting or that the clinician feels may contribute to perceptions that don't fit the client's self-image, we recommend that the clinician offer feedback in these areas.

Rather than attempting to memorize lists of qualifiers or artificially adopt set phrases, we recommend that modification of language and discourse be based on the client's own observations of gender markers in the specific environmental context of concern to the client (e.g., work, home, cultural community, social setting). To facilitate the determination of contextually appropriate speech and voice norms, the client should be encouraged to weigh research findings and the clinician's suggestions against her or his lived experience. Clients with strong beliefs about "appropriate" language may benefit from clinician assistance to compare stereotypical ideas of behaviour to the actual observed behaviour of peers.

Non-verbal communication. Norms relating to posture, gestures, and other non-verbal aspects of communication are strongly influenced by cultural, class, and age norms. Generally, in the dominant culture of North America, maintenance of eye contact, increased smiling, nodding and inclining toward others, increased use of hand and arm gestures, and occasional touching of the listener are associated with feminine communication patterns (Andrews, 1999; Gold, 1999). While it is not within the typical scope of practice of a speech-language pathologist to provide a detailed assessment of non-verbal communication behaviours, anything that is striking to the clinician or to the client should be noted as part of the subjective evaluation.

Subjective Third-Party Evaluation

In some cases it may be helpful to have one or more naïve listeners provide subjective impressions of a recording of the client's speech. This may be useful when clients are particularly concerned with passability, or when clients are unable to appreciate changes that have taken place. For example, one study found that MTF clients did not rate their speech as more feminine following therapy, but observers did (Soderpalm et al., 2004). To be considered "naïve," the listener should not be a speech clinician or student, and should also not be familiar with the client's goals. If passability is the goal, the listener should rate not only the cli-

ent's femininity or masculinity, but should also be asked to judge whether the speaker was male or female.

Assessing Potential for Speech and Voice Change

Clients vary in ability to achieve certain pitches, match a target pitch, and follow models of intonation or articulatory productions (Becklund-Freidenberg, 2002; Byrne et al., 2003; Dacakis, 2000, 2002; Soderpalm et al., 2004; Van Borsel et al., 2000). Using an exploratory diagnostic process helps determine how physically and psychologically easy or difficult it may be to effect change, and gives information about the sort of intervention that may be necessary in therapy. For example, if a client has difficulty matching pitches auditorily, using a visual pitch display will probably be necessary. If the pitch range appears restricted, a lower (MTF) or higher (FTM) frequency pitch target would be more appropriate, and specific exercises to increase vocal range such as Stemple's vocal function exercises (Sabol, Lee, & Stemple, 1995; Stemple, Lee, D'Amico, & Pickup, 1994) should be considered. If the MTF client has a seamless transition into falsetto, some falsetto notes may be available for widening the upper range of vocal inflections.

Speaking Pitch

There are a number of ways to explore average speaking pitch and speaking pitch range.

1. The client glissandos around in the upper (MTF) or lower (FTM) range, without moving into falsetto (MTF), then sustains a pitch and uses it to intone a word and short phrase. This is recorded and then evaluated for quality and ease of phonation. This is repeated several times throughout the range. The client is also asked to intone words and phrases in higher pitches (MTF) or lower pitches (FTM) to ensure there is room for vocal inflections (Kujawski, 2003).
2. An arbitrary target pitch is set by the clinician and the client matches it. Then, choosing pitches above or below that one, they decide on an initial target. It

should be noted that this pitch is for practice purposes only and can be changed at any time.

3. A pitch that is one fourth of an octave above (MTF) or below (FTM) the habitual speaking pitch is set by the clinician and the client matches it. The initial interval in *Auld Lang Syne* or *Here Comes the Bride* can be used to help the client understand the pitch change that is sought.

4. The clinician models a frequency within the lower range of female norms (MTF) or upper range of male norms (FTM) on a visual display in a computer voice analysis program, and the client produces a pitch that stays above (MTF) or below (FTM) it.

5. The client says a phrase in her most feminine (MTF) or his most masculine (FTM) voice.

For MTFs with low pitch, diagnostic therapy should be done to see if facilitation techniques enable higher pitches. Using sounds that facilitate efficient vocal fold vibration such as /m/, /z/, lip trilling, and tongue trilling, the client phonates in a higher pitch, either randomly or matching a pitch set by the clinician. The goal is to produce the sound at the desired pitch without any feeling of strain in the throat, emphasizing a strong feeling of vibrating or buzzing in the front of the face. For FTMs with high pitch, it may be useful to explore facilitation techniques that give sensations of ease and resonance in the lowest register of the voice.

If the client is unable to produce a higher or lower pitch without throat sensation or fatigue, the clinician may want to start with some standard voice therapy exercises to reduce inappropriate habits. Referral to an otolaryngologist may also be indicated.

Inflections

A short sentence is read by the client and examined for its inflectional variation. The target is an inflectional pattern consistent with the gender norms for the client's language. For English-speaking MTFs who are seeking to feminize speech, the goal is an inflectional pattern that is wide but still natural-sounding; for FTM English-speakers seeking to masculinize speech, the goal is an inflectional pattern that is narrower but not "flat" sounding. If the pattern is consistent with the client's goals relating to feminine or masculine speech norms, this is noted; if not, the clinician can model a more consistent inflectional pattern and the client can copy it. The result is played back for the client to hear the effect. This exercise gives information on the client's ability to hear and model vocal inflections, and also gives the client feedback about how the voice may sound if a different inflectional pattern is adopted.

Other Parameters

Changes to other parameters such as tongue carriage, articulatory productions, vocal quality, and vocal loudness can be considered if either the client or clinician thinks they may be important to address. In the initial session, useful information can be gleaned by exploring a number of speech/voice parameters from the trans-competent clinician's repertoire.

Assisting the Client to Determine Therapeutic Goals

To help the client determine fully informed, considered, and achievable therapeutic goals, it is useful for the clinician to provide a synopsis of the client's baseline speech and voice characteristics, physiologic limitations and estimated potential for change, and an informed professional opinion about the parameters that would be beneficial to address to achieve the client's stated objective (Dacakis, 2002; Hooper, 1985; Neumann et al., 2002b; Oates & Dacakis, 1983, 1997; Pausewang-Gelfer, 1999; Wollitzer, 1994). For example, if an English-speaking MTF client presents with the primary concern that her voice is not perceived as female, it may be appropriate to target a higher fundamental frequency if her habitual speaking pitch is 100 Hz; if her average pitch is higher than 150 Hz, it may be more appropriate to target resonance, inflection, and other speech characteristics that are believed to have a greater influence on gender perception when pitch is above the English-language norms for male speech.

Table 1 summarizes aspects of speech that are associated with sex and gender attribution, and associated English-language norms. Norms

TABLE 1. English-Language Norms of Speech and Voice Associated with Gender

Considered Highly Salient to Gender Attributions		
Element of Speech	Female/Feminine Norms	Male/Masculine Norms
Pitch	Mean =196-224 Hz, range = 145 Hz-275 Hz; higher upper and lower limits of range	Mean = 107-132 Hz, range = 80 Hz-165 Hz
Formant frequencies	Higher	Lower
Intonation	More variable in intonation, more upward glides	More level intonation, more downward glides
Weaker Evidence to Support Role in Gender Attributions		
Element of Speech	Female/Feminine Norms	Male/Masculine Norms
Loudness	68-74 dBA	68-76 dBA
Breathiness	Perceived as mildly breathy, softer speech onsets	Not perceived as breathy, harder speech onsets
Articulation	Clear, light	Forceful onsets; dropped phonemes, reduced use of voiced "th"
Duration	Longer mean duration of phrases and isolated words, lingering on vowels	Staccato speech style

should be considered as a spectrum rather than two isolated poles, to encourage speech professionals and clients to carefully consider therapeutic goals that fit with sense of self.

Assisting the Client to Understand Therapeutic Options

Some transgender individuals have sophisticated knowledge about gender-related speech parameters and therapeutic options, and come to the initial assessment with a clear direction they wish to pursue. Others have no knowledge and expect guidance from a professional. During the initial evaluation it is important to assess the individual's knowledge of speech and voice. Consumer education materials have been developed as part of the Trans Care Project to help promote consistent and accurate information about transgender speech change and treatment options (Davies & Goldberg, 2006). In all cases, care should be taken to ensure that clients understand potential benefits and risks relating to both non-surgical and sur-

gical voice change, and recommendations to prevent vocal fatigue or voice disorder (Dacakis, 2000, 2002; Hooper, 1985; Kaye et al., 1993; Kunachak et al., 2000; Oates & Dacakis, 1997, 1983; Thomas, 2003; Yang et al., 2002).

Because changes to specific acoustic voice characteristics affect numerous perceptual variables, a well-rounded speech treatment plan will target "constellations of related voice characteristics rather than independent acoustic variables" (Wollitzer, 1994, p. 99). For example, raising pitch may increase laryngeal tension and vocal tract constriction, influencing shimmer, jitter, signal-to-noise ratio, and resonance (and thus subjective perceptions of voice quality). For this reason, an optimal speech therapy program should target all parameters of speech, not just those related to pitch.

Preparing for the Process of Speech Modification

Speech feminization or masculinization is a long process requiring considerable work on the client's part. While therapy outcomes cannot be predetermined, the estimated amount of daily practice time and expected duration of the course of therapy should be discussed, as should the factors that can influence the course of therapy (Byrne et al., 2003). As changing speech requires altering deeply ingrained communication habits and behaviors that can be difficult to modify, it may be useful to use the "Stages of Change" model (Prochaska, DiClemente, & Norcross, 1992; Zimmerman, Olsen, & Bosworth, 2000) or other behavioral change tools to assist in anticipating and addressing barriers to implementing change.

If pitch-changing surgery is sought, there should be discussion of the parameters of speech that may still need work after surgery, such as intonation and format frequency. Clients should also be informed of the estimated healing time involved and the time required to stabilize the new pitch (Dacakis, 2002; Neumann et al., 2004; Wagner et al., 2003).

Treatment Options and Techniques to Feminize or Masculinize Speech and Voice

Non-Surgical Treatment (Speech Therapy)

Speech Therapy Goals

As discussed earlier, we recommend that the clinician assist the client to determine therapeutic goals, recognizing that transgender individuals have diverse identities and objectives regarding feminization or masculinization and that the clinician should not be directive in promoting specific goals. The range of therapeutic goals may include any or all of the following.

Speech assessment, information, and other preparation for speech therapy. Some clients are interested primarily in a speech assessment and a professional opinion on what would be involved in changing elements of speech. Information about therapeutic options can help with decisions regarding the timing of gender transition. One program described in the literature offered three to four introductory sessions that provided information about gender differences in communication, information about vocal hygiene and prevention of voice disorders, and

exercises to increase flexibility of voice production (Dacakis, 2002).

Enhanced observation and awareness of speech patterns of self and others. While transgender individuals are often highly skilled at observing others, practice may be needed to understand, observe, and analyze the specific components of speech (Hooper, 1985).

Changes to speech. Average speaking pitch, pitch range, inflections, formant frequency, breathiness, loudness, articulation, tongue position, language, facial expressions, and gestures may be targeted to feminize or masculinize speech (Bralley et al., 1978; Brown et al., 2000; Dacakis, 2000, 2002; de Bruin et al., 2000; Gold, 1999; Hooper, 1985; Kalra, 1977; Kaye et al., 1993; Kujawski, 2003; Mount & Salmon, 1988; Oates & Dacakis, 1997; Pausewang-Gelfer, 1999; Soderpalm et al., 2004). Specific objectives relating to voice modification depend on what is feasible to produce without strain, what fits with the client's self-image, and how important passability is to the client; some clients may be comfortable with gender-neutral speech, while others will want to aim for a voice that is perceived by listeners as male or female. For clients who are concerned about "fitting in" or about passability, rather than adopting an artificial set of speech norms it is recommended that clients observe communication patterns in their social, cultural, and work environments to develop a context-specific set of norms (Oates & Dacakis, 1997).

Prevention of vocal fatigue. Use of the vocal tract in non-habitual ways can cause strain. Important therapeutic goals are the maintenance of efficient and easy speech, establishing appropriate practice, and informing the client about how best to maintain vocal health (Dacakis, 2000, 2002; Gold, 1999; Kaye et al., 1993; Mount & Salmon, 1988; Oates & Dacakis, 1983, 1997; Soderpalm et al., 2004).

Treatment Format

Traditionally, speech therapy has emphasized one-to-one work to facilitate the personalized intervention necessary to modify and monitor change in target behaviours. However, speech therapy groups–typically comprised of four to six clients–are commonly used to work with specific populations (e.g., individuals with aphasia, people recovering from traumatic brain injury, clients with fluency disorders). Group therapy can facilitate peer support and encouragement, and reduce self-consciousness that may be experienced when the client is working alone with the therapist.

It has been our experience that both individual and group therapy are important components of transgender speech care. We recommend that both formats be made available, with the option for a client to take part in either or both depending on therapeutic needs and goals.

Components of a transgender speech therapy program that can be done well in a group include:

1. Education and information. Clients undergoing speech feminization or masculinization need to understand how the voice is produced; how physiological differences in male and female voice production system affect the voice and listener perception; physiologic and social norms relating to gender and speech; treatment options, outcomes, and risks; and techniques to prevent strain associated with voice change. While some transgender individuals are extremely well-informed about speech, others have no knowledge or have been exposed to inaccurate information via the internet or peer groups.
2. Discussion. Group format is ideal for participants to share observations, insights, and practical advice. In the *Changing Keys* speech and voice feminization groups developed by the lead author (discussed later in this article), participants have commented on how useful they found these discussions.
3. Speech therapy exercises. There are several advantages to using a group setting to offer those components of a therapy program that are required by all individuals. These would include relaxation exercises, basic exercises in efficient vocal technique, and ear training (using listening exercises to train a heightened perception of differences in speech). For individuals who feel self-conscious about doing speech exercises, participating in a group can have a normalizing effect.

Role-playing is more easily done in a group, and the opportunity to observe others can give valuable insight into participants' own practice. Additionally, the group provides a safe setting to learn listening skills, and to practice observing speech in a way that will not be intrusive in a real-world setting.

The necessary repetition of training exercises can be done in a group as long as the therapist is able to monitor the progress of all the participants and give individual input and feedback as required. The group can be divided into pairs to give practice time in both talking and listening.

Some interventions require one-to-one work with a therapist, including: (a) determining appropriate target pitch, (b) training target pitch if the individual has difficulty matching pitches auditorily, (c) significantly changing individual characteristics associated with "feminine" or "masculine" speech, and (d) individualized, specific input on anything the individual has difficulty understanding or doing in the group setting. Individualized input is especially important in training an efficient voice that is resistant to vocal fatigue or dysphonia.

Length of Treatment Time

Treatment time varies greatly depending on the degree of change sought, the client's vocal abilities, and psychosocial issues. There is no professional consensus on the optimal length of treatment for maximal treatment efficacy. One study reported a modest correlation between the number of therapy sessions and mean pitch achieved at the end of therapy (Dacakis, 2000); however, another reported that client satisfaction was not related to the number of therapy sessions, and that clients tended to become frustrated and discouraged when therapy continued over a long period of time (Soderpalm et al., 2004). It has been our experience that treatment generally ranges from a minimum of 15 hours to a maximum of 1 year of weekly sessions, and that shorter, more intensive treatment times encourage motivation and accommodate changes to life circumstances more readily than prolonged treatment.

Psychosocial adjustment is an important part of changing speech. Participants may require time to get in touch with what sort of voice best matches the person within. This is by necessity a process that takes time and professional input as to what is possible. Many transgender individuals begin with the goal of having a pitch that is unrealistically high (MTF) or low (FTM); only with experimentation and practice will it become apparent that this is probably not achievable, necessary, or even desirable. Additionally, it can take time to feel that an altered voice is an authentic expression of self rather than an artificial "mask." If psychosocial issues are significantly impacting treatment, referral to a trans-competent mental health professional may be useful.

Therapeutic Techniques

In an extensive review of speech literature, we did not find any published protocols for speech therapy with FTMs. We recommend that speech-language pathologists working with FTMs be clear that they are using a trial protocol, and seek client permission to record, evaluate, and publish information on the efficacy of the protocol.

There are numerous published protocols for speech feminizing therapy with MTFs (Andrews, 1999; Becklund-Freidenberg, 2002; de Bruin et al., 2000; Gold, 1999; Hooper, 1985; Kujawski, 2003; Mount & Salmon, 1988; Oates & Dacakis, 1997; Pausewang-Gelfer, 1999). As an example of a local protocol, the *Changing Keys* program–a mix of group and individual therapy–is discussed in Appendix A.

Evaluating the design of treatment protocols. Although treatment protocols must be flexible enough to address each client's goals, physiologic parameters, and psychosocial needs, therapy should be grounded in current knowledge of best clinical practice of speech and voice therapy. In the absence of empirical evidence testing the efficacy of specific techniques to feminize or masculinize speech, we evaluated speech therapy protocols on the basis of *clinical rationale*–a clearly articulated, logical, and valid reason for choosing a specific protocol or technique. On this basis, we feel the following strategies are supportable:

1. Imitation of non-transgender people observed in daily life (de Bruin et al., 2000; Gold, 1999; Hooper, 1985; Kujawski, 2003; Mount & Salmon, 1988; Neumann, 2000b; Oates & Dacakis, 1997). This input from the real world is useful in helping clients develop spontaneous speech habits that "fit" in their particular community.

2. Progressively complex practice while maintaining good voice quality (Hooper, 1985; Kujawski, 2003; Mount & Salmon, 1988; Oates & Dacakis, 1997; Pausewang-Gelfer, 1999). Integration of pitch, pitch range, and inflections is typically done in progressively complex practice (vowels, monosyllabic words, phrases, sentences; reading, answering questions, interactive dialogue). Motor learning theory suggests that, initially, simple behaviours are acquired more easily than complex ones (Kent & Lybolt, 1982). However, behaviours that are to be done together must be learned together.

3. Vocal flexibility exercises to maintain vocal range and voice quality (Pausewang-Gelfer, 1999). Vocal range and flexibility exercises are a standard part of a voice therapy protocol.

4. Motor training (Oates & Dacakis, 1997). As speech is a motor act, input is most useful when it is given at the motor-sensory level. Matching a sensory target (e.g., "Does your voice feel easy or stuck? In the face or in the throat?") is a more effective method of training the desired production than giving verbal instructions such as, "Do this with your jaw" (Titze & Verdolini, in press).

5. Identifying and altering voice qualities when coughing, laughing, and clearing the throat (Andrews, 1999; Dacakis, 2002; de Bruin et al., 2000; Oates & Dacakis, 1997). These vegetative and spontaneous laryngeal functions may be higher or lower in pitch than the client desires and may respond to therapeutic input.

6. Experimentation with a broad range of voice styles (Gold, 1999). Experimentation with a broad range of voice styles, including ones that might be considered far

beyond what the client would actually want to use, expands the range of possibilities, and makes smaller changes–ones the client may actually use–feel less extreme.

Non-Verbal Communication: Facial Expressions, Posture, and Movement

Some transgender individuals are keen observers of non-verbal behavior and are acutely attuned to gendered norms relating to non-verbal communication. Others may require assistance from a speech therapist. While recognizing that non-verbal communication is extremely important, some speech-language pathologists feel unqualified to offer input; others may feel more comfortable doing so. Depending on an individual clinician's expertise in this area and the client's financial resources, options can include:

1. Focusing on strengthening the client's observational skills. Experimentation and observation are more useful than learning and following rigid patterns of behaviour.
2. Offering general feedback on the client's self-defined parameters for change. Based on observation of community peers, the client can identify desired parameters for change, practice these changes in the therapy session, and receive subjective feedback from the clinician. Parameters for change may include smiling, eye contact, facial expressions, posture, and gestures while speaking and listening. Feedback depends on the desired goal (e.g., did the client smile more or less? When?) and also the clinician's subjective sense of whether the change seemed appropriate.
3. Offering general feedback about social conventions relating to masculine or feminine expressions and movement. The client should be informed of the culturally-specific nature of non-verbal communication norms and the limits of the clinician's expertise in this area. It can be helpful to discuss the difference between stereotypes, norms, and observed behavior, and to remind the client to consider the clinician's input in light of their own experience and perspective.
4. Referring to peer support resources. While the level of knowledge about non-verbal communication varies greatly among peer support providers, individual or group peer support may offer experiential insights and an arena for practice. As peer knowledge often has strong currency, it can be important to remind clients to weigh the suggestions of peers against their own experience.
5. Referring to a trans-competent clinician who has training in non-verbal communication. In some regions, workshops specifically for transgender women are available, such as the "Give Voice" program run by Sandy Hirsch in Seattle. Movement coaches in theatre training programs may be able to assist in finding or developing local resources.

Habituation

As with any speech therapy, habituation and generalization of feminized or masculinized communication is both challenging and necessary. There is a profound difference between being able to maintain a pitch change on a prolonged vowel in a clinical setting and sustaining changes throughout speech in everyday life, particularly when making offhand remarks in casual conversation when self-monitoring may not be as vigilant, or when the client is under stress or fatigued (Becklund-Freidenberg, 2002). Strategies to promote carryover into everyday life may include (a) practicing words that are typically part of daily conversation, such as, "Hi," "Bye," "Yes," and "No"; (b) focusing practice of conversational speech on situations or topics related to the client's life; (c) simulating real-life situations that the client feels pose the most difficulty, such as a job interview or interaction in a coffee shop (Goodnow, 2001; Hooper, 1985); (d) experimenting with emotional intensity by practicing sentences expressing joy, sorrow, irritation, and anger; and (e) practicing with the clinician outside the clinic setting, in telephone and in-person interactions.

Follow-Up Sessions

A small study of MTF transsexuals ($N = 10$) reported a significant correlation between a longer treatment time and stable elevation of pitch over time (Dacakis, 2000). In view of this finding, follow up sessions after the initial treatment has finished, or facilitated support groups for ongoing practice, may be important in maintaining change. Clinically supervised followup also provides an excellent opportunity to gather much-needed data about the effectiveness of a protocol over time.

Clinical group or individual followup sessions. There is not yet any empirical evidence regarding the optimum frequency for followup sessions, the optimum content, or the criteria for termination. In the absence of data, we suggest that refresher sessions be initially offered 3 months after treatment and then at 4 to 6 month intervals, or as the clinician and client deem appropriate.

Followup sessions should include a discussion of successes, problems, strategies, and difficulties the client has experienced since the end of therapy; a review of the core exercises of the program (to ensure the client is practicing correctly and to determine if the exercises are still appropriate); and time to address any concerns that have arisen since the end of treatment. Ideally, followup would include re-evaluation of the same parameters measured in the pre-treatment assessment, both to assess the maintenance of the desired changes and also to evaluate the effectiveness of refresher sessions.

If the initial therapy was provided in a group setting, a group setting is a natural forum for refresher sessions. As with group format for initial therapy, group format for refresher work offers valuable opportunities for clients to compare experiences. In our experience this can be most useful and encouraging, especially for those in the early stages of gender transition. Individualized followup may be more appropriate than group format if the client has numerous concerns or unusual concerns that require individual attention, or if the client feels uncomfortable in a group setting.

Client-run speech support groups. Self-help groups are commonly organized for individuals with speech and language disorders such as aphasia and stuttering, and may also be useful for transgender individuals who have completed clinical treatment and are seeking peer support to maintain or strengthen speech changes. Client-run speech groups can provide motivation to maintain practice, a forum to practice and to share ideas and concerns, and an opportunity to socialize and do specific role-playing. Client-run groups can also foster the client's sense of ownership and control of speech and voice production, rather than feeling dependent on the therapist.

In any self-help group there is a danger that an individual may inappropriately assume a professional clinical role. In a speech group, this could be circumvented by providing group facilitation training to members, having the speech-language pathologist as guest visitor from time to time, and having self-help sessions along with therapist-run refresher sessions.

Modification to Improve Accessibility and Utility to Clients with Access Barriers

Protocols must be flexible enough to address diversity of service needs and issues relating to access. In the transgender speech literature reviewed for this project, there was little discussion of modification to address the needs of clients who have difficulty accessing the typical setting or format of speech service, such as individuals who have speech, hearing, cognitive, or learning disabilities; are not highly fluent in English or are not literate; or are geographically isolated or cannot leave a residential long-term care facility or prison. Without empirical evidence to guide practice, we offer the following suggestions based on our experience providing services to a diverse range of transgender clients.

Distance services. Individuals who are physically unable to attend speech therapy or are awaiting speech therapy services could benefit from an information package available through the mail or internet. This kind of "distance learning program" is currently under development at La Trobe University in Australia (G. Dacakis, personal communication, March 7, 2005). Such a distance learning program could include information on the mechanics of speech and voice production, gendered aspects of speech and voice, tips on observing and listening to conversations of men and women in the client's own community, evaluation of commercial speech training programs available on the Internet, and phonosurgery risks and benefits–similar to the consumer education materials described earlier (Davies & Goldberg, 2006).

"Telehealth" is increasingly being explored for distance delivery of speech therapy services (Duffy, Werven, & Arons, 1997; Haynes & Kully, 2005; Jessiman, 2003; Mashima et al., 2003; Myers, 2005). Speech therapy cannot be done by telephone or email as therapy requires a comprehensive evaluation, regular monitoring of the client's performance, and specific training input. However, clients can use telephone or email to consult with a clinician and receive general information. Video hookup connecting a rural health unit with an urban speech program can be used to train rural practitioners and to provide a partial level of service to geographically isolated clients.

Multilingual services. For individuals who do not speak the dominant language, a basic information package can be translated into a variety of languages. Interpretation or translation of more in-depth information is challenging in speech services, as the clinician must speak the client's language well enough to be aware of subtleties of inflections, inflectional range, word stress, and semantic and syntactic choices. In cases where the speech therapist and client do not speak the same language, the only direct therapeutic input that could perhaps be given would be in changing the average speaking pitch. SLPs who are multilingual should be encouraged and supported to take trans-specific training, perhaps working in consultation with a more trans-experienced clinician to provide service in the client's primary language.

If the client is partially fluent in the language spoken by the therapist, wishes speech therapy in this language, and will be speaking this language in everyday life, therapy delivered in the client's secondary language can be beneficial as the client has the opportunity of learning more feminine or masculine patterns of speech as she or he acquires the language. For individuals who are only partially fluent in the language spoken by the therapist, the therapeutic process will likely be longer and will require much more individualized input.

Access for individuals with disabilities. Transgender clients with speech or hearing disabilities who are able to attend speech therapy sessions may find great benefit from using visual input during speech therapy. This has been used with good success with other populations–for example, palotography and ultrasound have been used in work with people who are hard of hearing and have phonological disorders (Bernhardt, Bacsfalvi, Gick, Radanov, & Williams, 2005; Bernhardt, Gick, Bacsfalvi, & Adler-Bock, 2005; Bernhardt, Gick, Bacsfalvi, & Ashdown, 2003). For transgender clients, there are a number of software programs that record fundamental frequency and allow the creation of a "model wave." The clinician could record a desired average speaking pitch or an intonation pattern and the client could then use the visual input to copy it; alternatively, the clinician could record the lowest (MTF) or highest (FTM) desirable frequency and the client could use the visual input to keep the speaking pitch above (MTF) or below (FTM) this line.

If a client has cognitive or learning disabilities, depending on the nature of the disability it may be useful to include a loved one or care aid in the therapeutic process. This person could help the client establish a regular practice schedule and give input to the exercises, under the guidance of the speech-language pathologist. A different format may be useful for the client who has difficulty processing the information necessary to change speech habits. Rather than using an approach that requires introspection (e.g., "How does that sound? Am I feeling my voice in my face?"), the clinician may be more directive in determining which exercises would be most useful and could be done appropriately by the client; the clinician and client together would draw up a practice schedule, and the client would simply practise the motor movements outlined. Individualized attention is likely more effective than group work to provide the client with more intensive input. To be successful, this kind of format would require regular clinical intervention and support outside the therapy room.

Self-Guided Speech Feminization

There are a variety of videos, websites, and other materials available for self-guided speech feminization. We cannot comment on the efficacy of these materials, but we are concerned that (a) many are not produced by speech professionals, and (b) there are risks associated with attempting to change voice without professional assistance. Speech feminization or masculinization involves substantial changes in habitual production and so has the potential to cause a voice disorder or aggravate an existing one. We strongly recommend that anyone seeking to feminize or masculinize speech first be assessed by a speech-language pathologist, that a speech clinician be involved in monitoring progress, and that a speech clinician be consulted if there are any symptoms of vocal fatigue or negative changes to vocal quality. Additionally, we recommend that consumers be cautious of any materials promoting a rigid set of speech norms, as speech is too individually and culturally driven to be guided solely by a set of generic rules.

Surgical Treatment: Pitch-Elevating Surgery

Surgical techniques to elevate pitch are based on the physiological components of pitch:

$$F_0 = (\text{vibrating length of vocal folds}/2) \times (\text{mean vocal fold tension/vocal fold density})^{1/2}$$

(Kunachak et al., 2000). Fundamental frequency can thus be raised by shortening the folds, decreasing the total mass of the folds, or by increasing the tension of the folds (Neumann et al., 2002a; Pickuth et al., 2000; Yang et al., 2002). Surgical techniques to achieve this include (a) anterior commissure advancement, (b) creation of an anterior vocal web, (c) cricothyroid approximation, (d) induction of scarring along the vocal folds, or (e) reduction of vocal folds by intracordal steroid injection, laser evaporation of the vocal fold, or composite reduction or reconstruction of the vocal fold (Brown et al., 2000; Donald, 1982; Kunachak et al., 2000; Neumann et al., 2002a, 2002b; Orloff, 2000; Pickuth et al., 2000; Thomas, 2005; Wagner et al., 2003; Yang et al., 2003). To date, we feel that cricothyroid approximation is the only method that has been assessed with sufficient rigor to be considered a viable treatment option (Brown et al., 2000; de Jong, 2003; Neumann et al., 2002b; Oates & Dacakis, 1997; Soderpalm et al., 2004; Wagner et al., 2003; Yang et al., 2002).

Thyroid chondroplasty may be performed at the same time as vocal surgery to reduce the laryngeal prominence (Brown et al., 2000; Kunachak et al., 2000; Neumann et al., 2002a; Neumann & Welzel, 2004; Wagner et al., 2003). This is a cosmetic procedure that should not affect the voice.

Risk-Benefit Ratio of Pitch-Elevating Surgery

There is a paucity of outcome data for pitch-elevating surgery, particularly longitudinal data to monitor outcomes over time, but there are concerns that the outcome is highly variable and that initial results tend to diminish over time (Koufman, n.d.). In addition, reported negative effects of pitch-elevating surgery include compromised voice quality, diminished vocal loudness, adverse impact on swallowing or breathing, sore throat, wound infection, and scarring (Brown et al., 2000; Dacakis, 2002; Koufman, n.d.; Lawrence, 2004; Oates & Dacakis, 1997; Neumann & Welzel, 2004; Petty, 2004; Thomas, 2003, 2005; Wagner et al., 2003; Yang et al., 2002).

In general, professional opinion is mixed about pitch-elevating surgery, with some clinicians stating that it is not a viable treatment option (Andrews, 1999; Koufman, n.d.), and others recommending that surgery be considered a treatment of last resort for MTFs who have not experienced satisfactory increase in voice pitch following speech therapy (Lawrence, 2004; Oates & Dacakis, 1997; Wagner et al., 2003). Other clinicians are more enthusiastic about pitch-elevating surgery, suggesting that surgery can protect the voice from damage caused by strain to elevate pitch through non-surgical means (Brown et al., 2000; Neumann & Welzel, 2004; Thomas, 2005; Yang et al., 2002). While there are clear risks of vocal surgery and the decision to pursue vocal surgery should be carefully considered, we feel the decision about risk-benefit ratio and preferred technique is best left to the patient, with input from both a trans-experienced surgeon and a trans-experienced speech-language pathologist.

Pre-Surgical Assessment

In addition to the standard screening performed prior to any surgery, such as assessment for risks relating to anesthesia and infection, assessment prior to pitch-elevating surgery should include anatomical and functional assessment of the larynx, subjective auditory assessment by both a speech-language pathologist and the surgeon, and computer recording and analysis of pitch range (Neumann & Welzel, 2004; Yang et al., 2002). Care should be taken to ensure the patient understands the risks and anticipated outcome of the technique that will be used.

After finding that some subjects have strained and unnaturally elevated voices following surgery, attributed to habitually speaking at an artificially elevated pitch for sustained periods of time prior to surgery, one surgical group reported testing for ability to phonate at a pitch within the masculine range as part of pre-operative consultation (Yang et al., 2002). Clients who are unable to do this were felt to have the equivalent of a muscle tension dysphonia, and were referred for preoperative voice therapy to recover the ability to produce relaxed phonation.

Estrogen is associated with risk for deep vein thrombosis and pulmonary embolism (Dahl, Feldman, Goldberg, & Jaberi, 2006). If the patient will be immobilized for a prolonged period during or following pitch-elevating surgery, consultation with the prescribing physician is necessary to discuss the advisability of tapering estrogen use before surgery (Bowman & Goldberg, 2006).

Smoking increases the risk of complications from anesthetic and impairs healing, and there is evidence that smoking following pitch-elevating surgery can negatively impact on voice quality and pitch (Wagner et al., 2003). Patients should be informed of the risks associated with smoking and of smoking cessation resources, and strongly encouraged to not smoke prior to or immediately following surgery.

Post-Surgical Care

Post-surgical care depends on the specific surgical technique employed. The surgeon should review aftercare instructions with the patient as part of informed consent prior to surgery. The surgeon should also be accessible for questions relating to post-operative complications. The patient's local primary care provider should consult with the surgeon to determine appropriate followup.

Immediately following surgery, temporarily decreased pitch, diminished voice quality, and edema were commonly reported in the literature, with spontaneous recovery in most cases. Less common complications that required medical intervention included mild emphysema, neck abscess, negative response to the sutures or plates used in cricothyroid approximation (requiring removal of the material), and loosening of the sutures used in cricothyroid approximation, requiring further surgery (Neumann & Welzel, 2004; Wagner et al., 2003).

For most pitch-elevating surgical techniques, it is recommended that patients not use the voice at all for one to seven days after surgery, and then use the voice cautiously until any discomfort due to postoperative edema has passed (Brown et al., 2000; Neumann & Welzel, 2004; Orloff, 2000). For the more invasive combined thyroid cartilage and vocal fold reduction, two weeks vocal rest is suggested (Kunachak et al., 2000). Following cricothyroid approximation, steam inhalation may be recommended to hydrate and lubricate the vocal cords, to promote healing (Brown et al., 2000).

Speech therapy is recommended following surgery to help the patient adapt to and stabilize the new voice (Neumann & Welzel, 2004; Wagner et al., 2003). If pitch-elevating surgery was performed before other components of speech had been satisfactorily altered, resonance, articulation, and other components may also need to be addressed via speech therapy (Dacakis, 2002; Neumann & Welzel, 2004).

OUTCOME EVALUATION

Evaluation is a continuous process in speech care, with various informal and formal methods that may be used to determine progress and shape the direction of future treatment (Hooper, 1985; Mount & Salmon, 1988; Soderpalm et al., 2004). We recommend that at minimum the baseline assessment be repeated immediately following the end of therapy, and post-treatment data compared to pre-treatment findings. If the client is agreeable to long-term followup, given the paucity of long-term data it would be ideal for the client to be re-evaluated 6 months, 1 year, 5 years, and 10 years after treatment; for transient clients this degree of followup may not be possible, but even data at 6 and 12 months would be a significant contribution to the field.

In addition to re-evaluating objective and subjective impressions of speech as per the initial assessment, we recommend that clients be invited to evaluate satisfaction with the outcome of treatment (Bralley et al., 1978; Byrne et al., 2003; Kujawski, 2003; Mount & Salmon, 1988; Pausewang-Gelfer, 1999; Soderpalm et al., 2004). Several trans-specific studies reported a discrepancy between subjective satisfaction and objective or subjective changes to voice, with some clients pleased with the outcome despite minimal objective change, and others perceiving less change than that reported by naïve listeners (Bralley et al., 1978; Dacakis, 2000; Soderpalm et al., 2004; Spencer, 1988). This raises the question of what is considered a "successful" intervention. Some authors interpreted the findings as evidence that clients cannot accurately judge "successful" voice change (Bralley et al., 1978); others felt that discrepancy between subjective satisfaction and objective changes to voice may have stemmed from increased passability in other dimensions (e.g., from hormones or electrolysis), a good working relationship with the clinician, or satisfaction with the availability or cost of the service (Dacakis, 2000). It is also possible that client goals shifted over time or that clients' goals for speech did not center on pitch or passability, the typical measures employed for evaluation.

Earlier we suggested that the primary goal of speech feminization or masculinization is to decrease discrepancy between speech and the client's sense of self; it is, we think, highly relevant to ask about the client's feelings about "fit" between speech and identity as part of post-treatment assessment, even if the client did not explicitly state this as an objective at the start of treatment (Soderpalm et al., 2004). Another relevant measure might be the client's report of being able to use the desired speech consistently in the settings that were identified as the targets at the outset of therapy (Kujawski, 2003; Pausewang-Gelfer, 1999).

We also encourage clinicians to invite clients to evaluate the quality of service provided. In some cases the clients may be very satisfied with the clinician's performance despite minimal changes to speech; whatever the outcome, clients may have constructive critical feedback to offer the clinician regarding the ability to relate information clearly and accurately, sensitivity and respect in communication, overall familiarity with transgender concerns, efficient coordination with other clinicians, and accessibility of treatment.

If long-term followup is feasible, in addition to the standard re-evaluation of speech it may be useful to inquire about clients' continuation of therapeutic exercises and symptoms of vocal fatigue (Dacakis, 2000; Soderpalm et al., 2004). Three of five participants in one long-term study reported that after speech therapy had ended, they attempted further change through techniques learned from the internet or in books (Soderpalm et al., 2004). It may be useful to offer consumer education regarding risk prevention and ongoing monitoring to clients who are interested in pursuing techniques outside a professional setting.

CONCLUDING REMARKS

Speech and voice change services for transgender individuals are an important element of transgender care. Treatments to feminize and masculinize speech and voice can help reduce discomfort for the dysphoric client, improving confidence and comfort in day-to-day communication interactions. As self-directed speech and voice change can result in vocal strain we strongly recommend that professional speech services be included in transgender health programs and made available not only to transsexuals but also crossdressers, bi-gendered people, androgynous people, and others who desire to feminize or masculinize their speech and voice.

There is currently an insufficient data base to determine evidence-based best protocols in transgender speech and voice modification. We hope that this article will both assist speech professionals in adapting and modifying existing protocols to address a client's individual needs, and also stimulate interest in evaluation of practice protocols for MTFs and FTMs. Further research in this area is strongly recommended.

NOTE

1. Published transgender speech research focuses on transsexual women, with only a few studies involving male crossdressers or female-to-male transsexuals. In this document we use "male-to-female" (MTF) broadly unless otherwise noted, to describe a spectrum of people who were assigned "male" at birth and who wish to feminize or de-masculinize their speech (including male crossdressers, transsexual women, and bi-gendered or androgynous people born male). Similarly, "female-to-male" (FTM) refers to people who were assigned "female" at birth and who wish to masculinize or de-feminize their speech. This breadth of terminology is used to promote inclusion of non-transsexual clients who may seek speech feminization or masculinization services.

REFERENCES

Andrews, M. L. (1999). Voice and psychosocial dynamics: Gender presentation. In M. L. Andrews (Ed.), *Manual of voice treatment: Pediatrics through geriatrics* (pp. 432-446). San Diego, CA: Singular Publishing Group.

Andrews, M. L., & Schmidt, C. P. (1997). Gender presentation: Perceptual and acoustical analyses of voice. *Journal of Voice, 11*, 307-313.

Andrianopolous, M. V., Darrow, K., & Chen, J. (2001). Multimodal standardization of voice among four multicultural populations: Formant structures. *Journal of Voice, 15*, 61-77.

Becklund-Freidenberg, C. (2002). Working with male-to-female transgendered clients: Clinical considerations. *Contemporary Issues in Communication Science and Disorders, 29*, 58.

Bernhardt, B., Bacsfalvi, P., Gick, B., Radanov, B., & Williams, R. (2005). Exploring electropalatography and ultrasound in speech habilitation. *Journal of Speech-Language Pathology and Audiology, 29*, 169-182.

Bernhardt, B., Gick, B., Bacsfalvi, P., & Adler-Bock, M. (2005). Ultrasound in speech therapy with adolescents and adults. *Clinical Linguistics and Phonetics, 19*, 605-617.

Bernhardt, B., Gick, B., Bacsfalvi, P. & Ashdown, J. (2003). Speech habilitation of hard of hearing adolescents using electropalatography and ultrasound as evaluated by trained listeners. *Clinical Linguistics and Phonetics, 17*, 199-216.

Bralley, R. C., Bull, G. L., Gore, C. H., & Edgerton, M. T. (1978). Evaluation of vocal pitch in male transsexuals. *Journal of Communication Disorders, 11*, 443-449.

Brown, M., Perry, A., Cheesman, A. D., & Pring, T. (2000). Pitch change in male-to-female transsexuals: has phonosurgery a role to play? *International Journal of Language and Communication Disorders, 35*, 129-136.

Bowman, C., & Goldberg, J. M. (2006). Care of the patient undergoing sex reassignment surgery. *International Journal of Transgenderism, 9*(3/4), 135-136.

Byrne, L. A., Dacakis, G., & Douglas, J. M. (2003). Self-perceptions of pragmatic communication abilities in male-to-female transsexuals. *Advances in Speech Language Pathology, 5*, 15-25.

Challoner, J. (2000). The voice of the transsexual. In M. Freeman & M. Fawcus (Eds.), *Voice disorders and their management* (pp. 244-267). Philadelphia: Whurr Publishing.

Coleman, R. O. (1983). Acoustic correlates of speaker sex identification: Implications for the transsexual voice. *Journal of Sex Research, 19*, 293-295.

Dacakis, G. (2000). Long-term maintenance of fundamental frequency increases in male-to-female transsexuals. *Journal of Voice, 14*, 549-556.

Dacakis, G. (2002). The role of voice therapy in male-to-female transsexuals. *Current Opinion in Otolaryngology & Head and Neck Surgery, 10*, 173-177.

Dahl, M., Feldman, J. L., Goldberg, J. M., & Jaberi, A. (2006). Physical aspects of transgender endocrine therapy. *International Journal of Transgenderism, 9*(3/4), 111-134.

Davies, S., & Goldberg, J. (2006). *Gender transition: Changing speech.* Vancouver, BC: Vancouver Coastal Health Authority. Available online at http://www.vch.ca/transhealth/resources/library/tcpdocs/consumer/speech.pdf

de Bruin, M. D., Coerts, M. J., & Greven, A. J. (2000). Speech therapy in the management of male-to-female transsexuals. *Folia Phoniatrica et Logopaedica, 52*, 220-227.

de Jong, F. (2003). *Surgical raise of vocal pitch in male to female transsexuals.* Paper presented at the XVIII Biennial Symposium of the Harry Benjamin International Gender Dysphoria Association, Ghent, Belgium.

Delph-Janiurek, T. (1999). Sounding gender(ed): Vocal performances in English university teaching spaces. *Gender, Place and Culture: A Journal of Feminist Geography, 6*, 137-153.

Donald, P. J. (1982). Voice change surgery in the transsexual. *Head and Neck Surgery, 4*, 433-437.

Duffy, J.R., Werven G.W., & Aronson, A.E. (1997). Telemedicine and the diagnosis of speech and language disorders. *Mayo Clinic Proceedings, 72*, 1116-1122.

Elert, C-C., and Hamrnarberg, B. (1991). Regional voice variation in Sweden. In *Actes du XIIème Congres International des Sciences Phonétiques*, Vol. 4 (Université de Provence, Service des Publications, Aix-en-Provence), 418-420.

Gold, L. (1999). Voice training for the transsexual. *VASTA Newsletter, 13*. Retrieved January 1, 2005, from http://www.vasta.org/newsletter/99/summer03.html

Goldberg, J. M. (2006). *Recommended framework for training in speech feminization/masculinization.* Vancouver, BC: Vancouver Coastal Health Authority. Available online at http://www.vch.ca/transhealth/resources/library/tcpdocs/training-speech.pdf

Goldberg, J. M., & Lindenberg, M. (Eds.) (2001). *Trans-Forming community: Resources for trans people and our families.* Victoria, BC: Transcend Transgender Support & Education Society.

Goldberg, J. M., Matte, N., MacMillan, M., & Hudspith, M. (2003). *Community survey: Transition/crossdressing services in BC–Final report.* Vancouver, BC: Vancouver Coastal Health and Transcend Transgender Support & Education Society.

Goodnow, C. (2001, February 12). Speech therapy helps transgender women develop a feminine sound. *Seattle Post-Intelligencer.* Retrieved January 1, 2005, from http://seattlepi.nwsource.com/lifestyle/transgender.shtml

Graddol, D., & Swann, J. (1989). *Gender voices.* Oxford: Basil Blackwell Ltd.

Gross, M. (1999). Pitch-raising surgery in male-to-female transsexuals. *Journal of Voice, 13,* 246-250.

Günzburger, D. (1993). An acoustic analysis and some perceptual data concerning voice change in male-female trans-sexuals. *European Journal of Disorders of Communication, 28,* 13-21.

Hasegawa, Y. & Hata, K. (1995). The function of F_0-peak delay in Japanese. In J. Ahlers, L. Bilmes, J. S. Guenter, B. A. Kaiser, & J. Namkung (Eds.), *Proceedings of the 21st Annual Meeting of the Berkeley Linguistics Society* (pp. 141-151). Berkeley, CA: Berkeley Linguistics Society.

Haynes, E., & Kully, D. (2005). The use of telehealth in the treatment of stuttering. *Communiqué: The Newsletter of the Canadian Association of Speech-Language Pathologists and Audiologists, 19*(3), 4.

Hearing, Speech & Deafness Center (2005). Voice feminization. Seattle, WA: Author. Retrieved January 1, 2005, from http://www.hsdc.org/You/Speech/voicefem.htm

Hirano, M. (1981). Clinical examination of voice. In G. E. Arnold, F. Winckel, & B. D. Wyke (Eds.), *Disorders of human communication* (5th ed., pp. 81-84). New York: Springer-Verlag.

Hooper, C. R. (1985). Changing the speech and language of the male to female transsexual client: A case study. *Journal of the Kansas Speech-Language-Hearing Association, 25,* 6.

Jessiman, S. (2003). Speech and language services using telehealth technology in remote and underserved areas. *Journal of Speech-Language Pathology and Audiology, 27,* 45-51.

Kalra, M. A. (1977). Voice therapy with a transsexual. In R. Gemme & C. Wheeler (Eds.), *International Congress on Sexology* (pp. 77-84). New York: Plenum Press.

Kaye, J., Bortz, M. A., & Toumi, S. I. (1993). Evaluation of the effectiveness of voice therapy with a male-to-female transsexual subject. *Scandinavian Journal of Logopedic and Phoniatrics, 18,* 105-109.

Kent, R. D., & Lybolt, J. T. (1982). Techniques of therapy based on motor learning theory. In W. H. Perkins (Ed.), *General principles of therapy* (pp. 13-25). New York: Thieme-Stratton.

King, J. B., Lindstedt, D. E., Jensen, M., & Law, M. (1999). Transgendered voice: Considerations in case history management. *Logopedics Phoniatrics Vocology, 24,* 14-18.

Kohnert, K., Kennedy, M. R. T., Glaze, L., Kan, P. F., & Carney, E. (2003). Breadth and depth of diversity in Minnesota: Challenges to clinical competency. *American Journal of Speech-Language Pathology, 12,* 259-272.

Koschkee, D. L., & Rammage, L. (1997). *Voice care in a medical setting.* San Diego, CA: Singular Publishing Group.

Koufman, J. (n.d.). *Call for a moratorium on voice feminization surgery for the M-to-F transsexual in the United States.* Winston-Salem, NC: Center for Voice and Swallowing Disorders. Retrieved January 1, 2005, from http://www.inbroaddaylight.net/moratorium.htm

Kujawski, C. (2003). *The transsexual voice.* Unpublished manuscript, Michigan State University. Retrieved January 1, 2005, from http://www.msu.edu/course/asc/823c/2003%20Powerpoint%20Presentations/The%20Transsexual%20Voice.ppt

Kunachak, S., Prakunhungsit, S., & Sujjalak, K. (2000). Thyroid cartilage and vocal fold reduction: A new phonosurgical method for male-to-female transsexuals. *Annals of Otology, Rhinology and Laryngology, 109,* 1082-1086.

Lawrence, A. A. (2004). Voice feminization surgery: A critical overview. Seattle, WA: Author. Retrieved January 1, 2005, from http://www.annelawrence.com/voicesurgery.html

Linville, S. E. (1998). Acoustic correlates of perceived versus actual sexual orientation in men's speech. *Folia Phoniatrica et Logopaedica, 50,* 35-48.

Mashima, P.A., Birkmire-Peters, D.P., Syms, M.J., Holtel, M.R., Burgess, L.P., & Peters, L.J. (2003). Telehealth: Voice therapy using telecommunications technology. *American Journal of Speech-Language Pathology, 12,* 432-439.

Mikos, V. A., & Pausewang-Gelfer, M. (2001, November). *The relative contribution of speaking fundamental frequency and formant frequencies to gender identification of biological males, biological females, and male-to-female transgendered individuals based on isolated vowels.* Presented at the Convention of the American Speech-Language-Hearing Association, New Orleans, LA.

Moran, M. J., McCloskey, L., & Cady, B. (1995). Listener age estimates of elderly African American and Caucasian male speakers. *Journal of Cross-Cultural Psychology, 26,* 751-758.

Morris, R. J., & Brown, W. S. (1994). Age-related differences in speech variability among women. *Journal of Communication Disorders, 27*, 49-64.

Mount, K. H., & Salmon, S. J. (1988). Changing the vocal characteristics of a postoperative transsexual patient: A longitudinal study. *Journal of Communication Disorders, 21*, 229-238.

Myers, C. (2005). Telehealth applications in head and neck oncology. *Journal of Speech-Language Pathology and Audiology, 29*, 125-129.

Neumann, K., & Welzel, C. (2004). The importance of the voice in male-to-female transsexualism. *Journal of Voice, 18*, 153-167.

Neumann, K., Welzel, C., Gonnermann, U., & Wolfradt, U. (2002a). Cricothyroidopexy in male-to-female transsexuals: Modification Type IV. *International Journal of Transgenderism, 6*(3). Retrieved January 1, 2005, from http://www.symposion.com/ijt/ijtvo06no03_03.htm

Neumann, K., Welzel, C., Gonnermann, U., & Wolfradt, U. (2002b). Satisfaction of MtF Transsexuals with operative voice therapy: A questionnaire-based preliminary study. *International Journal of Transgenderism, 6*(4). Retrieved January 1, 2005, from http://www.symposion.com/ijt/ijtvo06no04_02.htm

Núñez, A. E. (2000). Transforming cultural competence into cross-cultural efficacy in women's health education. *Academic Medicine, 75*, 1071-1079.

Oates, J. M., & Dacakis, G. (1983). Speech pathology considerations in the management of transsexualism: A review. *British Journal of Disorders of Communication, 18*, 139-151.

Oates, J. M., & Dacakis, G. (1997). Voice change in transsexuals. *Venereology: Interdisciplinary, International Journal of Sexual Health, 10*, 178-187.

Oates, J., & Russell, A. (1997). Perceptual Voice Profile. In *A sound judgment: A CD-ROM to teach perceptual voice analysis* [CD-ROM]. Campbelltown, Australia: Clear Digital Vision.

Orloff, L. A. (2000). *Disorders of pitch*. San Diego, CA: Division of Otolaryngology–Head and Neck Surgery, University of California, San Diego. Retrieved January 1, 2005, from http://www.surgery.ucsd.edu/ent/PatientInfo/voi_pitch.html

Pausewang-Gelfer, M. (1999). Voice treatment for the male-to-female transgendered client. *American Journal of Speech-Language Pathology, 8*, 201-208.

Pausewang-Gelfer, M., & Mikos, V. A. (2005). The relative contributions of speaking fundamental frequency and formant frequencies to gender identification based on isolated vowels. *Journal of Voice, 19*, 544-554.

Pausewang-Gelfer, M., & Schofield, K. J. (2000). Comparison of acoustic and perceptual measures of voice in male-to-female transsexuals perceived as female versus those perceived as male. *Journal of Voice, 14*, 22-33.

Petty, B. (2004, April). *The vocal instrument: How it works and how to take care of it*. Paper presented at Transgender Voices Festival, Minneapolis, MN.

Perez, K. (2004). *Voice feminization for transgender women*. Denver, CO: Exceptional Voice, Inc. Retrieved January 1, 2005, from http://exceptionalvoice.com/transgender.html.

Pickuth, D., Brandt, S., Neumann, K., Berghaus, A., Spielmann, R. P., & Heywang-Kobrunner, S. H. (2000). Spiral computed tomography before and after cricothyroid approximation. *Clinical Otolaryngology, 25*, 311-314.

Prochaska, J. O., DiClemente, C. C., & Norcross, J. C. (1992). In search of how people change: Applications to addictive behaviors. *American Psychologist, 47*, 1102-1114.

Rose, P. (1991). How effective are long term mean and standard deviation as normalization parameters for tonal fundamental frequency? *Speech Communication, 10*, 229-247.

Sabol, J. W., Lee, L., & Stemple, J. C. (1995). The value of vocal function exercises in the practice regimen of singers. *Journal of Voice, 9*, 27-36.

Soderpalm, E., Larsson, A., & Almquist, S. A. (2004). Evaluation of a consecutive group of transsexual individuals referred for vocal intervention in the west of Sweden. *Logopedics Phoniatrics Vocology, 29*, 18-30.

Spencer, L. E. (1988). Speech characteristics of male-to-female transsexuals: A perceptual and acoustic study. *Folia Phoniatrica, 40*, 31-42.

Stemple, J. C., Lee, L., D'Amico, B., & Pickup, B. (1994). Efficacy of vocal function exercises as a method of improving voice production. *Journal of Voice, 8*, 271-278.

Titze, I. R. (1997). Are the corner vowels like primary colors? *Journal of Singing, 5*, 35-37.

Titze, I. R., & Verdolini, K. (in press). *Vocology*. Iowa City, IA: National Center for Voice and Speech.

Thomas, J. P. (2003). *Cricothyroid approximation and laryngeal reduction: Information on risks specific to this pitch altering surgery and reduction of the external appearance of the voice box*. Portland, OR: Author. Retrieved January 1, 2005, from http://www.voicedoctor.net/surgery/consentform/pitchconsent.html

Thomas, J. P. (2005). *Male to female vocal surgery*. Portland, OR: Author. Retrieved October 31, 2005, from http://www.voicedoctor.net/media/cases/pitch/index.html

Tom, K. (2004, November). *Fundamental frequency characteristics of Mexican-American speakers of English and Spanish*. Paper presented at the Annual Convention of the American Speech-Language-Hearing Association, Philadelphia, PA.

Van Borsel, J., De Cuypere, G., & Van den Berghe, H. (2001). Physical appearance and voice in male-to-female transsexuals. *Journal of Voice, 15*, 570-575.

Van Borsel, J., De Cuypere, G., Rubens, R., & Destaerke, B. (2000). Voice problems in female-to-male transsexuals. *International Journal of Language & Communication Disorders, 35*, 427-442.

Wagner, I., Fugain, C., Monneron-Girard, L., Cordier, B., & Chabolle, F. (2003). Pitch-raising surgery in fourteen male-to-female transsexuals. *Laryngoscope, 113*, 1157-1165.

Wilson, J. A., Webb, A., Carding, P. N., Steen, I. N., MacKenzie, K., & Deary, I. J. (2004). The Voice Symptom Scale (VoiSS) and the Vocal Handicap Index (VHI): A comparison of structure and content. *Clinical Otolaryngology, 29*, 169-174.

Wiltshire, A. (1995). Not by pitch alone: A view of transsexual vocal rehabilitation. *National Student Speech Language Hearing Association Journal, 22*, 53-57.

Wolfe, V. I., Ratusnik, D. L., Smith, F. H., & Northrop, G. (1990). Intonation and fundamental frequency in male-to-female transsexuals. *Journal of Speech & Hearing Disorders, 55*, 43-50.

Wollitzer, L. C. (1994). *Acoustic and perceptual cues to gender identification: A study of transsexual voice and speech characteristics.* Unpublished master's thesis, University of British Columbia, Vancouver, British Columbia, Canada.

Yang, C. Y., Palmer, A. D., Murray, K. D., Meltzer, T. R., & Cohen, J. I. (2002). Cricothyroid approximation to elevate vocal pitch in male-to-female transsexuals: Results of surgery. *Annals of Otology, Rhinology and Laryngology, 111*, 477-485.

Yardley, K. M. (1976). Training in feminine skills in a male transsexual: A pre-operative procedure. *British Journal of Medical Psychology, 49*, 329-339.

Zimmerman, G. L., Olsen, C. G., & Bosworth, M. F. (2000). A 'Stages of Change' approach to helping patients change behavior. *American Family Physician, 61*, 1409-1416.

doi:10.1300/J485v09n03_08

APPENDIX. The *Changing Keys* Program

Changing Keys (CK) is an English-language speech feminization program offered in Vancouver, British Columbia, Canada. CK was created by a speech-language pathologist (Shelagh Davies) as part of the Transgender Health Program's services. The program consists of (a) a one-hour individual speech and voice evaluation at the start of the program, (b) weekly two-hour speech and voice therapy group sessions, for seven weeks, (c) individualized sessions midway through the seven weeks, (d) speech therapy exercises to be done between groups ("homework"), (e) a one-hour individual speech and voice evaluation at the end of the program, and (f) a refresher session held 3 to 4 months after the course has ended. CK is held at a multidisciplinary inner city community health centre that serves large numbers of transgender clients and houses the Transgender Health Program and a transgender peer support group.

The program is limited to six self-identified transgender women who want to feminize their voice, don't have coverage for speech therapy through Extended Health or other benefits, can commit to coming to all of the sessions and doing practice sessions between groups, feel comfortable working on voice in a group setting, and are able to read and speak comfortably in English (individual speech therapy is recommended for clients who are only partially fluent in English, to allow more clinician attention). It is not necessary that participants be living as women, be taking hormones, or have had surgery. Participants are asked to present as women or gender-neutral at the therapy sessions, as this is felt to facilitate practice of feminine voice.

The program is subsidized by the Vancouver Coastal Health Authority, a health governance body responsible for delivery of health services in the Vancouver-Coast region of British Columbia, to make it possible for low-income transgender women to participate. Participants are asked to pay what they feel they can afford within a sliding scale of $0-$100 for the entire program. This funding structure was key in making the program accessible as there are high rates of poverty among transgender women (Goldberg et al., 2003).

APPLICATION PROCEDURE AND CLIENT SCREENING

CK is advertised extensively by notices and posters to service providers who work with transgender women, announcements in community peer support groups, and online announcements to community mailing lists. Interested participants are asked to apply to the Transgender Health Program by providing contact information and answering seven questions relating to eligibility:

1. What is your goal for taking part in Changing Keys?
2. This pilot is restricted to people who self-identify as transgender women/male-to-female. Does this fit for you?
3. This pilot is restricted to people who don't have coverage for speech therapy through Extended Health or other benefits. Do you have benefits that pay for speech therapy? If so, we recommend you use those benefits to pay for private sessions.

4. Have you read over the dates, and can you commit to coming to all the sessions?
5. What are your preferred times for the pre- and post-group assessment?
6. Are you comfortable listening to information about voice and doing practice exercises with other transgender women in a group?
7. Are you able to read and speak comfortably in English? If not, please contact the Transgender Health Program to discuss options. (The Transgender Health Program can explore possible referral to a multilingual speech therapist in private practice, or arrange funded interpretation service for individualized sessions with an English-speaking speech therapist.)

PROGRAM STRUCTURE

Initial Assessment

The assessment provides an opportunity to evaluate the client's current speech and voice production habits, determine how well the speech matches the inner sense of self, consider what changes would be beneficial, and evaluate how easy or difficult the changes would be. Speech and voice parameters assessed include average speaking pitch, speaking pitch range, impression of vocal inflectional patterns, and voice quality. If vocal loudness subjectively appears to be outside normal female range it is objectively evaluated by measuring the average, maximum and minimum speaking loudness. Speech and voice are assessed in oral reading, picture description, and spontaneous conversation. Discrepancies of parameters among tasks are noted. The assessment is audiotaped so it can be reviewed at the end of the program and compared with the follow-up evaluation.

A subjective evaluation is also done. The client describes three specific things she would like to change about her speech and voice or three situations in which she would like to sound more feminine. She also fills in a questionnaire describing how her current speech and voice affect her life.

The client is asked to identify real-life situations–ranging from easy to difficult–in which she can practice generalizing what was learned in the sessions. This helps her try things out while still having the support of the group. It also allows participants to take ownership of the techniques as they are learning them and can be a powerful motivator to continue practice.

The assessment includes trial therapy to determine how easily the client is able to make changes in her speech and voice. Parameters assessed may include producing voice at a higher pitch, varying vocal inflections, changing voice quality, and modifying characteristics of articulation.

At the end of the assessment the results are discussed with the client, and together the client and the therapist establish goals for specific therapy. The therapy process is explained to the client, the expected commitment is described, and any questions about the therapy program are answered. The client should leave the evaluation with a clear idea of what changes are possible and useful, and have a sense of the processes involved.

Weekly Sessions

Six 2-hour group sessions are held weekly. Sessions are divided into four parts: (a) checking in on previous week's practice, observation and carry-over activities–what worked, what didn't, and what needs to be modified in group exercises or the individual's practice, (b) voice training, with the goals of producing an easy, resonant voice at the target pitch and generalizing it into speech of increasing complexity, (c) exercises directed at a specific topic, such as increasing vocal inflections, and (d) information and discussion: e.g., pitch-raising surgery, gender markers in communication.

Individualized Sessions

Halfway through the program there are 30-minute individual sessions with each participant. These are used to give one-to-one input into particular areas of difficulty and to modify exercises to suit each client. For example, if the client has difficulty sustaining the voice at a target pitch, specific voice training is given or a more suitable pitch is used. These sessions are often client-driven, with the client providing the focus for the session.

Homework

As this is a short, intensive program, participants are expected to do substantial practice between sessions. Although homework requires substantial commitment, clients are often highly motivated and diligent in practice. Homework consists of three parts:

1. Basic vocal training exercises. These exercises are taught the first day of therapy and are to be done for 10 minutes twice a day. Instructions are written in the course manual and recorded on a CD or tape.
2. Weekly topics of practice. These include specific practice of the speech parameters discussed in the weekly therapy session, such as transferring a higher speaking pitch into different real life situations (e.g., asking for a

transfer on a bus or answering the phone), using wider vocal inflections, and being an active listener.

3. Observations. Becoming familiar with gendered differences in communication is essential to making changes, but unstructured observation can be overwhelming and ineffective. Each week, participants are asked to observe a specific aspect of women's speech. For example, questions relating to inflection may include: How does a woman's voice move around during speech? How are inflections different among women? Do inflections vary with the age of the speaker, the speaking situation, how the woman may be feeling emotionally, her conversational partner? Other topics have included: Do women laugh or smile at different times than men? How do women take turns in conversation? What do women do when they are listening? What is it about speech that makes it sound feminine or masculine?

Final Assessment

The parameters measured in the initial assessment are re-measured and the client again completes the subjective evaluation form. The pre- and post- measurements and the tape recordings are compared and changes noted. Suggestions for modification and continuation of practice are discussed. The client's input about the course is sought.

Refresher Session

A 2 hour refresher session is held 3 to 4 months after the completion of the program. Participants bring a completed self-evaluation questionnaire and vocal parameters are reassessed. The basic exercises of the program are reviewed and there is time to discuss successes and challenges of using their new voice in the real world. This session serves as both a motivator for continued practice and an opportunity for the clinician to provide guidance on difficulties experienced by the client.

VOICE TRAINING

One of the aims of the Changing Keys program is to develop the production of a higher speaking pitch range that is efficient and easy to produce–a common goal of most course participants. The protocol used is based on the Lessac Marsden Resonant Voice Therapy (LMRVT) program, developed by Katherine Verdolini (Titze & Verdolini, in press).

Verdolini developed this therapy protocol for treating voice disorders, using input from both traditional singing and speaking voice pedagogy and current concepts in voice science and psychology. Although the protocol was not developed specifically to train transgender women, the twin focuses of ease and forward resonance sensations train efficient voice production that helps protect the vocal folds from damage. The forward focus may also help increase vowel formants, helping the voice to be perceived as female (Becklund-Freidenberg, 2002).

The core exercise program is taught in the first session and includes stretching, relaxing exercises, and producing the voice at a target pitch. Specific sounds that have been shown to encourage efficient vocal fold vibration and maximize forward resonance sensations are used to train the higher pitch. Voice training takes approximately 60 minutes in the first session, and then 20-30 minutes in subsequent sessions. Participants are instructed on how to monitor their practice. Difficulties that occur in practice, such as throat tightness or effortful production, are addressed in subsequent sessions and individual instruction is given as necessary.

Core Exercise Program

Relaxation

We begin with standard general relaxation exercises to relax the head and neck area, jaw, tongue, face, and mid-body respiratory muscles; additional exercises may be suggested for individual participants as needed. A goal during this time is to increase general awareness of how the mind and body feel at this particular point in this particular day: tired or rested, anxious or calm, focused or scattered, tight shoulders, breath-holding, etc.

Facilitating Production in the Upper Pitch Range

Using a voiced bilabial fricative ("raspberry") or a tongue trill (Spanish "r") the clients glide the voice around in the middle to upper pitch range. This technique is used in both voice therapy and singing pedagogy and has been described in Joseph Stemple's Vocal Function Exercises (Sabol et al., 1995; Stemple et al., 1994). According to Stemple, going to the end ranges of the voice has a similar effect as stretching a muscle to end range; the exercise facilitates ease and efficiency in the middle ranges. For our purposes, we are exploring the sensations of producing a higher-pitched voice easily and efficiently.

Sensations during the exercise are carefully monitored. The voice should feel resonant and easy in the throat at all pitches. If the throat begins to tighten in the higher pitches, voice therapy facilitation techniques are used. The goal is to produce a resonant, easy sound throughout the upper pitch range. Going into falsetto register is fine in this exercise. Although the target speaking pitch should be in modal rather than falsetto register, some transsexual women are able to use the falsetto occasionally when using a wide pitch range, and this can sound acceptable as long as it is well blended with the rest of the voice.

After this voice training program, the voice should not feel tired: it should feel warmed up and ready to use. If the voice begins to feel tired or if there is throat sensation, this is a signal that some intervention needs to be done in the way of modifying voice production technique. The exercise of gliding around in the upper part of the voice is then expanded into vowels.

Producing a Higher-Pitched Voice

Raising the average speaking pitch is a common goal among group participants, and is supported in the literature and by experienced clinicians. However, there is a wide range of clinical opinion about how to train a higher pitched voice and what pitch is optimal to target. Most clinicians agree that a goal for English-language speakers is to train a voice that is somewhere in the "middle range" between non-transgender English-speaking men's and women's voices–between 155 and 185 Hz. However, transsexual women frequently prefer a higher target pitch, so some experimentation may be necessary to establish what is both possible and optimal.

Once the body and voice have been "warmed up" using the previous exercises, we start the voice on a 2 to 3 second /m/ at F3 or 185 Hz. Because this is a group program, we use one pitch for practice; in one-to-one sessions it would be possible to choose a target pitch that matches a client's individual goals and existing vocal capacity. F3 (185 Hz) is a training pitch, not a target for average speaking pitch: it is higher than what most transsexual women will use in everyday speech. However, it is beneficial for participants to experience the sensations of producing a voice without strain that is much higher than their accustomed pitch. If this pitch produces strain for any participants, we lower the target pitch to one that can be produced with feelings of ease. A number of CK participants have commented that F3 (185 Hz) is too low and they use a higher one when doing this practice at home.

In accordance with the LMRVT protocol, clients are asked to monitor two things as they practice: Does the voice feel easy to produce, and does the sound feel like it is going up and out (or does it feel like it is getting caught–in the throat or anywhere else)? If the client does not have these sensations of ease, we do specific facilitation exercises. We then use the LMRVT protocol to expand this sensation of easy, resonant voice production into sounds and words. The goal is to generalize this easy, resonant, higher-pitched voice, first in structured speech and then into spontaneous speech in increasingly difficult situations.

Extending the Higher-Pitched Voice into Speech

Generalizing the use of higher pitch follows standard speech and voice therapy protocols, starting with easier tasks and gradually working into more challenging ones. Speech tasks are those that are common in speech and voice therapy, progressing from single words to short phrases, greetings, short oral reading tasks, picture descriptions, and structured questions and answers. While the voice is first produced at only one pitch (chanting), as soon as possible regular speech inflections are introduced.

Maintaining elevated pitch in a resonant voice that feels easy to produce is a vocally athletic task; the client is sustaining a pitch that the vocal mechanism was not constructed to produce. It must be done efficiently, both to sound like natural female speech and also to avoid the development of voice problems. Transferring this easy, resonant, efficient method of producing a higher pitched voice into everyday life is both challenging and important.

In doing these exercises the client begins to develop a physical sense of how she can produce a feminine voice and an aural sense of what it sounds like. It will necessarily sound very different from her male voice. This altered perception can be quite disorienting and it is essential to have a time period of adjustment to play around with what is possible and what may be the best fit with the participant's personality and sense of self.

As pitch work progresses, the average speaking pitch is checked periodically. There is no expectation that the average pitch will remain at the target training pitch of 185 Hz, but if it drops below 155 Hz there needs to be further work producing a higher voice in sustained sounds. At this point, practice in vocal inflections is begun, along with practice in producing the higher pitches.

Vocal Inflections

This phase of treatment begins with a discussion about English-language vocal inflections and associations with "femininity" and "masculinity," to determine clients' perceptions and existing knowledge. In feminizing vocal inflections among English-language speakers the goals are to decrease flat inflections, increase inflectional range, and increase vocal flexibility (the amount the voice moves around within a phrase, rather than the extent of pitch excursions).

As with other topics, we start work on vocal inflections by listening. For this purpose I use a tape of eight speakers describing a picture. The speakers are males and females of different ages and cultural backgrounds. We listen specifically to the vocal inflections used by the speakers, paying particular attention to different patterns used by men and women. Clients are also instructed to listen to conversations in their community and pay particular attention to vocal inflections.

Individuals who have habitually used little vocal inflection in speech often find that expanding the inflectional range feels embarrassing and artificial. In exploring vocal inflectional range clients are encouraged to go "over the top," far beyond what they would realistically use in speech. This can have a freeing effect and also allow the client to experiment without being restricted by what would be considered appropriate; refinements happen at a later stage of the program.

Exercises initially use limited vocabulary so the client must use a range of vocal inflections to convey meaning and emotional expression. As in any standard speech therapy protocol, the complexity of the task increases as the person's performance improves. Carryover into everyday life can be facilitated by choosing a specific phrase or sentence that the client uses frequently.

Work with inflections continues throughout the program, as this is an important aspect of speech and also one that usually takes time to change and habituate. As with pitch, clients frequently report they need to monitor these vocal parameters constantly during conversation. For this reason it is useful in the early stages of therapy to choose specific practice times when the client will be conscious of speech and voice production and use the techniques learned in therapy. The client is asked to begin with a person or place that is "comfortable" or "easy," and gradually extend the practice rather than confronting very difficult situations right away. Building confidence in the new speech and voice is an important part of the therapy program.

Vocal Quality: Breathy versus Resonant Speech

Among English-language speakers, mildly breathy speech is associated with feminine voice. Many transgender women have already adopted a breathy voice by the time they seek therapy. Mild breathiness also has the advantage of automatically modifying hard attacks on consonants and vowels, giving speech a softer quality. However there is a contradiction between resonant voice, which is the focus of CK, and breathy voice. A breathy quality is produced with less efficiency so the voice may be more prone to vocal fatigue and not be heard against background noise.

This contradiction is discussed as part of the group sessions and participants generally report intuitively finding their own ways of dealing with voice quality issues. For participants experiencing throat pain or vocal fatigue, the resonant voice works best as it lasts longer and is louder; other participants feel more comfortable with a breathier quality as it better conveys the impression they want. Some participants adopt a resonant voice in loud situations and a breathier one in quiet ones. This ability to change vocal qualities requires good control over voice production and may be a reasonable goal for some transgender women who are concerned about voice quality issues.

Vocal Loudness

CK participants typically struggle more with achieving adequate loudness in a noisy environment than an inappropriately loud speaking voice. Using a resonant voice increases loudness in an efficient and effective way, and can be trained specifically to be used where there is a lot of background noise. If loudness is a concern for participants, the group does a vocal exercise involving repetition of a phrase with differing levels of loudness. The goal is to increase the loudness by increasing resonance sensation, not by pushing from the throat. If the resonant voice is judged as too loud, there are specific training exercises that reduce loudness while maintaining forward focus; as discussed earlier, adopting a breathy quality will automatically reduce loudness.

Motor Speech Characteristics

Hard onsets on initial vowels and consonants are generally considered a masculine speech characteristic among English-language speakers (Andrews, 1999; Gold, 1999). Adopting a breathy voice quality may be enough to soften the onsets so they are no longer perceived as abrupt; conversely, softening the onsets may give a softer, breathier quality to the voice. As it is easier to modify a general feature of voice production than to specifically change each production of an initial phoneme, paying attention to voice quality may be the easier way to achieve a cluster of goals. We discuss articulation as we are experimenting with voice quality so participants are aware of the interaction.

Encouraging more connected speech production can also help reduce the abrupt interruptions in speech flow that hard onsets create. This technique is similar to vocal prolongation used in fluency therapy; however, in this instance, the speech rate is maintained at a normal or near normal level.

In working with articulation we listen to examples of "feminine" and "masculine" patterns or listen to the speech of a group participant who already uses connected speech and gentle onsets. The group then repeats specific phrases or words, to get the feeling of that kind of production. Due to time constraints the group generally does not spend a significant length of time on articulation; if it is of particular concern to an individual, intervention may take place in a private session.

Language and Discourse Pragmatics

Although language choice and speaker-listener interaction during conversation are influenced by many factors other than gender, there is a body of work in the sociolinguistics and popular literature specific to gender influences on communication. We discuss this literature in CK, both to give a point of reference and to stimulate debate and observation skills. Participants then see whether or not what is written in textbooks is actually happening in their own communities. This encourages context-specific norms that are flexible and can easily be adapted to suit the client's personality and situation. Also, since word choice and interaction in conversation vary greatly from person to person and situation to situation, training specific behaviours is too rigid. The participants are encouraged to consider what women and men in their own communities are doing, and to determine which patterns feel comfortable to them.

Topics discussed include in this phase of the program include: (a) the use of qualifiers and tags, such as "isn't it," "sort of," "kind of," "don't you think," "I think that," and "could you possibly," (b) sharing difficulties and problems as a means of establishing connection, (c) confirming the speaker's emotional messages, (d) making comments about another woman's clothing or appearance, (e) direct versus indirect confrontation, (f) listening styles and behaviors, and (g) cues relating to conversational turn-taking and interruptions.

Role playing is typically used for therapy exercises that target language choice and discourse pragmatics. For example, if the purpose of the exercise was to use words that convey more emotional content, the participants could describe a picture, focusing on its emotional impact. For exercises focusing on development of active listening skills, participants may practice in pairs; the listener is instructed to encourage the speaker and actively show that she is paying attention, while the speaker must seek the listener's opinion and involvement in the conversation. If the goal was to make a casual connection with another woman in a public place, two participants could role-play having a casual conversation in a public setting, such as chatting in a lineup at a cashier, trying on clothes, or waiting at a bus stop. To facilitate carryover, participants are asked to practice the issue addressed in the group in real-world situations, as homework.

PRELIMINARY EVALUATION OF CHANGING KEYS

CK is a new program, and evaluation of its effectiveness is still in the early stages. Preliminary results suggest a range of outcomes, with some participants experiencing more significant change than others. On a self-evaluation questionnaire most participants noted positive changes in their speech and voice, and expressed increased confidence when speaking. Further evaluation is needed to assess the program's effectiveness and refine the CK protocol.

Social and Medical Transgender Case Advocacy

Catherine White Holman
Joshua M. Goldberg

SUMMARY. While some clients are confident self-advocates, many transgender individuals and loved ones find it difficult to advocate for themselves and turn to a trusted clinician for assistance. This article discusses the role of the health and social service clinician in transgender case advocacy. Although the setting, circumstances, and client needs vary greatly, the overarching goal of clinical advocacy is to address the societal barriers that interfere with clients' functionality and well-being. We suggest a protocol for advocacy assessment in the clinical setting and discuss trans-specific advocacy concerns relating to financial assistance, employment, changing identification, general advocacy, and outline concerns of specific populations within the transgender community. doi:10.1300/J485v09n03_09 *[Article copies available for a fee from The Haworth Document Delivery Service: 1-800-HAWORTH. E-mail address: <docdelivery@haworthpress.com> Website: <http://www.HaworthPress.com> © 2006 by The Haworth Press, Inc. All rights reserved.]*

KEYWORDS. Transgender, transsexual, crossdressing, gender variance, advocacy

Advocacy is part of the scope of practice for health and social service clinicians working with transgender people and loved ones. Although the setting, circumstances, and client needs vary greatly, the overarching goal of clinical advocacy is to address the societal barriers that interfere with clients' functionality and well-being.

Case advocacy refers to support of an individual client by (a) increasing the client's ability to be self-determining, (b) conveying the client's wishes in circumstances where the client cannot speak for themselves, and (c) making recommendations based on the client's best interests, when the client's wishes are not known and cannot be determined (Blackmore, 2001). In our combined 20 years experience as advocates within community health settings, case advocacy is the level of advocacy most typically engaged in by health and social service practitioners who provide direct client care.[1]

Catherine White Holman is Community Counselor, Three Bridges Community Health Centre, Vancouver, BC, Canada. Joshua M. Goldberg is Education Consultant of the Transgender Health Program, Vancouver, BC, Canada.

Address correspondence to: Catherine White Holman, 1292 Hornby Street, Vancouver, BC, Canada V6Z 1W2 (E-mail: Catherine.WhiteHolman@vch.ca).

This manuscript was created for the Trans Care Project, a joint initiative of Transcend Transgender Support & Education Society and Vancouver Coastal Health's Transgender Health Program, with funding from the Canadian Rainbow Health Coalition. The authors thank Bronwyn Barrett, Jael Emberley, Dianne Goldberg, Gail Knudson, Fraser Norrie, Megan Oleson, Lukas Walther, and Nadine Wu for their comments on an earlier draft, and Donna Lindenberg, Olivia Ashbee, A. J. Simpson, and Rodney Hunt for research assistance.

Available online at http://ijt.haworthpress.com
© 2006 by The Haworth Press, Inc. All rights reserved.
doi:10.1300/J485v09n03_09

While some clients are confident self-advocates, many transgender individuals and loved ones find it difficult to advocate for themselves due to overwhelming life circumstances, fear of reprisal resulting from a direct challenge to an individual in power, or physical or financial barriers to self-representation (Simpson & Goldberg, 2006). In these circumstances clients may seek advocacy assistance from loved ones, community peers, health or social service professionals, or professional advocates who are not clinicians.

Although health and social service clinicians are not usually advocacy experts, in some circumstances the health or social service clinician is, by virtue of their professional standing and expertise, best positioned to assist in case advocacy. Many government systems require a medical or mental health clinician to provide documentation to support an application (e.g., disability or health benefits, change to legal sex designation, refugee claim). In other cases, advocacy is requested to navigate the health and social service system, or to help deal with transphobic discrimination within health and social services.

Case advocacy is most often considered part of social work scope of practice, and social workers do provide many of the types of advocacy assistance outlined in this article. However, physicians, nurses, and mental health professionals may also be asked by transgender people or loved ones to provide case advocacy. We have therefore written this article for an interdisciplinary audience, indicating areas where a specific type of clinician is more likely to be involved.

In all areas of clinical practice, but particularly in advocacy, it is imperative that the clinician be attentive to issues of power and privilege, and seek to understand how the broader historical and social contexts influence clinician-client interactions. Advocates can have a significant positive influence on clients' access to resources and choices, but there is also the potential for an advocate to misrepresent a client's wishes or best interests, or to remove the client's agency by making decisions for the client (Goldsmith & Reid, 1997). It is important to ensure that even when a clinician is representing a client, the clinician is still acting on the client's behalf and under the client's instructions (Simpson & Goldberg, 2006).

INITIAL ADVOCACY ASSESSMENT

Assessment of advocacy needs may be done by semi-structured interview, standardized questionnaire, or a combination of both. It has been our experience that a significant number of transgender people did not complete school and are not functionally literate (this is also a concern for people who are not fluent in English); others find verbal interviews very difficult due to speech disability or anxiety about interacting with a clinician. For this reason we strongly recommend offering the client a choice of completing any forms or applications by verbal interview or by writing, and offering translation or interpretation for any clients who need assistance.

The content of advocacy assessment depends largely on the work setting (e.g., institution vs. community, rural vs. urban), client group (e.g., youth vs. adults), and the priorities of each client. We recommend using a flexible staged process that first identifies immediate risks to health and safety–such as abuse or violence, unsafe working or living conditions, hunger, suicidality, untreated physical or mental health conditions, or acute substance use detoxification–and then considers broader health and psychosocial issues. Immediate goals may include strengthening the support network, reducing isolation, building resiliency and self-esteem, assistance with system navigation, stabilizing housing (e.g., by referring to shelters and/or affordable housing), or facilitating referral to medical or mental health services.

As discussed in a later section of this article, many transgender people in North America live in poverty and often have difficulty paying for daily costs of living as well as the costs of health care. Early in the assessment process it is important to determine how clients financially survive (e.g., work income, social assistance, family help) and to assess whether they are receiving the benefits to which they are entitled.

Assessment of support should include friends, family of origin, chosen family, ethnocultural community, faith community, social community, relationship to the transgender community, and professional supports. Care should be taken not to assume a particular family structure either in family of origin or chosen family, and to be inclusive of any loved ones the client feels are important. For example, pets can be an important support to people who have social anxiety or who are socially isolated.

In addition to assessing social supports, we also routinely assess grief and loss. It has been our experience that transgender people and loved ones have often experienced multiple losses related to social stigma. Losses may include rejection by family, friends, and community, following disclosure of being transgender or the loved one of a transgender person; loss of work; and loss of housing.

While it is important to gain an accurate sense of areas of concern, care is needed to ascertain strengths as well. Determining personal strengths and positive supports is necessary, not only to bolster a client's sense of competency and ability to be self-determining, but also to create a complete picture of the client's life.

TRANS-SPECIFIC CONSIDERATIONS IN CASE ADVOCACY

General advocacy skills utilized with other clients in clinical settings are the same advocacy skills needed for work with the transgender community, but there are trans-specific concerns that clinicians should be familiar with. In all work with the transgender community, clinicians should be familiar with basic transgender psychosocial issues, and are expected to be respectful and non-discriminatory. In trans-specific advocacy, expertise is needed beyond basic awareness and sensitivity: clinicians must know how to effectively navigate the systems their clients are encountering, and must be able to provide effective and appropriate advocacy assistance.

In our experience, the systems commonly encountered by transgender clients and loved ones are often poorly integrated and poorly documented, creating significant frustration both for the client and the clinician. It is imperative that clinician advocates understand the systems their clients are engaged with, and keep informed of changes to these systems. In British Columbia, the Transgender Health Program and Transcend Transgender Support & Education Society have created online "how to" guides that explain systems and processes to

clinicians and clients (Goldberg & Lindenberg, 2001; White Holman & Goldberg, 2006). We encourage clinicians to work with transgender community organizations, which often have strong experiential systems knowledge, to develop practical guides for clinician advocates specific to other regions.

Service Referrals

Client assessment includes consideration of resources to address issues that are beyond the clinician's scope of practice. Referrals for transgender individuals and loved ones often require advocacy, and it is important to be cognizant of this in developing a care plan.

Most transgender people and many loved ones have had the experience of being refused services outright, either being told, "We don't serve people like you" or, "We don't know how to help you." Before making a referral it is important to contact the referral source to ensure that the service is accessible to transgender people. In many cases it is necessary to actively advocate as part of making a referral, to educate agency staff about transgender sensitivity protocols and trans-specific accommodations that may be required.

We often try to gauge the overall trans-sensitivity and competency of a program by asking about previous experience working with transgender people, and routinely share this information with our clients so they know what to expect and can discuss any education or preparation they feel is needed as part of the referral process. Depending on client concerns and the scope of the services sought, we may also inquire about trans-specific accommodations. Safe access to washrooms is often a key issue regardless of the type of service. If the referral involves a residential program, we often ask about bathing facilities, sleeping arrangements, and safe storage of wigs, prosthetics, and medical equipment such as hormones and dilators. Residential concerns are discussed further below.

Because transgender people often have difficulty accessing gender-specific services, we are particularly careful to inquire about client inclusion and exclusion criteria, transgender experience, and trans-specific protocols before making a referral to an agency or program that is specifically for women or for men. In addition to considering the issues for residential services discussed below, the clinician should determine whether the content of service (e.g., counseling relating to childhood trauma) is so specific that it excludes participation of transgender women and men. Bi-gender, multi-gender, and androgynous individuals who want to access a gender-specific service may require more concerted advocacy to facilitate the referral.

In these sorts of preliminary inquiries no identifying information about the client should be shared unless the client requests it to promote continuity of care. If there is no immediate risk to the client's safety, explicit consent is needed prior to the sharing of information.

Reducing Barriers to Accessing Services

In a survey of rural and urban transgender community members ($N = 179$), 72% reported difficulty accessing health care services related to gender transition or crossdressing, with financial expense the most commonly reported barrier to access (55% of respondents, n = 130) and 43% of respondents reporting services were not available in their region (Goldberg et al., 2003). Individuals living in rural and remote areas, those living in prison or residential care facilities, and those who are housebound as a result of chronic illness or disability may have particular difficulty accessing community services. Goldberg and Lindenberg (2001) suggest that clinician advocates can help address financial and geographic barriers by advocating with government programs for assistance with service, transportation, and accommodation fees, and arranging in-residence visits for individuals who cannot travel. Telehealth advocacy services may be more accessible for some clients than in-person office visits (Davies & Goldberg, 2006).

Societal binary norms of gender create unique barriers for individuals who are bi-gendered or multi-gendered, androgynous, or have fluid gender identity or expression. This is problematic in terms of the bureaucratic requirements transgender individuals may have to negotiate (e.g., filling out paperwork that asks "M or F") and also in accessing sex- and gender-segregated facilities such as public washrooms or addiction treatment services. The clinician advocate working in an agency can take an active role in internal systemic advocacy, making forms and facilities welcoming for people who do not fit within binary gender norms.

Language barriers are a concern for individuals with disabilities that affect communication or those with low literacy due to learning disabilities, lack of educational opportunity, or limited knowledge of the dominant language. Clinicians can advocate for funding to translate consumer materials into large print and audio format for individuals with visual disabilities, and can assist in creating graphics-based information for individuals with low reading literacy. In North America, many trans-specific print and peer support resources are available only in English (although there are also francophone groups in some areas of Canada, and Spanish groups in some areas of the U.S.). It has been our experience that interpreter services may not be an option for people who are not fully out as transgender, as there are privacy and confidentiality concerns for people in small, tightly-knit communities where an interpreter may know a transgender person's family or social peers. Additionally, interpreters must be familiar enough with transgender issues to accurately translate; this is particularly crucial for medical information. While interpretation and translation services do not replace multilingual clinical services, both are important services in areas where multilingual services are not readily available. Clinician advocates can assist by lobbying for coverage of interpreter and translation services so the financial burden does not fall on the client.

While all transgender people and loved ones can benefit from clinical advocacy to reduce barriers to accessing services, some populations are particularly vulnerable to the social inequities that make advocacy necessary. Transgender youth and elders, migrants, people with disabilities, people of colour, sex trade workers, people who use illicit drugs, and homeless people face both transphobia and additional economic and social oppression. Clinicians must actively engage in reaching out to transgender individuals who experience multiple forms of marginalization and oppression, and must be particularly attentive to the multiple barriers that exist for these populations in accessing care.

Common Issues of Concern in Transgender Case Advocacy

Transgender people and loved ones present with a wide variety of advocacy needs. The following areas, in our experience, are relatively frequent concerns for clients and also for clinicians who are unsure of how to provide the best possible care. However, our experience is specific to community work in British Columbia, and should not be considered universally representative. The issues discussed below are not prioritized in order of importance: immediate needs vary from client to client. As discussed in the previous section, the first task should be a thorough assessment that determines the client's immediate situation and priorities.

Financial Assistance

Daily Costs of Living

A number of studies in North American cities have documented high poverty and unemployment rates among transgender individuals (Goldberg et al., 2003; Lombardi, Wilchins, Priesing, & Malouf, 2001; Nemoto, Operario, Keatley, & Villegas, 2004). In the study by Goldberg et al. (2003), 31% of 179 participants reported income from social assistance (i.e., provincial or federal government benefits), non-government pension, or long-term disability funds. Accordingly, clinicians working with the transgender community should be familiar with social assistance programs. It has been our experience that people applying for government benefits often need help to complete the initial application and, in some cases, to initiate appeals and advocate throughout the appeal process. Clinicians without poverty advocacy experience should consider consulting with or referring to experienced poverty law advocates.

Health Care Benefits

As part of assessment, clinician advocates should determine whether their transgender clients have the full health coverage to which they are entitled. In some regions, health care costs may be covered by individuals paying directly, by government bodies, or by private insurance companies; in other regions direct client payment is the only option. In regions where clients qualify for health benefits, assistance may be needed with application for coverage or submission of claim forms, and advocacy required if benefits are denied.

The clinician advocate should be familiar with general public health coverage and knowledgeable about which types of care are excluded. In regions where there is public health coverage for feminizing or masculinizing medical interventions (hormone therapy, electrolysis or laser hair removal, speech therapy, and sex reassignment surgery), the clinician should be aware of specific eligibility criteria and any required assessments. Clients may need assistance to understand the process of applying for coverage and to coordinate the collection of required documentation. Clinicians may also be asked to provide collateral information in the form of a letter to the assessors to confirm that the client meets eligibility criteria.

In many regions transition-related expenses are not fully covered by public or private benefit plans, and the client may have to pay directly not only for medical services but also costs relating to changes in clothing and identification. Referral to a trans-positive debt counselor, financial planner, credit union, or other financial aid resource may be appropriate.

Assistance with the Costs of Child Care

The needs of transgender parents are often not recognized as it is assumed that transgender people do not have children. It has been our experience that many transgender parents are single parents with low incomes, and we therefore strongly recommend inquiring about child care needs as part of general assessment. In some regions, child care subsidies are available as part of social assistance.

Housing Assistance

In studies of transgender communities in several regions of North America, 20-25% of participants reported unsatisfactory housing conditions (Goldberg et al., 2003; Minter &

Daley, 2003; Risser & Shelton, 2002; Xavier & Simmons, 2000). As with any population that is disproportionately poor, transgender people may need assistance to find affordable long-term housing. Transgender people may also need assistance to find safe emergency housing or shelter (Mottet & Ohle, 2003).

With both long-term and short-term housing, advocacy may be needed to address discrimination by landlords or harassment by neighbours. In North America, transgender or Two-Spirit Aboriginal people and transgender people of colour, youth, elders, individuals who do not have legal status in the country they are living in, people with disabilities, and injection drug users are particularly at risk due to the intersection of oppressions that increase risk for poverty, violence, and discrimination in housing.

Emergency housing and shelter needs depend on the client's circumstances. For some transgender people and loved ones, poverty relating to employment discrimination or inability to work leads to homelessness. Others are fleeing violence by a family member, current or former romantic partner, co-worker, or neighbour, and need both shelter and trauma support services. Homelessness may be the result of eviction by a prejudiced landlord, or abandonment by loved ones upon disclosure of personal transgender identity or a relationship with a transgender person.

In North America, many emergency housing facilities and shelters are sex-segregated and lack adequate private access to showers, bathrooms, and sleeping facilities. Some residential facilities make placement decisions based on genitals rather than gender identity. Surgery-based policies are not only profoundly disrespectful of transgender people's sense of self but also expose transgender people to harassment and assault by other residents. Strategies for residential advocacy and accommodation are further discussed in a later section.

Systemic advocacy is necessary to promote agency-wide policy changes that remove barriers to transgender people. However, case advocacy is also useful, as many shelters have a transgender access policy that involves case-by-case decisions about whether or not the person is "appropriate" as a client. In our experience, shelter intake staff who lack experience

with transgender people often overestimate the complexity of integrating transgender clients into their service and are, as a result, hesitant to allow transgender people in. Advocates can offer examples of the practical, simple strategies used by other shelters to successfully accommodate transgender needs, such as a curtain across a shower stall or access to a single-user bathroom. An excellent resource manual available online can be used to help emergency shelters design policy and practice guidelines for the accommodation of transgender clients (Mottet & Ohle, 2003).

In regions where crisis social services are available, there have been cases of authorization of coverage for a transgender adult to temporarily stay at a motel when no emergency shelter facilities were available. This is not the preferred option as it makes access to ancillary shelter services (laundry, food, etc.) more difficult and promotes segregation of transgender clients, but in some cases a motel may be the safest or only option.

Employment Advocacy

It is not uncommon for transgender individuals to experience discrimination and harassment at work (Lombardi et al., 2001). In regions with human rights legislation, blatant discrimination can be addressed by human rights complaints. Union grievance may be feasible if the employee works in a unionized workplace. The clinician's role in both instances would be to help the client find appropriate legal advocacy resources, with referral to peer or professional support services if there is emotional distress.

In some cases proactive employment advocacy can be useful in preventing harassment or discrimination. For example, transgender people intending to "come out" or transition on the job can be assisted to develop a plan that includes education for the employer about the practical aspects of on-the-job transition and the legal rights of transgender employees (Horton, 2001; Walworth, 1998). Health and social service clinicians can provide useful information that frames the transition as a carefully considered process necessary to improve quality of life, rather than a frivolous choice.

In some cases transgender people may seek vocational assistance to explore career options or obtain retraining. If referral to specialized employment services is appropriate, care should be taken to ensure that vocational counseling resources are trans-competent prior to referral.

Changing Identification and Records

Transgender people who use a name that is different than their legal name or prefer a different pronoun than their legal sex designation may require assistance to advocate for use of preferred name and pronoun at work, school, and health and social service settings. It is not only considered disrespectful to use the wrong name or pronoun to address a transgender client, but in some jurisdictions is legally considered harassment if done intentionally and persistently (San Francisco Unified School District, 2000). Employers, teachers, health and social service professionals, and other public service personnel are expected to use the name and pronoun that a transgender person has indicated is preferred. Clinicians can assist with case advocacy when there are institutional barriers to implementation.

Some transgender people may seek assistance to legally change name or sex designation. Clinicians or community advocates can help with the application process, obtaining updated identification, and change of government, work, school, bank, and other institutional records. As there are multiple fees to legally change identification and obtain new identification, advocacy with the issuing agency or social services may be necessary to make it possible for transgender people living in poverty to complete the process.

Name Change

Many transgender people change their names informally or formally to better match their sense of self. Some people may be satisfied with informally asking others to use their preferred name; others want to legally change their name. In some cases name change is done not only to be consistent with felt sense of self, but also to mark a transition, to distance oneself from the past, or to protect privacy (e.g., fear of violence by former partners).

In industrialized countries, virtually all institutions require recording of legal name. Advocacy to enable recording of *preferred* name both validates a client's autonomy and right to self-define identity, and also makes it easier to ensure consistent use of the preferred name. If a worksite, school, health clinic, or other institution uses a computerized system that cannot be changed to include a field for preferred name, alternative accommodation should be sought, such as noting preferred name in a "notes" field.

Procedures for legal change of name vary greatly from region to region. Transgender clinical advocates should become familiar with the institution that handles name change, the process to change name, and any associated costs. A sample letter from a physician presenting name change as a medical necessity is available as an online supplement at http://www. vch.ca/transhealth/resources/library/tcpdocs/ guidelines-advocacy.pdf

Pronoun Change

Assumptions are often made about a preferred pronoun based on name or, in some cases, on legal sex designation. As most institutions do not track a client's preference for gender pronoun (she, he, or a gender-neutral pronoun such as "zie"), we recommend advocacy for discontinuation of gender-specific forms of address (e.g., "Mr." or "Ms." on letters) and use of the client's name instead of gender pronouns. If the client prefers that a specific pronoun be used, advocating for inclusion of gender pronoun preference in a "notes" field or on the inside front cover of a client's paper file is appropriate.

Change of Legal Sex Designation

Legal sex is the designation "M" or "F" that appears on legal records and some forms of identification. There is no consistent policy across jurisdictions regarding criteria for change of legal sex designation, and it is not possible in some countries. As part of the advocacy assessment the clinician should find out whether legal sex designation can be changed, and if so, contact specific issuing agencies as needed to determine eligibility criteria and the change procedure. A sample letter from a physician requesting change of legal sex designation is available as an online supplement at http://www.vch.ca/

transhealth/resources/library/tcpdocs/guidelines-advocacy.pdf

Medical care includes the recording of the client's sex on the medical chart and on lab requisitions. For accuracy in care and interpretation of lab results, we recommend that either "FTM" or "MTF" be used, and if this is not possible that the decision be made based on the criteria discussed by Feldman and Goldberg (2006). If the sex used on a lab requisition form is contrary to the client's identity, the rationale should be explained to the client.

Family and Parenting Concerns

Disclosure Planning and Conflict Relating to Disclosure

In numerous instances we have been asked to help a transgender individual or loved one negotiate a conflict with another family member. This most often happens when transgender issues are disclosed to a loved one who is not supportive.

Ideally, the method and timing of disclosure will be within the client's control. If the client has not yet disclosed their transgender status to family members but is considering doing so, the clinician advocate can facilitate disclosure planning (Bockting et al., 2006). For parents, this includes consideration of age-appropriate ways to disclose to children (Goldberg & Lindenberg, 2001). The clinician advocate can assist the parent to consider some of the practical issues that can arise, such as changes of identification in the child's school records (Minter, Keegan, & Funatake, 2002).

Bockting and colleagues (2006) describe a range of possible counseling interventions for loved ones of transgender individuals following disclosure. When family members are not willing to engage in counseling, the clinician advocate may assist in other ways. For example, the client may ask the clinician for written materials to be given to family members following disclosure, or referrals for mediation or other dispute resolution services. The clinician advocate can also provide perspective on typical family processes of adjustment (Ellis and Eriksen, 2002; Emerson & Rosenfeld, 1996).

Transgender people with a cognitive disability or mental illness, youth, and others who are dependent on family members for care are particularly vulnerable following disclosure, as families often provide both financial and social support. In many cases family caregivers have, with support and information, come to actively support their transgender loved one; however, the client should be made aware of the possibility of withdrawal of support, with economic and social considerations explored as part of decision-making.

Child Custody, Adoption, and Foster Parenting

Transgender parents are not intrinsically more likely to have difficulty parenting than non-transgender parents (Green, 1998). However, the stereotype of transgenderism being associated with sexual deviance may cause problems for transgender parents, particularly in family court proceedings or interactions with child protection services. As an example, one of our clients, a long-time foster parent, lost custody of foster children and was removed from the foster parent roster when child protection services became aware of his transgender identity. In investigation of allegations of abuse or neglect, child protection workers may also evaluate transgender parents more harshly than non-transgender parents in similar circumstances. Lack of legal recognition of transgender marriage and legislation prohibiting adoption by gay and lesbian couples can also complicate custody and adoption proceedings for transgender parents (Marksamer & Daley, n.d.).

Family law advice is outside the scope of practice for most health and social service clinicians. However, in our experience, family law concerns can significantly impact transgender parents' health, and the clinician advocate can be a significant resource in assisting the transgender parent to cope with stress and find appropriate resources. Transgender parents at risk of losing custody to another parent or to the state often feel hopeless and helpless (Minter et al., 2002), and may lack confidence to pursue or defend custody. In some cases, parents have internalized transphobia, saying their child would be "better off" without them. It can be helpful to ensure that parents are aware of positive legal precedents relating to transgender parents' custody rights (Owens, 2001), and are informed of their rights. For social workers in child protection services, it is important to include trans-specific resources in the types of support services offered to families at risk.

In custody proceedings, clinician advocates may help educate the transgender individual's legal counsel about transgender issues, either by informal conversation or the preparation of an information package that counsel may present to the custody judge. A formal clinical report may be helpful in establishing that (a) the client is psychologically stable, and that (b) transgender issues will not, in the clinician's opinion, affect the parent's ability to care for their child (Israel, 1999).

Reproductive Options

The World Professional Association for Transgender Health's *Standards of Care* advise that prior to hormonal or surgical sex reassignment, transgender individuals should be warned about reproductive impacts (i.e, reduced fertility and possible permanent sterility) and reproductive options such as sperm banking for MTFs (Meyer et al., 2001). If reproductive counseling is sought, the clinician advocate can assist with referral and, with the client's permission, contact prospective counselors to determine their level of transgender knowledge and experience. The clinician may also assist the MTF client to find a sperm bank and facilitate education for staff, so the MTF who is already cross-living will be treated in a respectful manner when she goes for a consultation, or to make sperm deposits (Feldman & Goldberg, 2006).

FTMs may need similar assistance in finding a trans-competent fertility specialist, obstetrician, midwife, or other reproductive health expert. The FTM who has questions about fertility, or is seeking assisted reproduction services, needs a clinician who is not only trans-sensitive, but knowledgeable about possible impacts of sex steroids on fertility (if there is a history of testosterone use). For FTMs who wish to conceive but are dysphoric, the clinician advocate can work with the client to consider strategies to manage dysphoria during examination, insemination, pregnancy, and childbirth.

Human Rights and Discrimination

Social stigma leads to mistreatment of transgender people and loved ones by health and social service providers, employers, landlords, or others in positions of power. There is a difference between substandard care and discrimination: standards of care for professionals are governed by regulatory associations and involve judgment against the actions of professional peers (e.g., Is a physician acting outside the bounds of commonly accepted medical practice?), while discrimination involves the negative treatment of a person based on their membership in a specific group, and is judged based on general societal standards for professional interactions.

Clinicians can help transgender people and loved ones understand their rights and options for filing a complaint if they feel their rights have been violated. Depending on legislation and resources in the client's region, complaints relating to substandard care may be made to an employing agency, professional association, or government regulatory body; discrimination complaints may be made to provincial or federal human rights tribunals if these exist. In some cases, civil suits or criminal charges may be initiated if there is sufficient legal support.

It has been our experience that it is helpful for clients to record all of the details of an incident involving mistreatment whether or not they intend to pursue an informal or formal complaint. Recording the information allows the person who experienced it to clarify what happened in their own mind, and also facilitates reporting at a later date if this is the route they so choose. Clinician advocates can assist the client in recording these details.

There is seldom explicit protection for transgender individuals in existing human rights legislation, but in many regions across North America transgender people have succeeded in complaints based on discrimination on the grounds of sex, disability, or sexual orientation. In many cases these decisions have rested on the legal concept of *accommodation*. In North American human rights law, services and employers are legally required to take substantial and meaningful steps to address barriers to inclusion and participation. Changes may include altering rules or policies that are discriminatory, or changing the physical structure of a facility. To justify the denial of a request for accommodation, an institution must typically be able to prove that the cost and disruption, impact on workplace collective agreements, or health and safety concerns are substantial (Goldberg, 2006).

While definitions of accommodation vary across jurisdictions, within North America accommodations are typically required to respect the autonomy, comfort, self-esteem, and confidentiality of the person to protect their dignity. For example, offering a person in a wheelchair the use of a freight elevator at the back of a building is not considered a dignified accommodation. Similarly, segregation of transgender people is objectionable because it disrespects their dignity (Goldberg, 2006).

Most clinicians are not legal experts and should not give legal advice. However, clinician advocates should be generally familiar with human rights protection for transgender individuals and loved ones, and particularly: (a) definitions of discrimination and harassment in human rights legislation, (b) procedures for filing human rights complaints, (c) possible outcomes of a human rights complaints process, and (d) peer and professional resources to assist individuals who wish to make human rights complaints.

Violence and Abuse

Like non-transgender people, transgender people may be abused by a family member, partner, acquaintance, person in position of power (e.g., teacher, law enforcement personnel, health professional), or stranger. One American study of transgender adults reported that approximately 50% of respondents were survivors of violence or abuse (Courvant & Cook-Daniels, 1998), and another reported that 25% of transgender respondents had experienced hate-motivated physical/sexual assault or attempted assault (Lombardi et al., 2001). In a survey of rural and urban transgender community members ($N = 179$), 26% of participants stated a need for anti-violence services (Goldberg et al., 2003).

Violence against transgender individuals is reflective not only of societal transphobia but also the intersections of racism, homophobia, sexism, and class oppression. In examining reports of hate crimes against transgender people, Currah and Minter (2000) found that 98% of all "transgender" violence was perpetrated specifically against people in the male-to-female spectrum. Of the 38 murders of transgender people reported internationally in 2003, 70% were women of colour, with a disproportionate number involved in the survival sex trade (Goldberg & White, 2004).

Key advocacy issues in work with transgender survivors of violence include advocating for access to anti-violence services, working with hospital staff to ensure appropriate levels of support during physical examination, assisting in safety planning, and legal advocacy relating to the criminal justice system (Goldberg, 2006). Safety planning and legal advocacy may also be sought by loved ones of transgender individuals, who are also vulnerable to social stigma and violence and experience difficulty accessing anti-violence services (Cook-Daniels, 2001). Transgender people or loved ones who are fleeing abusive relationships or are unable to work as a result of trauma may also need assistance to apply for social assistance (where available).

Advocacy with Child Protection Services

In regions with child protection programs, transgender people may ask the clinician for advocacy assistance with child protection services, either as parents whose children are at risk of removal or have been removed, or as youth who have been neglected or abused. The clinician advocate should have a general understanding of child removal procedures and advocacy resources for parents and youth.

To date there has been no systematic documentation of transgender individuals' experiences with child protection systems, and it is therefore not clear whether transgender individuals are disproportionately engaged with the child protection system as are some other marginalized populations in North America (e.g., Aboriginal people). However, transgender children are at increased risk for abuse and violence (Goldberg, 2006), and compared to our non-transgender youth clients, a disproportionately high number of our transgender youth clients have been engaged with the child protection system. Issues for youth in care are discussed in detail later in this article.

We strongly encourage community-based clinicians with clients who are engaged with child protection services to try to develop a positive working relationship with the child protection staff involved in the client's case. Child protection workers have the power to significantly affect the client's life, both negatively and positively. We have worked with numerous caring and conscientious child protection workers who, with a bit of assistance and information about transgender needs, have been able to be strong advocates within their agency, with external institutions (schools, youth-serving agencies, legal system), and with members of the client's immediate and extended family. We have also worked with child protection workers who have been actively transphobic and have made it very difficult for their clients within the system. When a child protection worker is actively transphobic and resistant to working with community-based advocates, we have found it useful to try to involve trans-positive staff in other areas of the child protection agency. Child protection staff sometimes are, in our experience, more receptive to working with people they perceive as direct colleagues.

Advocacy with Specific Populations

Transgender Youth

Elsewhere, we discuss the range of psychosocial issues transgender youth may seek assistance with (White Holman & Goldberg, 2006). Below, we discuss three areas that our transgender youth clients often ask for advocacy assistance with: schools, access to hormone therapy, and child protection services.

Schools

In North America, transgender youth face widespread harassment and violence at school. A 2001 American study of self-identified lesbian, gay, bisexual, and transgender students in grades 6-12 ($N = 881$) found that transgender youth reported higher frequency of verbal harassment and physical assault compared to non-transgender participants, and that 90% of the transgender participants reported feeling unsafe in school (Kosciw & Cullen, 2001). Transgender youth are also reported as having higher risk of dropping out of school (Marksamer & Vade, n.d.). Transgender and butch youth interviewed about their experiences of violence described school as "hell" and reported that the violence experienced in school had negatively impacted their self-esteem, academic achievement, drug and alcohol use, and sexual health (Wyss, 2004).

Some North American school boards have attempted to address transphobia in schools by amending existing anti-discrimination, anti-harassment, and anti-bullying policies to provide explicit protection for transgender people. For example, the Vancouver (Canada) School Board's Lesbian, Gay, Bisexual, Transgender and Questioning (LGBTQ) Policy and Action Plan seeks to "provide a safe environment, free from harassment and discrimination, while also promoting pro-active strategies and guidelines to ensure that lesbian, gay, transgender, transsexual, two-spirit, bisexual and questioning students, employees and families are welcomed and included in all aspects of education and school life and treated with respect and dignity."

Explicit anti-discrimination and anti-harassment policies are important. But when transgender issues are only framed in a lesbian/gay/bisexual ("LGB") context, the specific accommodations required by transgender people may not be well understood. School policies should not only explicitly address responses to instances of verbal or physical harassment, but should also address trans-specific accommodation relating to: (a) sex-segregation in bathrooms, showers, locker and change rooms, sports teams, gym classes, field trips, support and counseling groups, sex education classes, and dress codes; (b) records that include legal name and sex designation; (c) protocols relating to preferred pronoun and name; (d) privacy and confidentiality; (e) inclusion of trans-positive content in school curriculum; and (f) training and resources for school staff (Cho, Laub, Wall, Daley, & Joslin, 2004; Marksamer & Vade, n.d.). Staff who are working with youth who are undergoing medically assisted transition should also have access to information about hormonal and surgical modification. To our knowledge the San Francisco Unified

School District is the only school board in North America that covers these details in its transgender policy (San Francisco Unified School District, 2000). North American post-secondary schools are also just beginning to initiate policies to accommodate transgender students (Beemyn, 2003).

In the absence of such policies, case advocacy has been useful in helping school professionals understand and accommodate the needs of transgender students, employees, and staff. In many instances, clinicians working within the school system–such as social workers, counselors, and nurses–have been strong advocates to ensure fair treatment of students by staff and also to facilitate connection with community-based resources. We encourage community-based clinicians to liaise with school-based clinicians, and vice versa.

It has been our experience that elementary schools have a more difficult time with decisions relating to transgender students than secondary and post-secondary schools. There is often concern that by supporting a younger gender-variant child in their self-defined gender identity or gender expression, the school will be inadvertently creating a psychological pathology in the child. This is reflective of the general debate in psychiatry about the appropriate response to cross-gender identification in young children (Cohen-Kettenis & Pfäfflin, 2003; Pickstone-Taylor, 2003) and is made more complex when the parents or guardians are strongly opposed to their child being allowed to explore and express cross-gender identity and behavior. Generally, we advocate that elementary schools create environments that normalize gender diversity, find age-appropriate ways to counter gender stereotypes, and support gender exploration (including cross-gender role playing, experimentation with different names and pronouns, etc.). For youth who are distressed about their sex or gender, clinicians can help coordinate referrals to trans-competent child or adolescent clinicians (de Vries, Cohen-Kettenis, & Delemarre-van de Waal, 2006). Counseling for family members may also be useful (Bockting et al., 2006).

Hormone Therapy During Adolescence

For transgender youth with *gender dysphoria*– a conflict between physical characteristics or social role and felt sense of self–pubertal development of facial and body hair, breasts, and other secondary sex characteristics can intensify distress. Puberty-delaying hormones may be recommended in some cases; masculinizing or feminizing hormones are not recommended until age 16, and surgery is not recommended before age 18 (de Vries et al., 2006).

While hormonal therapy during adolescence is supported in the World Professional Association for Transgender Health's *Standards of Care* (Meyer et al., 2001), not all clinicians support this position, and some will not prescribe hormones before age 18 (de Vries et al., 2006). Even in regions where adolescent hormone therapy is supported in principle, there are few mental health practitioners who transgender adolescents can access at no cost, for the in-depth screening required prior to initiation of hormone therapy. Additionally, if parents are not supportive it can be very difficult for transgender youth to obtain clinician approval to proceed with hormone therapy, as parental approval and consent is strongly recommended even if the adolescent is considered sufficiently mature to make treatment decisions. In these cases the clinician may be an important advocate in helping parents or legal guardians understand the importance of hormonal therapy, and in helping the youth to fully consider all options and consequences of early treatment.

Legal consent issues are particularly complex for gender dysphoric youth who are under state guardianship. Youth who are not legally considered mature enough to make their own decisions regarding health care will need intervention by child protection staff to liaise between birth parents and foster parents or other guardians prior to any medical intervention. If the state-appointed guardian supports treatment, it may be possible to proceed even in the absence of consent by birth parents. In 2004, the Family Court of Australia ruled that a 13-year-old FTM, who was a ward of the court, should be approved for hormonal treatment of Gender Identity Disorder. In this case the biological father was deceased, and the biological mother did not attend the court hearing, but the guardian (the biological aunt) was supportive of treatment; there have not yet been test cases involving active opposition to treatment by birth parents. However, some jurisdictions include a provision for application for a judicial order to provide health care if a parent refuses to consent to health care "that, in the opinion of two medical practitioners, is necessary to preserve the child's life or to prevent serious or permanent impairment of the child's health."

Transgender Youth in Care

The term "youth in care" refers to children and adolescents who are under the care of the state, and are living in a group or foster home. Legislation and procedures for voluntary or involuntary placement in state-supervised care vary regionally. The clinician advocate should have a protocol in place for report of abuse or neglect by a legal minor, and should also have a basic understanding of options for youth who, for reasons other than reportable abuse, cannot live at home.

Like all youth in care, transgender youth enter the child protection system for a variety of reasons and in a variety of ways. Parental abuse or neglect may be directly connected to disclosure of transgender identity or a child's visible gender variance; in other cases the parents are not transphobic, but are not able to provide adequate care for other reasons such as mental illness or addiction. Some youth are "out" to their parents as transgender, while others may not start questioning their gender or may not disclose transgender identity until they are in care.

Whatever the circumstances that leads a transgender youth to be in care, once in care the youth faces risks to safety and privacy similar to those in emergency shelters. A study of youth in care in New York cautioned that transgender youth were "frequent targets for abuse," with reports of violence by group home staff, foster parents, and age peers (Pazos, 1999). Sullivan, Sommer, and Moff (2001)'s review of the American foster care system found widespread neglect, harassment, stigma, and abuse of lesbian, gay, bisexual, and transgender youth in care.

It is imperative that transgender youth in care be allowed to live as they feel themselves to be, including support of client autonomy regarding clothing, makeup, hairstyle, name, and pronoun. Advocacy may be needed with sex-segregated group facilities to ensure this. In *Jean Doe v. Bell*, a 17-year-old MTF living in a group

home for boys won a discrimination case against a foster care agency whose clothing policy forbade her to wear "female attire"–including skirts and dresses–to "protect the safety and welfare" of other residents. The judge found that the policy discriminated against Doe and ordered accommodation of her preferences (Jean Doe v. William C. Bell, 2003).

The Child Welfare League of America recommends that youth-serving agencies support adolescents in foster care who ask for "help on gender orientation issues, as well as the foster parents and birth parents who care for them" (DeCrescenzo & Mallon, 2002, p. 18). As discussed earlier, "help" may include facilitation of access to trans-competent psychotherapy and medical assistance to change the body.

While most clinicians are not legal experts and cannot offer legal advice, the clinician advocate should have a general understanding of legal concerns of youth in care as part of understanding the psychosocial concerns of youth under state guardianship. The clinician advocate should also ensure that transgender youth in care are aware of peer support and legal advocacy resources.

Transgender Elders

Transgender elders are marginalized by widespread societal assumptions that gender diversity does not exist among seniors. Some transgender seniors have identified as transgender for many years or transitioned as young adults; others start questioning their gender, come to identify as transgender, or seek to transition late in life (Witten, 2002). Many of the elders we have worked with kept their identity a secret for many decades, and were motivated to come out as transgender after the death of a partner, or with the diagnosis of a potentially terminal disease (as they felt there was less to lose at this point). While some seniors are very open about being transgender, others are fearful of disclosing that they are transgender–particularly in settings where others have great power over their lives, such as residential care settings) and may be deeply closeted. In our experience clinicians and family members can dismiss disclosure of transgender identity as being a sign of dementia or confusion, and advocacy may be needed to create an environment that supports the senior to explore and express feelings relating to gender.

Historically, the North American psychiatric model for treatment of gender-variance focused on suppressing transgender feelings and behaviours. One report noted that transgender elders may have, as children or young adults, experienced the use of electroshock therapy, aversion therapy, and other invasive types of "conversion" therapy–with resulting tardive dyskinesia, severe depression, cognitive impairment, or other neurological damage (Minter, 2003). For individuals who lived through severe societal or medical repression as transgender people, there may be issues of rage, grief, or shame that intensify or surface with age.

There is no upper limit on the age at which a person may begin medically assisted transition, and seniors who are in good health have started hormones or undergone feminizing or masculinizing surgeries late in life. However, elders who are frail or have medical contraindications to hormones or surgery may not be able to undergo a medically assisted transition. This can lead to depression and despair for people who feel they will never be able to live as they know themselves to be. The clinician advocate can play an important role in referring to peer and professional counseling supports, and also in helping the client to explore non-medical options for gender transition (Bockting et al., 2006).

Financial needs may also be a concern for some transgender seniors. Where social benefits such as public pensions are available these should be discussed, and direct assistance or referral to a trans-competent senior agency offered if the client is struggling with the application.

Transgender Migrants

In North America, individuals who do not have citizenship status (including those with temporary work, student, or visitor visas; immigrants and refugees who have permanent resident status; people seeking asylum; and undocumented individuals) face multiple barriers to full societal participation. Institutionalized and interpersonal anti-immigrant bias, racism, xenophobia, and ethnocentrism can be a shock for newcomers who may only have seen materials portraying North America as an inclusive and tolerant society. Many of the transgender immigrants and refugees we have worked with have been particularly affected by obstacles to employment and resulting poverty. Provincial and federal assistance for refugees vary from region to region, but is often inaccessible or insufficient. Clinicians working with this population must have a strong working knowledge of migrant, immigrant, and refugee-serving agencies; ethnocultural community organizations; immigration and citizenship legislation and government programs; and transgender peer and professional resources.

For undocumented transgender individuals, life is often very difficult. Many essential services and benefits are not accessible to undocumented people: Without legal status it is typically not possible to get identification, to legally work, to obtain any type of social assistance or health benefits, to receive financial assistance with child care, or to attend school or training programs. Additionally, undocumented people live under constant fear of arrest and deportation. Despite this, in recent years we have seen increasing numbers of undocumented transgender people who do not meet the *Convention Relating to the Status of Regugees* definitions of refugees but feel Canada is a safer place than their country of origin. Clients who are undocumented may need substantial and repeated advocacy to facilitate access to health and social services, and possibly assistance to apply for refugee or immigrant status.

The quality of trans-specific health care varies greatly from country to country. Some migrants have had access to hormonal or surgical care that is far superior to that available in Canada; others have received substandard care and may present with serious medical problems. Referral to a trans-competent primary care provider is vital. Some community health centres welcome people who do not have health coverage, including newcomers and undocumented individuals.

Several of the transgender refugees we have worked with were imprisoned and tortured by prison or military personnel for being transgender. Specialized peer support and professional trauma counseling may be required.

Transgender individuals or their lawyers may ask health and social service clinicians to assist with refugee applications. Typically, the clinician is asked to provide a formal report outlining the reported persecution experienced by the refugee applicant, and evaluating the resulting impact on physical or mental health. When possible the clinician advocate should also include information about the specific conditions faced by transgender people in the country of origin. International transgender organizations may be able to assist with this research.

Transgender Individuals with Cognitive or Mental Health Concerns

Transgender people with cognitive or mental health concerns are vulnerable to social isolation, abuse, and violence. While some may be financially supported by family, those who are unable to work due to their disability are often living in poverty. Additionally, it has been our experience that people with cognitive disability or mental health concerns are sometimes infantilized by caregivers and thus disregarded when they try to express their felt sense of gender, a wish to crossdress, or desire to be perceived as a gender other than that assigned at birth.

For clients who are seeking medically assisted gender transition, advocacy is often needed to establish client competency to make medical decisions (Bockting et al., 2006). Clinicians can provide important collateral information in this regard. A sample letter is available as an online supplement at http://www.vch.ca/transhealth/resources/library/tcpdocs/guidelines-advocacy.pdf

Some clients with cognitive disability or mental illness are able to work with appropriate assistance. Advocacy with vocational and employment support organizations can be useful.

While we support clients' self-definition of gender (including use of preferred pronoun and name) in all circumstances, we have found that some advocates eager to demonstrate their trans-positivity have unconsciously pushed transgender people with cognitive disability and mental illness to make hasty decisions that posed great risk to safety. For example, we worked with one MTF client with borderline cognitive capacity whose counselor responded to her disclosure of "feeling like a woman" by strongly encouraging her to come out to family caregivers, start publicly presenting as a woman and asking strangers to use a female name and female pronouns, pursue legal name change, and initiate feminizing hormones. All of these changes were overwhelming to family members and also put the client at great risk as she was not able to distinguish between safe situations to come out and situations where it was not safe to disclose her identity.

The advocate's role is to help the client explore options, not to be directive or otherwise lead to the client to choose any particular option. Some clients who are cognitively impaired by developmental disability or mental health conditions–particularly those who have been taught to be compliant in institutional care–may be easily influenced by professionals' suggestions, and care is needed to avoid inadvertent influence. Having said this, we also note that some advocates can be so protective of the cognitively disabled person that they actively oppose decisions relating to pursuit of transgender identity or expression out of fear of the consequences. It is imperative that advocates not assume responsibility for decision-making for people with disabilities. The advocate should neither push for suppression nor for disclosure of transgender identity, but should assist the client to make an informed decision and help create a safety plan, if disclosure is desired. Clients who are able to live independently may need assistance to find suitable housing and to set up independent living support services.

Transgender Individuals Living in Residential Facilities

While client needs vary depending on the situation, typically our transgender clients in residential facilities have been concerned primarily about safety, lack of access to trans-competent health care, privacy, confidentiality, and social isolation. Mottet and Ohle's (2003) guide for emergency shelters, which is available online, can be adapted for use by longer-term residential facilities.

While systemic changes are needed, case advocacy is also important in promoting safety and accessibility of residential services. The clinician advocate should discuss the client's preferred arrangements for sleeping quarters, bathing facilities, and washroom access, as client needs vary. In residential facilities with group washrooms, changing areas, and showers, standing screens or hanging curtains can be used to create private spaces for any client who desires privacy. It is important that these types of accommodations be offered to all residents (not just those who are openly transgender), and that staff understand that these accommodations are not suggested to "protect" non-transgender residents from seeing the transgender person's body. We often suggest to residential facility staff that non-transgender residents who express discomfort with seeing a transgender person's body can be directed to use the screened off private area themselves, so the transgender client does not have to accommodate other clients' transphobic views.

Although there are some co-ed residential facilities, it has been our experience that many residential services are sex-segregated. This is intrinsically problematic for: (a) transgender people who do not identify with binary concepts of men and women, (b) transgender people who do identify as men or women but do not fit the agency's definition of who a man or woman is, (c) male and female crossdressers or others whose gender expression does not match conventional norms, and (d) individuals who are not able to cross-live full time despite having a consistent cross-gender identity. Transgender people who do not "fit" with the system's structure may be refused services, placed in a facility that does not conform with their identity, or denied privileges accorded to other residents. Systemic advocacy is needed to create options that are not sex- or gender-specific; in the interim, case advocacy is important in ensuring respectful treatment of transgender individuals within sex- or gender-specific residential settings.

For people who are long-term institutional residents, there are additional concerns relating to social isolation and access to trans-competent health care. The clinician advocate can assist by determining needs that cannot be met within the facility, liaising with outside providers, and making arrangements for services to be delivered on-site or for clients to be brought out to access services in the community. In our experience, staff at residential facilities are often reluctant to make the arrangements themselves, but are often amenable to clinicians coming into a facility or clients being brought out to community services if someone else negotiates logistics such as transportation. As part of arranging logistics, institution security policies should be discussed so there is a clear understanding about procedures for visitors entering and leaving the facility.

It is not uncommon for individuals in residential settings to be transferred to a new facility, and this can happen repeatedly. Prior to such transfers, the clinician advocate should talk with the client and, with the client's permission, inform the new staff of trans-specific concerns so gains made from advocacy with the first facility are not lost in the transfer. In our experience advocacy is often needed with every transfer to educate staff and residents about transgender issues, help agency staff implement proactive anti-discrimination measures, and create plans to address general residential issues (placement, safety, etc.). For example, as part of the transfer of a transgender MTF from acute care to a continuing care facility we provided education sessions for staff and other residents, and care planning to discuss accommodation of the client's specific needs as a non-operative transsexual woman. In this case the client was completely open about her identity and wanted us to speak freely about her particular history and needs; in other circumstances the education would need to be managed carefully to avoid "outing" a transgender individual to other residents.

Hospitals and Hospices

Increasingly, hospitals and hospices are creating mixed-gender wards. However, individual rooms on a mixed ward are typically not mixed; i.e., rooms are designated for women or for men. If the facility has sex-segregated wards, floors, or rooms, advocacy may be needed to ensure that the transgender person is accommodated in a way that is respectful of their identity and also allows them privacy in washroom, bathing, dressing, and undressing. A single-patient room on a mixed ward is often the best option.

Advocacy may be required to ensure sensitive and respectful bathing, physical examination, or any other procedure involving the chest or genitals of transgender patients (whether in emergency or on the ward). For people who are dysphoric about these areas of their bodies, having them looked at or touched can be humiliating and traumatic. Additionally, individuals whose bodies have been altered by hormones or surgery may be fearful of the caregiver's response. There is a need to manage appropriate disclosure to ensure that staff are aware of any special considerations for examination, while still maintaining the privacy of the patient. Staff should not gossip about a transgender patient's body or include notes on the front of the chart where others could see the information. As not all transgender people are "out" to loved ones, discussions about a transgender person's medical or personal history should not take place in front of loved ones unless the patient has explicitly consented to this.

Examinations following a physical or sexual assault, a suicide attempt, or incidents of self-harm (including attempted autocastration) must be handled with particular sensitivity. Increased social work and counseling support is recommended to clients following trauma of any kind, including self-inflicted trauma, due to frequent lack of external support and vulnerability rooted in transphobia.

As in any facility or program, hospice and palliative care staff must create and ensure a safe environment for the patient, family, and supporters. "Chosen family" must be valued and have open access to their loved ones, as is traditionally offered to biological family members. Assistance with end-of-life directives or wills may be required.

Funeral or memorial planning can be a complex issue. In some instances, family members do not know a person is transgender, do not recognize their preferred name and pronoun, or clash with partners or other loved ones over burial or cremation decisions. In some instances family or religious leaders have opposed the burial of a transgender family member in a family burial plot or in consecrated ground. It may be helpful to try to find trans-positive spiritual, religious, and cultural leaders to help advocate with family members for a service that is in accordance with the deceased person's wishes.

It is our experience that community-based clinicians from the same discipline as the hospi-

tal staff are the most effective advocates in hospitals and hospices; nurses make a particular impact on other nurses, and physicians tend to listen to other physicians. We have, with clients' permission, involved colleagues in mental health, nursing, and family practice to advocate for our hospitalized clients when we feel other clinicians would be more effective advocates.

Long-Term Residential Care

Long-term residential care, sometimes described as *continuing care*, refers to long-term medically supervised housing for people unable to live independently, or with loved ones. As in hospitals and hospices, trans-specific protocols should be implemented to ensure respectful and sensitive personal care, particularly in bathing, physical examination, or any other procedure involving the chest or genitals of transgender patients. Privacy and confidentiality are also key concerns for many people in long-term care, as information can spread very quickly throughout a facility. As the majority of long-term care residents are elderly, advocacy relating to long-term care includes advocacy specific to transgender seniors (discussed in more detail in the section on work with specific populations).

Crossdressing or other gender-variant behaviour is seen by some residential care providers as "acting out" and is often actively discouraged. In our experience there is particular confusion within long-term care about crossdressing being an "inappropriate" expression of sexuality, as crossdressing is stereotypically considered a type of sexual fetish. We have found it useful to educate staff about the diversity of reasons people crossdress, and also to encourage frank discussion of the sexual needs of long-term care residents. Advocacy may include the filing of formal complaints if transgender residents are being punished for cross-gender expression.

Transgender people in residential care often experience severe isolation, complicated by barriers to accessing peer support. Community social workers may be able to assist by coordinating transportation planning and caregiver assistance to make it possible to access trans-specific community peer support groups and events, or to facilitate inpatient visits. Other clinicians in long-term care facilities can also proactively educate colleagues to help ensure that transgender visitors who are providing peer support to a resident are treated respectfully by all staff.

Prisons

There is little documentation of transgender individuals and incarceration. However, the high rates of poverty, addiction and economic discrimination experienced by transgender people in North America may increase involvement in the sex trade, drug trade, fraud, or theft for financial survival (Goldberg, 2004; Lee, 2003).

It has been our experience that it is very difficult for clinicians who are not in the prison system to effectively advocate for prisoners without the aid of clinicians who are inside the system. The prison system is extremely insular, with limits on how frequently outsiders are allowed access and what types of information can be shared. In some cases a community-based practitioner may be allowed in to provide specialized assistance relating to gender transition, but for general care, community-based practitioners will likely need to work with a point person inside the facility that the client is in, train that person in the specifics of transgender care, and relay needed information. Consultation with community organizations and individuals with experience in prison advocacy is often useful.

Placement and Safety. Placement policies vary, but individuals in the MTF spectrum are typically held in men's prisons unless they have had genital surgery. Reports from various countries suggest that violence against male-to-females (MTFs) imprisoned with men is the norm rather than the exception (Peek, 2004; Scott & Lines, 1998). In a study of MTFs held with men in Canadian prisons, Scott and Lines (1998) documented incidents of sexual assault and resulting transmission of sexually transmitted infections (including HIV), physical and verbal harassment, and coercion to provide sex in exchange for protection from other inmates.

Some prisons have attempted to deal with safety issues by placing MTFs in protective custody, involuntary segregation, or isolation (Daley, 2005; Goldberg, 2004; Lee, 2003). However, as protective custody is often used to segregate sexual offenders and sexual predators from the general population, this is an unsafe option for MTFs (Scott & Lines, 1998). As described by Lee (2003) and Daley (2005), placement in segregation or isolation units is further inappropriate as this practice results in transgender prisoners losing access to programs and privileges that are available to prisoners in the general population. It is imperative that people in the MTF spectrum be considered at high risk for abuse and appropriate measures taken to protect their safety, but measures should not be punitive. Rather than creating a system-wide placement policy, Lee (2003) suggests case-by-case placement decisions that considers each transgender prisoner's needs and local options.

FTM experiences in women's prisons have not been as extensively documented as the experience of MTF in men's prisons. However, according to Lee (2003), guards in American prisons often view transgender individuals in the FTM spectrum as lesbians and sexual predators, punishing suspected sexual contact through disciplinary infractions and refusing use of earned privileges, isolating FTMs from other prisoners, and subjecting the prisoners to harassment through verbal slurs and unjustified cell searches. Lee points out that the maltreatment of FTM prisoners (predominantly people of colour) by guards (predominantly white) is complex, with sexism, racism, homophobia, and transphobia intersecting to promote repression and violence. Such concerns can only be addressed through systemic advocacy.

Strip-Searching and Forced Nudity. There are documented incidents of prison guards, officers, and medical personnel using strip-searching and forced nudity to humiliate and harass transgender prisoners, or to satisfy curiosity about the body of a transgender prisoner (Daley, 2005). While systemic advocacy is needed to address these types of abuses of power, clinician advocates can contribute by conveying information about appropriate medical examination (Feldman & Goldberg, 2006) and by discussing options for human rights complaints with the client.

Access to Trans-Specific Services. Access to trans-specific information and services is a general problem in residential settings. Security considerations in prisons make it particularly challenging for transgender prisoners to access information, peer support, and professional care, particularly when prisons are located outside urban centres where transgender resources are typically concentrated.

Several publications offer recommendations for policy change and discussion of possible individual accommodations (Goldberg, 2004; Lee, 2003; Scott & Lines, 1998). Connection with trans-competent health and social service practitioners is a practical and reachable goal in many cases. The clinician advocate can assist by providing direct care, training staff within the system to provide basic care for individuals undergoing gender transition, and by donating books and other print resources to the prison library or to community programs that distribute reading material to prisoners. The clinician advocate can also raise awareness of prisoner concerns with transgender community groups, and potentially facilitate contact between community groups and incarcerated individuals.

General Prison Advocacy Considerations. Transgender prisoners struggle with the same issues as non-transgender prisoners: overcrowding; lack of access to needles, bleach, and safer sex supplies; separation from family and loved ones; geographic isolation; forced work in unsafe and underpaid conditions; substandard diet; systemic racism and homophobia; lack of access to cultural or faith community; limited phone access; poverty; and lack of privacy (Lee, 2003; Scott & Lines, 1998). Advocacy with transgender prisoners should be inclusive of the general issues of concern, not only trans-specific issues.

CONCLUDING COMMENTS

In our experience, clinician advocates benefit by having supportive collegial networks. The stigma associated with gender-variance can affect clinicians who are marginalized by colleagues for working with people commonly perceived as "perverts" or "freaks." This can be particularly challenging for clinicians who are advocating for change within their own work setting. We have found it useful to connect with

other advocates to build support to face these challenges, to share information about successful strategies we have used on behalf of our clients, and to discuss changes to the systems we are working in. We encourage clinicians to become actively involved in The World Professional Association for Transgender Health and to connect with transgender community groups as a way to build this network.

Case advocacy can be both challenging and rewarding. We have found engagement in advocacy to be a positive antidote to the frustration, anger, and cynicism that can result from repeatedly bearing witness to discrimination, harassment, and mistreatment experienced by transgender people and loved ones. Contributing to positive change, and witnessing the resulting impact on clients' quality of life, is tremendously satisfying. We hope that this article helps health and social service professionals value advocacy as part of clinical practice with transgender individuals and loved ones, and encourages clinicians to take an active role as client advocates.

NOTE

1. *Systemic advocacy* (sometimes referred to as *global advocacy*, *community advocacy*, or *class advocacy*) involves system-wide action that will benefit a group of people. Systemic advocacy includes efforts to change societal attitudes, legislation, institutional and organizational policy and procedures, and the way an individual conducts practice with all of their transgender clients (Multiple Sclerosis Society of Canada, 2004). While frontline health and social service practitioners are often involved in education of colleagues, influencing organizational and institutional policy, and providing expert opinion relating to legal cases, most clinicians are not funded to provide these kinds of services and systemic advocacy is therefore typically a much smaller area of practice.

REFERENCES

Beemyn, B. (2003). Serving the needs of transgender college students. *Journal of Gay and Lesbian: Issues in Education*, *1*(1), 33-50.

Blackmore, R. (2001). Advocacy in nursing: Perceptions of learning disability nurses. *Journal of Learning Disabilities*, 5, 221-234.

Bockting, W. O., Knudson, G., & Goldberg, J. M. (2006). Counseling and mental health care for transgender adults and loved ones. *International Journal of Transgenderism, 9*(3/4), 35-82.

Bowman, C., & Goldberg, J. M. (2006). Care of the patient undergoing sex reassignment surgery. *International Journal of Transgenderism, 9*(3/4), 135-165.

Cho, S., Laub, C., Wall, S. S. M., Daley, C., & Joslin, C. (2004). *Beyond the binary: A tool kit for gender identity activism in schools.* San Francisco, CA: Gay-Straight Alliance Network, Transgender Law Center, and National Center for Lesbian Rights.

Cohen-Kettenis, P. T., & Pfäfflin, F. (2003). *Transgenderism and intersexuality in childhood and adolescence: Making choices.* Thousand Oaks, CA: Sage Publications.

Cook-Daniels, L. (2001). SOFFA questions and answers. Milwaukee, WI: FORGE. Retrieved May 13, 2006, from http://www.forge-forward.org/handouts/SOFFA-QA.pdf

Courvant D., & Cook-Daniels, L. (1998). *Trans and intersex survivors of domestic violence: Defining terms, barriers, and responsibilities.* Portland, OR: Survivor Project.

Currah, P., & Minter, S. (2000). *Transgender equality: A handbook for activists and policymakers.* New York, NY: National Gay and Lesbian Task Force and The National Center for Lesbian Rights.

Dahl, M., Feldman, J., Goldberg, J. M., & Jaberi, A. (2006). Physical aspects of transgender endocrine therapy. *International Journal of Transgenderism, 9*(3/4), 111-134.

Daley, C. (2005). *Safety inside: Problems faced by transgender prisoners and common sense solutions to them–Testimony to National Prison Rape Elimination Commission.* San Francisco, CA: Transgender Law Center.

Davies, S., & Goldberg, J. M. (2006). Clinical aspects of transgender speech feminization and masculinization. *International Journal of Transgenderism, 9*(3/4), 167-196.

de Vries, A. L. C., Cohen-Kettenis, P. T., & Delemarre-van de Waal, H. (2006). Clinical management of gender dysphoria in adolescents. *International Journal of Transgenderism, 9*(3/4), 83-94.

DeCrescenzo, T., & Mallon, G. P. (2002). *Serving transgender youth: The role of child welfare systems–Proceedings of a colloquium.* Washington, DC: Child Welfare League of America.

Ellis, K. M., & Eriksen, K. (2002). Transsexual and transgenderist experiences and treatment options. *Family Journal: Counseling and Therapy for Couples and Families, 10,* 289-299.

Emerson, S., & Rosenfeld, C. (1996). Stages of adjustment in family members of transgender individuals. *Journal of Family Psychotherapy, 7,* 1-12.

Feldman, J., & Goldberg, J. M. (2006). Transgender primary medical care. *International Journal of Transgenderism, 9*(3/4), 3-34.

Goldberg, J. M. (2004). *Trans people in the criminal justice system: A guide for criminal justice personnel.* Vancouver, BC: Justice Institute of BC and Trans Alliance Society.

Goldberg, J. M. (2006). *Making the transition: Providing services to trans survivors of violence and abuse.* Vancouver, BC: Justice Institute of BC.

Goldberg, J. M., & Lindenberg, M. (2001). *TransForming community: Resources for trans people and our families.* Victoria, BC: Transcend Transgender Support & Education Society.

Goldberg, J. M., Matte, N., MacMillan, M., & Hudspith, M. (2003). *Community survey: Transition/crossdressing services in BC–Final report.* Vancouver, BC: Vancouver Coastal Health and Transcend Transgender Support & Education Society.

Goldberg, J. M., & White, C. (2004). Expanding our understanding of gendered violence: Violence against trans people and loved ones. *Aware: The Newsletter of the BC Institute Against Family Violence, 11,* 21-25.

Goldsmith, P., & Reid, G. (1997). *A guide for advocates: Knowing your rights* (2nd ed.). Vancouver, BC: Federated Anti-poverty Groups of BC. Retrieved May 13, 2006, from http://www.povnet.org/resources/fapgmanual.pdf

Green, R. (1998). Transsexuals' children. *International Journal of Transgenderism, 2.* Retrieved January 1, 2005, from http://www.symposion.com/ijt/ijtc0601.htm

Horton, M. A. (2001). *Checklist for transitioning in the workplace.* Retrieved January 1, 2005, from http://www.tgender.net/taw/tggl/checklist.html

Israel, G. E. (1999). *Child custody issues for the transgender parent.* San Francisco, CA: Author. Retrieved May 14, 2006, from http://www.firelily.com/gender/gianna/custody.html

Jean Doe v. William C. Bell, Commissioner, New York City Administration of Children's Services and New York City Administration for Children's Services, 194 Misc.2d 774, 775 754 N.Y.S.2d 846, 848 (Sup. Ct. 2003).

Kosciw, J. G., & Cullen, M. K. (2001). *The GLSEN 2001 National School Climate Survey: The school-related experiences of our nation's lesbian, gay, bisexual and transgender youth.* New York, NY: Gay, Lesbian and Straight Education Network.

Lee, A. L. (2003). *Nowhere to go but out: The collision between transgender & gender-variant prisoners and the gender binary in America's prisons.* Retrieved May 13, 2006, from http://www.srlp.org/documents/alex_lees_paper2.pdf

Lombardi, E. L., Wilchins, R. A., Priesing, D., & Malouf, D. (2001). Gender violence: Transgender experiences with violence and discrimination. *Journal of Homosexuality, 42,* 89-101.

Marksamer, J., & Daley, C. (n.d.) *Transgender family law 101.* San Francisco: National Center for Lesbian Rights and Transgender Law Center. Retrieved May

14, 2006, from http://www.transgenderlawcenter.org/pdf/tg_family_law_101.pdf

Marksamer, J., & Vade, D. (n.d.) *Transgender and gender non-conforming youth: Recommendations for schools.* San Francisco, CA: Transgender Law Center. Retrieved January 1, 2005, from http://www.transgenderlawcenter.org/tranny/pdfs/Recomendations%20for%20Schools.pdf

Meyer, W. J., III, Bockting, W. O., Cohen-Kettenis, P. T., Coleman, E., Di Ceglie, D., Devor, H., Gooren, L., Hage, J. J., Kirk, S., Kuiper, B., Laub, D., Lawrence, A., Menard, Y., Monstrey, S., Patton, J., Schaefer, L., Webb, A., & Wheeler, C. C. (2001). *The standards of care for Gender Identity Disorders* (6th ed.). Minneapolis, MN: Harry Benjamin International Gender Dysphoria Association.

Minter, S. (2003). *Legal and public policy issues for transgender elders.* San Francisco, CA: National Center for Lesbian Rights.

Minter, S., & Daley, C. (2003). *Trans realities: A legal needs assessment of San Francisco's transgender communities.* San Francisco, CA: National Center for Lesbian Rights & Transgender Law Center.

Minter, S., Keegan, J., & Funatake, P. (2002, November). *Child's best interests: Transgender parent issues workshop and discussion.* Paper presented at the National Gay and Lesbian Task Force's 15th Annual Creating Change Conference, Portland, OR.

Mottet, L., & Ohle, J.M. (2003). *Transitioning our shelters: A guide to making homeless shelters safe for transgender people.* New York, NY: National Coalition for the Homeless & National Gay and Lesbian Task Force Policy Institute.

Multiple Sclerosis Society of Canada–BC Division (2004). *Advocacy.* Vancouver, BC: Author. Retrieved May 13, 2006, from http://www.mssociety.ca/bc/PDF/advocacy.PDF

Nemoto, T., Operario, D., Keatley, J., & Villegas, D. (2004). Social context of HIV risk behaviours among male-to-female transgenders of colour. *AIDS Care, 16,* 724-735.

Owens, A. M. (2001, February 1). Father's sex change does not alter custody, court says: Girl, 6, calls parent Mommy and Daddy; cautious in public [Electronic version]. *National Post Online.* Retrieved January 1, 2005, from http://www.pfc.org.uk/news/2001/custody.htm

Pazos, S. (1999). Practice with female-to-male transgendered youth. In G. P. Mallon (Ed.), *Social services*

with transgendered youth (pp. 65-82). Binghamton, NY: The Haworth Press, Inc.

Peek, C. (2004). Breaking out of the prison hierarchy: Transgender prisoners, rape and the Eighth Amendment. *Santa Clara Law Journal, 44,* 1211-1248.

Pickstone-Taylor, S. (2003). Children with gender non-conformity. *Journal of the American Academy of Child & Adolescent Psychiatry, 42,* 266.

Risser, J., & Shelton, A. (2002). *Behavioral assessment of the transgender population, Houston, Texas.* Galveston, TX: University of Texas School of Public Health.

San Francisco Unified School District (2000). *Board of Education administrative regulation: Non-discrimination for students and employees* (Reg. R5163). Retrieved January 1, 2005, from http://www.transgenderlaw.org/college/sfusdpolicy.htm

Scott, A. V., & Lines, R. (1998). HIV/AIDS in the male-to-female transsexual and transgendered prison population: A comprehensive strategy. *Canadian HIV/AIDS Policy & Law Newsletter, 4*(2/3), 55-59.

Simpson, A. J., & Goldberg, J. M. (2006). *An advocacy guide for trans people and loved ones.* Vancouver, BC: Vancouver Coastal Health Authority.

Sullivan, C., Sommer, S., & Moff, J. (2001). *Youth in the margins: A report on the unmet needs of lesbian, gay, bisexual, and transgender adolescents in foster care.* New York, NY: Lambda Legal Defense and Education Fund, Inc.

Walworth, J. (1998). *Transsexual workers: An employer's guide.* Bellingham, WA: Center for Gender Sanity.

White Holman, C., & Goldberg, J. M. (2006). Ethical, legal, and psychosocial issues in care of transgender adolescents. *International Journal of Transgenderism, 9*(3/4), 95-110.

Witten, T. M. (2002). Geriatric care and management issues for the transgender and intersex populations. *Geriatric Care and Management Journal, 12*(3), 20-4.

Wyss, S. E. (2004). 'This was my hell': the violence experienced by gender non-conforming youth in US high schools. *International Journal of Qualitative Studies in Education, 17,* 709-730.

Xavier, J., & Simmons, R. (2000). *Final report of the Washington Transgender Needs Assessment Survey.* Washington, DC: Administration for HIV and AIDS, District of Columbia Department of Health.

doi:10.1300/J485v09n03_09

Training Community-Based Clinicians
in Transgender Care

Joshua M. Goldberg

SUMMARY. Community-based care of transgender individuals can help promote access for individuals whose needs are not well met by a centralized, institution-based system. As there is wide variability in transgender expertise and familiarity among community-based practitioners, practice guidelines and clinical training are needed to promote consistency and quality of care. This article suggests frameworks for training clinicians working in the community setting. Suggested core competencies are followed by an outline for basic, intermediate, and advanced levels of clinical training, and a discussion of education priorities. doi:10.1300/J485v09n03_10 *[Article copies available for a fee from The Haworth Document Delivery Service: 1-800-HAWORTH. E-mail address: <docdelivery@ haworthpress.com> Website: <http://www.HaworthPress.com> © 2006 by The Haworth Press, Inc. All rights reserved.]*

KEYWORDS. Transgender, education, training, cultural competence, clinical competence

For several decades multidisciplinary specialty university- or hospital-based gender clinics have been considered the *sine qua non* of transgender care. However, in recent years there has been increasing interest in creating community-based networks of care to improve access for transgender individuals whose needs are not well met by a centralized, institution-based system (Kopala, 2003; West Sussex Health and Social Care NHS Trust, 2005).

As there is wide variability in expertise and familiarity with transgender care among community-based practitioners, for a community-based network of care to be viable there is a need for practice guidelines and clinical training to encourage consistency and quality of care. To be effective training must not only address trans-specific sensitivity and awareness, but also the skills and experience needed to be clinically competent.

In 2006, four education frameworks were developed to guide the Vancouver Coastal Health Authority in creating systematic training for health and social service students as well as professionals already in practice. The frameworks are based on (a) review of course outlines

Joshua M. Goldberg is Education Consultant of the Transgender Health Program, Vancouver, BC, Canada.

This manuscript was created for the Trans Care Project, a joint initiative of Transcend Transgender Support & Education Society and Vancouver Coastal Health's Transgender Health Program, with funding from the Canadian Rainbow Health Coalition. The author thanks Trevor Corneil, Marshall Dahl, Shelagh Davies, Peter Granger, Afshin Jaberi, Gail Knudson, Marjorie MacDonald, Melady Preece, Linda Rammage, Marsha Runtz, Colleen Varcoe, and Julian Young for their comments on an earlier draft, and Donna Lindenberg, Olivia Ashbee, A. J. Simpson, and Barbara Suzanne Rouse for research assistance.

[Haworth co-indexing entry note]: "Training Community-Based Clinicians in Transgender Care." Goldberg, Joshua M. Co-published simultaneously in *International Journal of Transgenderism* (The Haworth Medical Press, an imprint of The Haworth Press, Inc.) Vol. 9, No. 3/4, 2006, pp. 219-231; and: *Guidelines for Transgender Care* (ed: Walter O. Bockting, and Joshua M. Goldberg) The Haworth Medical Press, an imprint of The Haworth Press, Inc., 2006, pp. 219-231. Single or multiple copies of this article are available for a fee from The Haworth Document Delivery Service [1-800-HAWORTH, 9:00 a.m. - 5:00 p.m. (EST). E-mail address: docdelivery@haworthpress.com].

Available online at http://ijt.haworthpress.com
© 2006 by The Haworth Press, Inc. All rights reserved.
doi:10.1300/J485v09n03_10

from British Columbia post-secondary undergraduate and graduate programs in counseling, medicine, nursing, psychology, social work, and speech; (b) interviews with 10 clinicians who provide clinical training in transgender care; (c) a review of international transgender training programs; and (d) feedback by local clinicians involved in training of community clinicians.

This article summarizes the elements of the training frameworks that are relevant to an international audience, in the hopes of stimulating development of clinical education programs in other regions. Suggested core competencies for community-based clinicians providing transgender care are followed by an outline for basic, intermediate, and advanced levels of clinical training, and a discussion of education priorities.

A THREE-TIER APPROACH TO TRANSGENDER CARE AND CLINICAL EDUCATION

Within the Trans Care Project we classify community-based transgender care as basic (Tier 1), intermediate (Tier 2), or advanced (Tier 3). Each tier has specific competencies needed to provide various types of services. Table 1 compares this three-tier model in transgender care to models of addiction and HIV care in the primary care setting.

Tier 1, basic care, involves sensitive, respectful, inclusive, and welcoming service. The Tier 1 clinician will be familiar enough with transgender issues to respond appropriately should a client or patient disclose transgender identity, cross-gender behaviour, or gender concerns, or express confusion or concern about a transgender loved one. Appropriate response includes non-judgmental attitude, facilitation of discussion of transgender issues, and referrals as needed to peer and professional resources. As this level of competence is required for all community-based clinicians, the target audience for training is broad, including students, postgraduates, and clinicians already in practice. Tier 1 training may also be relevant for office staff or other non-clinical personnel who interact with the transgender client or patient in a clinical setting, with an appropriate

focus on respectful communication, charting, privacy, and other administrative issues.

Tier 2, intermediate care, involves modification of standard protocols to address trans-specific needs. For example, the Tier 2 mental health professional would be able to skillfully explore how societal stressors may impact the transgender client who presents with depression; in the primary medical care setting, the Tier 2 family physician or nurse practitioner would modify standard medical protocols to address trans-specific needs relating to health promotion, disease prevention, diagnosis and assessment, treatment, and medical advocacy. The focus of Tier 2 training is the clinician who is already sensitive to transgender concerns and has had experience working with at least one transgender client or patient. Clinicians who do not have transgender experience but have completed Tier 1 training and are interested in expanding accessibility to the transgender community should also be recruited for this level of training.

Tier 3, advanced care, relates to trans-specific services such as assessment and evaluation of gender concerns, clinically assisted gender transition (e.g., endocrine therapy, speech and voice change, coordination of post-operative care), and treatment for compulsive cross-dressing. Although Tier 3 services are relatively specialized they are still deliverable within the community setting, and as such do not include surgical sex reassignment procedures that require hospitalization. This advanced level of care requires targeted recruitment of experienced clinicians with a suitable foundation in clinical practice, and a commitment to ongoing learning relating to developments in transgender care.

Core Competencies for Community-Based Clinicians Involved in Transgender Care

Tier 1 competencies are very general and thus applicable across disciplines. As Tiers 2 and 3 involve more clinically sophisticated levels of service, the core competencies at these levels are specific to the area of practice. Core competencies in endocrine care, mental health, primary medical care, and speech and voice change are summarized in Tables 2a, 2b, and 2c. In Tiers 2 and 3, clinicians are expected to

TABLE 1. Transgender Equivalents to Competencies in Treatment of Addictions and HIV in the Primary Medical Care Setting

Tier	Core Competencies		
	Addictions	HIV	Transgender equivalent
1: Basic (all primary medical care providers)	Understanding and awareness of addiction issues, able to respond appropriately if patient discloses substance use, able to screen for and recognize drug or alcohol concerns, ability to provide referrals for specialty evaluation or treatment if needed	Understanding and awareness of HIV transmission, able to respond appropriately if patient discloses behavior that is high-risk for HIV transmission, able to screen for HIV infection and counsel on risk reduction, able to provide referrals for specialty evaluation or treatment if needed	Understanding and awareness of transgenderism, able to respond appropriately if patient discloses transgender identity or gender concerns, able to screen for and recognize gender concerns, able to provide referrals for specialty evaluation or treatment if needed
2: Intermediate (primary medical care providers with a single or small group of patients needing trans-specific care)	Able to provide drug and alcohol assessment, including patient interview, physical exam, and lab investigation if needed; able to outline options for treatment, including pharmacologic options; provision of pharmacologic treatment; able to coordinate with other clinicians involved in care	Able to assess patient's position on continuum of HIV-related disease, including HIV-specific exam, history, and lab investigation; able to provide routine followup and medical monitoring; provision of prophylactic therapy; able to coordinate with other clinicians involved in care	Able to provide trans-specific assessment, including history, physical exam, and lab investigation if needed; able to consider trans-specific elements in provision of general primary medical care; able to outline options for feminizing or masculinizing endocrine therapy; able to coordinate with other clinicians involved in care
3: Advanced (primary medical care providers with more patient experience)	Licensed to prescribe methadone for opioid dependency	Sufficiently trained and experienced to be able to oversee antiretroviral therapy	Sufficiently trained and experienced to be able to initiate hormone therapy and provide care relating to sex reassignment surgery

have the knowledge and skills of the preceding tier(s), as well as additional skills, training, and experience.

Designing Transgender Clinical Training

Adult education is most effective when it is learner-centred, relevant to the learner's needs, and actively engaging (Candy, 1991). In medical practice, it has been established that passive learning such as reading clinical material or attending a clinical lecture is not effective in changing physicians' behavior (Freemantle et al., 1996; Grimshaw et al., 2001), and that learning activities which actively engage the clinician in problem-solving (e.g., case discussion, role-play), provide the opportunity to practice skills, are sequenced in an iterative work-learn-work cycle, and involve challenge by peers are most likely to result in change in clinical practice (Davis et al., 1999; Grimshaw, 1998; Pérez-Cuevas et al., 2000). Further,

multi-faceted interventions targeting different barriers to change in clinical practice are more likely to be effective than single interventions (Grimshaw et al., 2001). These principles should be understood when designing transgender clinical training, and effort made to employ a diversity of strategies to engage participating clinicians.

Tier 1: Basic Training

Basic training involves building transgender sensitivity and awareness. Cultural competency models used in health education (Campinha-Bacote, 1999; Juckett, 2005; Kim, 1995; McGarry, Clarke, & Cyr, 2000; Núñez, 2000; Ronnau, 1994; Reynolds, 2001; Sue, 2001; Tervalon & Murray-Garcia, 1998; Weaver, 1999) may be useful in developing this level of competency in transgender care. Cultural competence training aims not only to sensitize clinicians to interpersonal issues in the clinician-pa-

TABLE 2A. Core Competencies in Transgender Care: Tier 1 (Basic)

Area of Care	Core Competencies
All	1. Aware of differences between sex, gender, and sexual orientation
	2. Familiar with diversity of gender identity and gender expression in the general population
	3. Familiar with terms transgender patients are likely to use, including terms relating to gender transition
	4. Aware of health issues commonly of concern to transgender individuals
	5. Able to distinguish between non-problematic gender-variant identity or expression and gender concerns that may warrant clinical attention
	6. Aware of local patient and clinician resources
	7. Familiar with basic trans-sensitivity protocols such as use of preferred gender pronoun and name
	8. Able to communicate effectively with others involved in care

TABLE 2B. Core Competencies in Transgender Care: Tier 2 (Intermediate)

Area of Care	Core Competencies
Endocrine therapy	Provision of feminizing or masculinizing endocrine therapy (Dahl et al., 2006) is, as a trans-specific form of care, a Tier 3 service.
Mental health	Tier 1 requirements, plus:
	1. Familiar with common transgender psychosocial concerns and able to provide psychosocial supports to gender-variant clients and their families
	2. Able to provide supportive counseling to adolescents and adults who are: (a) seeking information about transgender issues, questioning their gender identity, curious about transgenderism, or exploring the possibility that they or a loved one may be transgender; (b) considering "coming out" as transgender; or (c) seeking support relating to adjustment issues in gender transition (at a level comparable to adjustment issues in other life transitions)
	3. Sufficiently knowledgeable about transgender issues to explore the mental health impact of societal marginalization and stigma
	4. Familiar with the basic processes of transgender identity development and gender transition
	5. Able to help clients explore options for gender identity and expression
	6. Aware of trans-specific clinical advocacy issues and able to address general advocacy concerns (e.g., referrals to gender-specific facilities)
Primary medical care	Tier 1 requirements, plus:
	1. Familiar with common transgender health concerns
	2. Able to explain to patients the general processes involved in gender transition
	3. Able to perform trans-specific assessment, including patient interview, physical examination, and lab investigations
	4. Able to appropriately chart and interpret sex-specific lab tests
	5. Able to offer trans-relevant health promotion and disease prevention services
	6. Aware of trans-specific medical advocacy issues, and able to complete required paperwork for patients needing medical letters
	7. Sufficiently knowledge to adapt screening protocols relating to cancer, cardiovascular disease, diabetes, and osteoporosis for patients who are taking feminizing or masculinizing endocrine agents
	8. Able to provide basic post-operative care following surgeries that are not trans-specific (e.g., breast augmentation, mastectomy, facial feminization, hysterectomy, salpingo-oophorectomy)

TABLE 2B (continued)

Area of Care	Core Competencies
Speech and voice	Tier 1 requirements, plus: 1. Sufficiently knowledgeable to assess whether problems with voice quality or other general speech/voice complaints are resulting from or complicated by transition-related speech change 2. Able to thoroughly evaluate the transgender client's speech and voice 3. Able to address trans-specific questions about preventive voice care 4. Able to provide information about surgical and non-surgical treatment options to feminize or masculinize speech and voice

TABLE 2C. Core Competencies in Transgender Care: Tier 3 (Advanced)

Area of Care	Core Competencies
Endocrine therapy	Tier 1 & 2 requirements, plus: Prescribing clinician[a] Prescribing to an adult patient: 1. Knowledgeable about transgender medical care, including trans-specific health history, physical examination, and interpretation of sex-specific laboratory tests 2. Knowledgeable about physiologic mechanisms involved in hormonal feminization and masculinization 3. Knowledgeable about endocrine agents that may be used 4. Aware of dosage considerations 5. Able to explain expected physical and psychological changes to patient 6. Able to explain potential adverse effects and health risks to patient 7. Aware of protocols for physical screening prior to initiation of endocrine therapy and protocols for long-term maintenance Prescribing to an adolescent patient: #1-7 above, and 8. Aware of protocols for staged use of GnRH analogues and cross-sex hormones 9. Able to explain expected effects of GnRH analogues to patient 10. Aware of potential impact of transgender endocrine therapy on aspects of pubertal development such as bone growth and density Clinician assessing psychological eligibility and readiness[b] Assessment of adult patients: 1. Masters degree or its equivalent in a clinical behavioral science field, granted by an institution accredited by a recognized national or regional accrediting board 2. Documented credentials from a proper training facility and a licensing board 3. Documented supervised training and competence in psychotherapy 4. Specialized training and competence in the assessment of the *DSM-IV/ICD-10* Sexual Disorders 5. Continuing education in the treatment of gender identity disorders—e.g., attendance at professional meetings, workshops, or seminars; participation in research related to gender identity issues Assessment of adolescent patients: #1-5 above, and 6. Training in childhood and adolescent developmental psychopathology 7. Competency in diagnosing and treating the ordinary problems of children and adolescents 8. Aware of developmental issues in assessing hormone eligibility and readiness 9. Aware of assessment tools specifically designed for use with this population

TABLE 2C (continued)

Area of Care	Core Competencies
Mental health	Tier 1 & 2 requirements, plus:
	If working with children
	1. Able to evaluate suspected gender concerns in children
	2. Able to provide psychosocial support to gender dysphoric children and their families
	If working with adolescents or adults
	1. Strong knowledge of transgender identity development and psychological issues in gender transition
	2. Able to evaluate and treat gender dysphoria and compulsive crossdressing
	3. Able to assess hormonal and surgical eligibility and readiness[b]
	4. Familiar with normal adjustment concerns prior to and following sex reassignment; able to provide counseling for individuals experiencing regret following sex reassignment
Primary medical care	Tier 1 & 2 requirements, plus:
	1. Aware of processes involved in determination of hormonal and surgical eligibility and readiness
	2. Able to provide hormone screening, initiate hormone prescription, and provide comprehensive hormone maintenance
	3. Able to provide basic post-operative care following genital surgery
Speech and voice	Tier 1 & 2 requirements, plus:
	1. Knowledgeable about theory relating to adult speech and voice production
	2. Substantial clinical experience assessing and treating typical speech and voice disorders in adults (recommend minimum 2 years clinical experience)
	3. Knowledgeable about gender differences in speech and voice
	4. Aware of the effects of hormones on speech and voice
	5. Knowledgeable about transgender speech parameters, and able to conduct trans-specific assessment, treatment, and post-treatment evaluation

[a]While pharmacists do not need to be knowledgeable about transgender endocrine therapy to fill a physician's prescription, as cross-sex hormone use is off-label pharmacists involved in transgender endocrine therapy will ideally have knowledge relating to administration, formulation, and potential adverse effects of feminizing or masculinizing endocrine therapy. The pharmacist should also be able to monitor potential drug interactions if additional medication is prescribed by another clinician.

[b]The World Professional Association for Transgender Health's (WPATH's) *Standards of Care* (Meyer et al., 2001) discuss in detail competency requirements for clinicians involved in assessing psychological eligibility and readiness to begin endocrine therapy. For transgender adults, feminizing or masculinizing endocrine therapy is typically initiated by a family physician, nurse practitioner, or endocrinologist upon the recommendation of a Tier 3 mental health practitioner. Physicians and advanced practice nurses with training and experience in behavioral health, gender identity concerns, and sexual issues may choose to have sole responsibility for all aspects of adult transgender endocrine care, including assessment of eligibility and readiness.

tient relationship, but also to raise clinician awareness of the broader sociocultural forces–within clinical disciplines and in society at large–that influence health and create disparities in access to care (Committee on Understanding and Eliminating Racial and Ethnic Disparities in Health Care, 2003; Raj, 2002; Wear, 2003).

Training in effective practitioner-patient interaction includes preparing the clinician to identify and reduce or eliminate barriers to ac-cessing care, to understand how to partner with patients in health care decisions, to communicate effectively with the patient and the patient's loved ones, and to be sufficiently skilled to function as the patient's health care advocate (Núñez, 2000; Sue, 2001). Applying the cultural competency model to transgender health, topics for Tier 1 training could include:

1. Awareness: personal and societal attitudes about gender diversity, gender

variance, and transgender behaviour and identity; common transphobic myths and stereotypes; the impact of transphobia on the provider-patient relationship and on access to health care

2. Knowledge: frequency of gender-variance, transgender concepts and terms, range of gender concerns, local resources

3. Skill: trans-specific clinical communication protocols, recognition of concerns requiring more advanced assistance

Núñez (2000) suggests using a combination of lectures, case discussions, problem-based learning cases, role playing, clinical reasoning exercises, self-awareness exercises, and communication skills workshops to improve cultural competence. To facilitate translation of knowledge, skills, and awareness into the clinical setting, Núñez recommends small group role-plays, simulated patient evaluations using trained lay volunteers (e.g., standardized patient examinations), interactive case seminars, and discussion of videotaped interactions.

As all clinicians are expected to have Tier 1 knowledge of transgender issues, ideally Tier 1 training would be incorporated into undergraduate education. Dedicating resources for practicum placements in community programs that serve transgender people may also facilitate Tier 1 learning at an undergraduate level.

As incorporation of transgender content into existing undergraduate curriculum is a long-term process involving ongoing discussion and advocacy with post-secondary institutions, in the interim Tier 1 training should be made available in formats that can be used by students and professionals already in practice. For example:

1. Self-paced online training: Lectures, problem-based learning cases, clinical reasoning exercises, and reflexive self-awareness exercises could be made available as a self-paced online module. Videos that emphasize the diversity of the transgender population (Burnham, 2001) could be included in the module to introduce facilitate exploration of personal attitudes and reactions to gender-variance.

2. Virtual classroom: WebCT or other educational software that combines computer-mediated communication (discussion groups, chat rooms, etc.) and the provision of didactic material could be used to support a facilitated virtual interest group of students and clinicians. The communication element would support case discussions and other interactive learning.

3. Interdisciplinary seminar: An introduction to transgender care could be delivered as an interdisciplinary half-day or full-day seminar. Ideally this type of training would be delivered by a transgender clinician (or co-delivered by a non-transgender clinician and a transgender layperson), with a panel of transgender speakers or small group facilitators to introduce participants to diversity within the transgender community. The seminar should not consist wholly of lectures, and should include interactive, problem-based learning. The seminar could be videotaped for use in future training.

4. Publications and presentations: Although printed material is insufficient to transform practice, awareness of transgender health can be raised by publication of transgender health articles in clinical journals and newsletters of health professional associations, and poster and paper presentations at meetings of professional associations. Clinically rigorous consumer education materials are also useful awareness-raising tools for clinicians who are unaware of basic transgender issues.

Evaluating existing transgender content in clinical education. In a review of undergraduate and graduate courses in clinical programs at universities throughout British Columbia, transgender content was noted in some psychology and psychiatry courses (Goldberg, 2006). However, the existing content was typically not consistent with the basic goal of Tier 1 training–promoting inclusive, respectful, and culturally competent treatment of transgender individuals in the community-based clinical setting. For example, gender-variance was usually depicted as a type of psychopathology, the terms "transgender" and "transsexual" were often conflated, and mental health practice with the transgender community typically portrayed as a highly specialized subset of sexual medicine. A detailed review of transgender content and teaching materials would be useful in determining resources that could help promote a consistently trans-positive framework for basic education. A "train the trainer" module based on the same principles of adult learning as in clinical practice (interactive, engaging, problem-based) would help post-secondary instructors teach transgender health content in a non-pathologizing, non-stigmatizing manner that facilitates service provision in the general community setting.

A "LGBT" approach to Tier 1 education. While there is political utility in bringing lesbian, gay, bisexual, and transgender (LGBT) individuals together to address issues of shared concern, the efficacy of an LGBT approach in teaching transgender clinical care should be carefully considered. Although there are some shared experiences between lesbian/bisexual women, gay/bisexual men, and transgender people (of all sexual orientations), there are significant differences between these three populations in terms of health promotion, disease prevention, screening, treatment, psychosocial concerns, clinical advocacy, and other clinical issues.

In the absence of evaluation of the validity of a LGBT approach in training relating to transgender clinical care, a trans-specific approach is recommended for clinical training. If a LGBT approach is pursued, the curriculum should also be structured in a way that addresses critical trans-specific concepts, not just issues that transgender individuals share with non-transgender lesbians, gays, and bisexuals (McCarthy, 2003). In addition, the instructor must have substantial clinical experience with all four groups, not just gays, lesbians, and bisexuals.

Tier 2: Intermediate Training

A quantum leap in awareness, knowledge, and skill is involved between Tiers 1 and 2. Tier 1 training aims to improve practitioner comfort in working with the transgender population and to provide basic cultural competence. Tier 2 training addresses issues of *clinical competence*: the ability to provide care that is not only sensitive and respectful of transgender individuals, but also clinically effective in health promotion, clinical assessment, and clinical treatment. Tier 2 training objectives include:

1. Awareness: understanding of the care protocols that should be modified in treatment of transgender individuals, and the issues to consider in adapting standard protocols; trans-specific clinical advocacy issues
2. Knowledge: health impacts of transphobia, treatment options for gender concerns (including psychotherapy, pharmacotherapy, surgery, and social role transition), health impacts of hormonal and surgical change, discipline-specific care protocols, resources for individuals undergoing gender transition
3. Skill: interviewing, physical examination, interpretation of sex-specific laboratory tests or other evaluative procedures, trans-specific documentation

In addition to didactic teaching techniques similar to those described in Tier 1, an experiential component is needed in Tier 2 training to facilitate development of skill in patient interview and patient examination. This may include critical reflection on videotaped interviews and examinations, observation of more experienced practitioners, role-plays, and simulations with trained volunteer patients. Green and Seifert (2005) suggest using structured case-level feedback when new information is first presented, context-based practice as knowledge is transformed from a theoretical concept to practice, and deliberative practice as procedural knowledge is starting to crystallize.

Role-plays with non-transgender colleagues have utility in initial practice of new terminology, patient questions, and patient education considerations that may be unfamiliar to the practitioner new to transgender health. However, for training of medical practitioners, role-plays with non-transgender colleagues are not sufficient. It is difficult to simulate the cognitive dissonance of working on a patient whose identity does not match their physiology in a role-play, and impossible to simulate the effects of hormones or surgery–both critical factors in clinician skill in the physical examination. However, use of transgender community volunteers as standardized patients for physical examination may be problematic as physical examination is often traumatic for people with gender dysphoria. Prospective volunteers should be carefully screened, and any simulated examinations carefully supervised. Existing standardized patient training programs should be consulted to determine appropriate training and support strategies.

Tier 3: Advanced Training

Clinicians who take Tier 3 training should already have substantial experience working with the transgender community. A self-learning assessment is recommended to determine areas where further training is required. For some clinicians, elements of Tier 1 and 2 training may be appropriate to include as part of Tier 3 training.

Tier 3 training should include direct experience working with advanced clinicians who provide care to a diverse group of transgender individuals. The opportunity to observe, discuss cases, and receive clinical supervision by a highly experienced provider is an important aspect of Tier 3 training.

As the target group for this level of training is relatively small, it may be most efficient to deliver didactic training through a virtual classroom (using interactive web-based technology) or real-time video technology. Didactic training should include complex case discussions, problem-based learning cases, clinical reasoning exercises, and other activities that engage the learner. Below are suggestions for development of didactic training in specific areas of transgender care.

Endocrine therapy. Clinicians from numerous disciplines may be involved in endocrine therapy. Consideration should be given to the advantages and disadvantages of discipline-specific training versus combined training for clinicians who may be collaborating in patient care.

In 2004 and 2005 the Transgender Health Program offered a series of training programs for clinicians involved in assessing hormone and surgery eligibility and readiness. A two-day Tier 2 mental health intensive was attended by 50 clinicians with varying levels of transgender experience, with an invitation for clini-

cians with a MD or Masters degree or higher in a clinical mental health discipline to take part in more advanced training relating to hormone assessment. A two-day followup was then held for 11 family physicians, clinical counselors, clinical social workers, and psychologists who had attended the intensive and were interested in further training relating to hormone assessment. A prior learning assessment and review of clinician credentials was conducted as part of the followup training. This group is now conducting hormone assessments, and is meeting monthly for clinical supervision and discussion of complex cases. Two Ph.D. psychologists in the group have completed additional training relating to assessment of eligibility and readiness to pursue SRS.

Training for prescribing clinicians could follow a similar structure: a day-long training intensive for a large group of clinicians, advanced training (with learning assessment and credential review) for a smaller group, and clinical supervision for graduates of advanced training. A sample curriculum for a day-long seminar orienting clinicians to the physical aspects of endocrine therapy is available as an online supplement at http://www.vch.ca/transhealth/resources/library/tcpdocs/training-endocrine.pdf. Experienced clinicians could offer a followup intensive covering more advanced topics such as steps in physical screening prior to initiation of hormones; interpretation of sex-specific laboratory tests; formulation and dosage considerations; regimen adjustment following gonadal removal; issues in cardiovascular, metabolic, and gynecologic care over the lifespan; hormone cycling; and transition of hormonally-treated adolescents into adult endocrine care.

Mental health. Tier 3 care involves specialty care in transgender mental health. Training focuses on evaluation and treatment of gender dysphoria (including assessment of eligibility and readiness for endocrine therapy or sex reassignment surgery), evaluation and treatment of compulsive crossdressing, and complex psychological issues in gender transition such as persistent regret following sex reassignment.

The American Academy of Clinical Sexologists, Columbia University Department of Psychiatry, and University of Minnesota Department of Family Medicine and Community Health offer Tier 3 programs for mental health professionals. As these all involve a commitment over 1-2 years, it may be beneficial to consider the creation of shorter fellowships for community-based clinicians who do not work exclusively with transgender individuals but have a large enough client group to warrant advanced training.

Primary medical care. For family physicians and nurse practitioners, the difference between Tier 2 and Tier 3 competence is not as significant as the gap between Tiers 1 and 2. Most of the knowledge and skills required for physical screening prior to hormone prescription, hormone initiation, and post-operative care following genital surgery will have already been developed in Tier 2 training. Additional didactic training relating to protocols for pre-hormone screening (including patient examination and laboratory examination), the initial changes that can be expected in the first 1-3 years of hormone treatment, and post-operative complications following genital surgery should be developed to support the knowledge component involved in Tier 3 care.

Tier 3 primary care training should also include detailed discussion of the processes involved in determination of eligibility and readiness for hormonal and surgical readiness. This includes discussion of differential diagnosis of gender concerns, assessment of co-existing conditions, the eligibility and readiness criteria outlined in the WPATH *Standards of Care*, and the role of a mental health practitioner in complex cases.

Speech and voice. The University of Iowa and the Provincial Voice Care Resource Program at Vancouver Hospital offer intensive voice science training programs for speech-language pathologists. A similar intensive approach could be used for training speech-language pathologists in transgender speech and voice change. Ideally, a combined didactic and experiential training intensive would be held in conjunction with an already-established transgender speech program. Drawing from the structure of the Provincial Voice Care Resource Program's voice disorders intensive, a week-long transgender speech intensive could include:

1. Pre-reading: Relevant research articles and protocols for speech and voice feminization or masculinization (Davies & Goldberg, 2006)
2. Didactic training (mornings): transgender basics, gendered aspects of speech and voice, trans-specific treatment options, trans-specific assessment and speech therapy techniques, and trans-specific outcome evaluation
3. Observation (afternoons): transgender speech and voice assessment, group and one-to-one therapy, outcome evaluation
4. Supervision for the first two transgender clients after completion of training

A suggested curriculum is available as an online supplement at http://www.vch.ca/transhealth/resources/library/tcpdocs/training-speech.pdf.

Ongoing Professional Development

The biennial WPATH conference and virtual networks such as the WPATH transgender medicine discussion listserv provide opportunities for clinicians across regions to discuss complex issues in care. Most community-based clinicians do not work exclusively with transgender individuals and find it impractical to spend large amounts of money or time on ongoing professional development. It may therefore be advantageous to focus on smaller-scale regional networks of clinicians who can meet periodically (every 12-18 months) to discuss training needs, coordination of care, outreach strategies to involve new clinicians, and emerging issues in the transgender health field. Funding could be sought to support one member from this group to attend the WPATH conference and bring back information for other network members.

PLANNING AND EVALUATION

Determining Education Priorities

The objective of transgender training for health and social service clinicians is improved access to quality care for transgender individuals and loved ones. A systematic education plan should therefore target education to have the maximum impact on care access, taking into consideration regional resources and needs.

For example, in developing an education plan for British Columbia, Trans Care Project staff used the Transgender Health Program's clinician directory to map out levels of service available in each region of the province, analyzed the program's client referral requests to determine which types of services were in high demand, and then set training targets for each discipline. Following the closure of the Vancouver Gender Dysphoria Program in 2002, the immediate priority was training of community-based hormone and surgery assessors; 3 years later, with training of adult assessors completed, Tier 2 and 3 training for family physicians and nurse practitioners and Tier 3 training for clinicians working with gender-variant children have become the main priorities.

Known service access barriers should be considered in determining priorities for training. For example, participants in a survey of transgender community members in British Columbia (*N* = 179) reported financial cost as the main barrier in accessing gender transition and crossdressing services (Goldberg, Matte, MacMillan, & Hudspith, 2003). Accordingly, while fee-for-service clinicians are welcome to attend training, recruitment is heavily focused on clinicians in the public health system. To improve service availability for transgender individuals who are not fluent in English, education subsidies and other financial incentives are being explored to encourage multilingual clinicians to take part in training.

Evaluating Transgender Clinical Training

Quality control and quality improvement measures should be included in the education plan. While it is useful to evaluate changes to knowledge and attitudes (e.g., by pre- and post-test), transgender clinical training should not only improve clinicians' knowledge; ultimately, training aims to transform clinical practice.

Michie and colleagues (2005) identify twelve psychological domains that influence implementation of change in clinical practice, and suggest specific interview questions to investigate clinician knowledge; clinician skills; social and professional role and identity; clinician beliefs about capabilities; clinician beliefs about consequences; clinician motivation and goals; memory, attention, and decision processes; en-

vironmental context and resources; social influences; emotion regulation; behavioural regulation; and nature of the behaviour. Ideally, education will include interactive or self-directed followup that helps clinician trainees identify barriers to change in practice and suggests strategies to facilitate change. Ongoing learning may include engaging clinicians in further training sessions, internal systems advocacy to address environmental barriers to clinical change, the creation of clinical peer support to motivate and push the clinician to change, or other activities that address the domains identified by Michie and colleagues (2005).

As improved access to quality care is the overarching goal of training, evaluation of the education plan should include an assessment of service quality and accessibility over time. Depending on the clinical setting, it may be possible to evaluate: (a) client satisfaction with the quality of service, (b) clinician utilization of a practice protocol (by self-report or chart audit), (c) the number of clinicians willing to be listed in a resource directory or referral guide, (d) the number of successful referrals (where the referring agency is able to find a suitable practitioner to meet the client's request), or (e) client reports of barriers to getting needed services.

CONCLUDING REMARKS

The training frameworks developed thus far by the Trans Care Project and summarized in this article are only a starting point for education of health and social service professionals who serve the transgender community. Further work is needed to develop training frameworks for clinicians working outside the community setting, including those in acute care, tertiary care, continuing care, palliative care, and the prison system.

There are many financial and logistical challenges in implementing transgender clinical education in regions where transgenderism is misunderstood, devalued, and highly stigmatized. When resources are scarce, it is tempting to centralize services. However, doing so creates a paucity of knowledge among community-based clinicians, limiting transgender access to health and social services. The Transgender

Health Program in British Columbia provides an example of the potential for development of community-based services, and the importance of collaboration between clinicians, educators, and community advocates in creating both practice guidelines and training to improve the quality and consistency of care.

REFERENCES

Burnham, C. W. G. (2001). *Gender Line* [film]. Vancouver, BC: Video Out Distribution.

Campinha-Bacote, J. (1999). A model and instrument for addressing cultural competence in health care. *Journal of Nursing Education, 38*, 203-207.

Candy, P. C. (1991). *Self-direction for lifelong learning: A comprehensive guide to theory and practice.* San Francisco: Jossey-Bass Publishers.

Committee on Understanding and Eliminating Racial and Ethnic Disparities in Health Care (2003). *Unequal treatment: Confronting racial and ethnic disparities in health care.* Washington, DC: National Academies Press.

Davies, S., & Goldberg, J. M. (2006). Clinical aspects of transgender speech feminization and masculinization. *International Journal of Transgenderism, 9*(3/4), 167-196.

Davis, D., O'Brien, M. A. T., Freemantle, N., Wolf, F. M., Mazmanian, P., & Taylor-Vaisey, A. (1999). Impact of formal continuing medical education: Do conferences, workshops, rounds, and other traditional continuing education activities change physician behavior or health care outcomes? *Journal of the American Medical Association, 282*, 867-874.

Freemantle, N., Harvey, E., Grimshaw, J. M., Wolf, F., Bero, L., Grilli, R., & Oxman, A. D. (1996). The effectiveness of printed educational materials in changing the behaviour of health care professionals. In Cochrane Collaboration, *Cochrane Library*, Issue 3. Oxford: Update Software, 1996.

Goldberg, J. M. (2006). *Recommended framework for training mental health clinicians in transgender care.* Vancouver, BC: Vancouver Coastal Health Authority.

Goldberg, J. M., Matte, N., MacMillan, M., & Hudspith, M. (2003). *Community survey: Transition/cross-dressing services in BC–Final report.* Vancouver, BC: Vancouver Coastal Health and Transcend Transgender Support & Education Society.

Green, L. A., & Seifert, C. M. (2005). Translation of research into practice: Why we can't "just do it." *The Journal of the American Board of Family Practice, 18*, 541-545.

Grimshaw, J. M. (1998). What have new efforts to change professional practice achieved? *Journal of the Royal Society of Medicine, 91*(35), 20-25.

Grimshaw, J. M., Shirran, L., Thomas, R. E., Mowatt, G., Fraser, C., Bero, L., Grilli, R., Harvey, E. L., O'Brien, M. A., & Oxman, A. D. (2001). Changing provider behaviour: An overview of systematic reviews of interventions. *Medical Care, 39*(S2), 2-45.

Juckett, G. (2005). Cross-cultural medicine. *American Family Physician, 72*, 2267-2274.

Kim, W. J. (1995). A training guideline of cultural competence for child and adolescent psychiatric residencies. *Child Psychiatry and Human Development, 26*, 125-136.

Kopala, L. (2003). *Recommendations for a transgender health program.* Vancouver, BC: Vancouver Coastal Health Authority.

McCarthy, L. (2003). What about the "T"? Is multicultural education ready to address transgender issues? *Multicultural Perspectives, 5*, 46-48.

McGarry, K., Clarke, J., & Cyr, M. G. (2000). Enhancing residents' cultural competence through a lesbian and gay health curriculum. *Academic Medicine, 75*, 515.

Meyer, W. J., III, Bockting, W. O., Cohen-Kettenis, P. T., Coleman, E., Di Ceglie, D., Devor, H., Gooren, L., Hage, J. J., Kirk, S., Kuiper, B., Laub, D., Lawrence, A., Menard, Y., Monstrey, S., Patton, J., Schaefer, L., Webb, A., & Wheeler, C. C. (2001). *The standards of care for Gender Identity Disorders* (6th ed.). Minneapolis, MN: Harry Benjamin International Gender Dysphoria Association.

Michie, S., Johnston, M., Abraham, C., Lawton, R., Parker, D., & Walker, A. (2005). Making psychological theory useful for approaching implementing evidence based practice: A consensus. *Quality & Safety in Health Care, 14*, 26-33. 10.1136/qshc.2004.011155

Núñez, A. E. (2000). Transforming cultural competence into cross-cultural efficacy in women's health education. *Academic Medicine, 75*, 1071-1079.

Pérez-Cuevas, R., Reyes, H., Guiscafré, H., Juárez-Díaz, N., Oviedo, M., Flores, S., & Muñoz, O. (2000). The primary care clinic as a setting for continuing medical education: Program description. *Canadian Medical Association Journal, 163*, 1295-1299.

Raj, R. (2002). Towards a transpositive therapeutic model: Developing clinical sensitivity and cultural competence in the effective support of transsexual and transgendered clients. *International Journal of Transgenderism, 6*. Retrieved January 1, 2005, from http://www.symposion.com/ijt/ijtvo06no02_04.htm

Reynolds, A. L. (2001). Multidimensional cultural competence: Providing tools for transforming psychology. *The Counseling Psychologist, 29*, 833-841.

Ronnau, J. P. (1994). Teaching cultural competence: Practical ideas for social work educators. *Journal of Multicultural Social Work, 3*, 29-42.

Sue, D. W. (2001). Multidimensional facets of cultural competence. *Counseling Psychologist, 29*, 790-821.

Tervalon, M., & Murray-Garcia, J. (1998). Cultural humility versus cultural competence: A critical distinction in defining physician training outcomes in multicultural education. *Journal of Health Care for the Poor and Underserved, 9,* 117-124.

Wear, D. (2003). Insurgent multiculturalism: Rethinking how and why we teach culture in medical education. *Academic Medicine, 78,* 549-554.

Weaver, H. N. (1999). Indigenous people and the social work profession: Defining culturally competent services. *Social Work, 44,* 217-225.

West Sussex Health and Social Care NHS Trust (2005). *Transgender services for the residents of Sussex.* Swandean, England: Author.

doi:10.1300/J485v09n03_10

Index